Clinical Handbook of

PSYCHIATRY

and the LAW

Second Edition

Clinical Handbook of
PSYCHIATRY
and the LAW

Second Edition

Paul S. Appelbaum, MD

A.F. Zeleznik Professor of Psychiatry
Department of Psychiatry
University of Massachusetts Medical Center
Worcester, Massachusetts

Associate Professor of Psychiatry
Massachusetts Mental Health Center
Harvard Medical School
Boston, Massachusetts

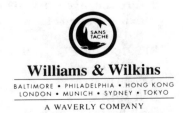

Williams & Wilkins

BALTIMORE • PHILADELPHIA • HONG KONG
LONDON • MUNICH • SYDNEY • TOKYO

A WAVERLY COMPANY

Editor: Michael G. Fisher
Associate Editor: Carol Eckhart
Copy Editor: Mary Kidd
Designer: Wilma E. Rosenberger
Illustration Planner: Lorraine Wrzosek
Production Coordinator: Charles E. Zeller

Copyright © 1991
Williams & Wilkins
428 East Preston Street
Baltimore, Maryland 21202, USA

Accurate indications, adverse reactions, and dosage schedules for drugs are provided in this book, but it is possible that they may change. The reader is urged to review the package information data of the manufacturers of the medications mentioned.

Printed in the United States of America

First Edition 1982 by McGraw-Hill Book Company

Library of Congress Cataloging in Publication Data

Appelbaum, Paul S.
    Clinical handbook of psychiatry and the law / Paul S. Appelbaum,
  Thomas G. Gutheil,—2nd ed.
        p. cm.
    Gutheil's name appears first on the earlier edition.
    Includes bibliographical references.
    Includes index.
    ISBN 0-683-0237-6
    1. Psychiatrists—Legal status, laws, etc.—United States.
2. Forensic psychiatry—United States.   3. Psychotherapist and
patient—United States.   I. Gutheil, Thomas G.   II. Title.
        [DNLM: 1. Forensic Psychiatry.   W 740 A648c]
    KF2910.P75G87   1991
    344.73'041—dc20
    [347.30441]
    DNLM/DLC
    for Library of Congress   90-13167
                                                                          CIP

94 95
3 4 5 6 7 8 9 10

To our parents

Preface to the Second Edition

Much has changed in the worlds of psychiatry and law since the publication in 1982 of the first edition of this work, which received the Manfred S. Guttmacher Award of the American Psychiatric Association and the American Academy of Psychiatry and the Law as the "outstanding contribution to the literature of forensic psychiatry." Even a brief sampling of the issues that mental health professionals must confront in the 1990s bears witness to the growth in the scope and complexity of legal impact on clinical practice.

Malpractice suits have multiplied, and awards have skyrocketed, based on once infrequently heard allegations concerning failure to protect victims of patients' violence, sexual misconduct with patients, and negligent supervision, among others. New rights for patients, including some version of a right to refuse antipsychotic medication, and recourse to rights' protection systems have become firmly established in most jurisdictions. Mental health professionals have been challenged by the complex dilemmas created by the AIDS epidemic. Attempts to control the cost of mental health care have exacerbated concerns about protecting confidentiality and preventing liability.

It has become clear to us over the years that for this book to retain its utility as a practical guide for clinicians and trainees alike, substantial updating would be required. We are pleased to be able to present the results of that effort. While retaining the highly accessible format of the first edition, we have revised and reorganized the text to reflect a decade's evolution of law and clinical practice. Many new case examples have been added, and the reference lists at the end of each chapter have been thoroughly updated. We acknowledge in this edition the development of child psychiatry and law as a separate subspecialty in its own right; our previous effort to address issues in child custody has been eliminated, and readers are referred to one of the excellent texts available that now address the full range of child psychiatry and law issues.

Our hope is that this second edition of the Clinical Handbook of Psychiatry and the Law will continue to meet the needs of mental health clinicians of all disciplines, as well as of trainees, students, attorneys, and researchers for the next decade.

Paul S. Appelbaum, M.D.
Thomas G. Gutheil, M.D.

How to Use This Book

"**I**'m a clinician, not a lawyer. All I want to do is help people. Why doesn't the law just let me do my job?"

This plaintive cry of the clinician, which can be heard these days echoing down hospital corridors, through the recesses of private offices, and in the interview rooms of outpatient clinics, expresses the raison d'être of this book. Decry it as they may, mental health professionals of every theoretical orientation and in all types of practice settings can no longer afford to be ignorant of the law. Court decisions, statutes, and administrative regulations have so affected clinical practice that few everyday decisions can be made without awareness of the legal rules governing such actions and, equally important, of the effect that those rules may have on the treatment of the patient.

The problems that arise from this situation are generically different from those with which clinicians (or lawyers) have been accustomed to dealing in the past. Rather than facing a dilemma that comes clearly labeled as "clinical" or "legal," clinicians now frequently confront problems in which the clinical and legal aspects are so intertwined that they seem nearly inseparable; neither the lawyer nor the clinician, using only the tools of his primary discipline, can take fully into account the complexities of such a situation. Only with an understanding that passes freely across disciplinary boundaries can one perceive the relation between the components of the problem and anticipate the impact on the problem as a whole of an intervention in either the legal or the clinical realm.

Of course, the ideal solution to the needs created by this radical change in the requirements for clinical practice would be for every clinician to have available for consultation an expert in legal psychiatry whose knowledge encompasses both worlds. Although such experts have assumed consultants' roles in some of our larger psychiatric teaching centers, there are too few of these individuals to make the goal of easy access for every clinician a realizable one.

We hope that this book provides the next best alternative: a manual for ready reference that will become the first point of departure when questions arise about the impact of law or regulation on the daily practice of psychiatric and psychological care. Mental health clinicians from all disciplines and from every level of training will find this work designed to respond to the questions both complex and mundane that develop in the customary course of practice. Psychiatrists who are unfamiliar with the area will find this handbook a useful study aid in preparation for the forensic psychiatry sections of the specialty board examinations. Lawyers and law students who want to understand—from the critical perspective of the clinician—the issues in mental health law will also be able to begin their researches here.

It is the firm conviction of the authors that textbooks or reference works that attempt to divorce the legal from the clinical, as so many do, are bound to fail in becoming a handy tool for the clinician who must, of necessity, relate *every* aspect of his work to its effect on patient care. Likewise, works that try to impart only a dry list of legal rules for the clinician to memorize and obey, without conveying an understanding of, or an appreciation for, the legal reasoning that underlies them, will be equally unsuccessful; legal rules apply only to a unique factual situation and often survive only until the next court ruling or session of the legislature. The clinician who is able to understand the basis for the rule will, on the other hand, be able to apply the basic concepts to unfamiliar circumstances and, when the law changes, to follow knowingly its evolution. Hence, this book consistently strives to accomplish two ends: (1) always to interrelate the legal and the clinical aspects of an issue; and (2) to convey, whenever possible, something of the history of the law's approach to a problem, in the recognition that today's rule is, in most cases, merely the most recent unstable equilibrium that the historically contending sides of the argument have attained.

A word is in order, too, about what this book is *not*. It is most emphatically not designed to give legal advice or to take the place of a consultation with a competent attorney. Rather, the information contained herein will help the clinician decide when to contact an attorney (and describe how to avoid coming to the pass where that becomes a necessary step). In addition, since the comments one elicits from an attorney are commonly as cryptic as those from one's physician, this book should help the clinician understand the basis for the legal advice she receives.

This is not, moreover, a comprehensive textbook of psychiatry and law. Not only would a work of that magnitude require several times the bulk of this volume, but in consequence, it would be so unwieldy as to frustrate the busy clinician in search of an accessible and easily understandable explanation. For similar reasons of convenience, we have chosen not to burden the reader with a profusion of footnotes. Instead, a representative bibliography follows each chapter, providing a means for those who wish to investigate the subject in greater depth to do so.

Finally, the clinician will not find enumerated in this work the particular details of law and regulation that govern practice in the 51 diverse jurisdictions of this nation. Even had we attempted such a task, the rapid changes of case law and statute would have made the work outdated before it reached the reader's hand. For specific features of the laws that govern their work, all clinicians should become familiar with the applicable statutes and regulations in their jurisdictions. A visit to the main branch of the public library in each city should uncover an up-to-date version of the state statutes. These volumes often appear unnecessarily intimidating to the non-lawyer but can yield much useful information if used in the manner in which one would use any other reference work: carefully locating the information desired in the index (e.g., mental health law, psychotherapist-patient privilege) and reading the relevant statutes. An alternative is to contact the local branch of the professional organization for each of the mental health disciplines to ask for their help in obtaining copies of the appropriate laws.

Now, something about the format of this work. Since most mental health clinicians need both to acquire a basic overview of legal issues in their work and to have a ready reference when future questions arise, this handbook has been designed with both purposes in mind. Those with little background in the field will want to read it through to acquaint themselves with the basic issues. Then, as needed, they can use the detailed table of contents of each chapter, with their numerous subheadings and the frequent cross-references in the text, to locate rapidly the information that they need.

Each chapter is divided into seven sections:

I. CASE EXAMPLES

These case summaries open each chapter on a clinical footing and attempt to frame the legal and clinical issues that will be discussed. Based on real (but thoroughly disguised) cases from the authors' consultative and supervisory experience, they are presented in two parts, this first part intended to give the reader a chance to think through the issues for himself before grappling with the solutions posed by the collective experience of the legal and mental health systems in the epilogue.

II. LEGAL ISSUES

This section reviews, highlights, and interprets the most important legal cases and statutes, while always attempting to convey the rationale that underlies the law's approach. Historical, ethical, and philosophical perspectives are also offered. Emphasis is placed on those legal issues most directly related to everyday clinical work, but special situations, such as criminal forensic evaluations, are covered as well.

III. CLINICAL ISSUES

In recognition of the impact of abstract legal doctrines on actual clinical practice and on the subjective experience of the patient, this section describes these effects and outlines practical means of coping with them within the treatment context. Also addressed are the clinical issues involved in more traditional forensic work, including evaluations performed for the courts, as well as the clinical effects of a variety of legal procedures.

IV. PITFALLS

"Pitfalls" addresses the psychological difficulties that clinicians face in attempting to deal with problems of a mixed clinical and legal nature. While the dynamic psychiatrist might label these pitfalls as manifestations of the countertransference, they represent obstacles to good patient care about which all clinicians, regardless of theoretical orientation, should be aware.

V. CASE EXAMPLE—EPILOGUES

Integrating the material contained in the preceding sections, these followups return to the cases described earlier in the chapter and outline their resolution. They also serve as a handy self-assessment of the reader's understanding of the chapter.

VI. ACTION GUIDE

A unique operational summary of the chapter, the Action Guide places the elements previously discussed into a condensed, action-oriented framework. It serves both as a quick-reference outline for appropriate responses to clinico-legal dilemmas and as a means for rapid review of the material in each chapter.

VII. SUGGESTED READINGS

Each chapter is followed by a selection from the most notable, provocative, and useful articles and books on the topic, designed to serve as an entry point into the literature for clinicians and lawyers alike.

It is our hope that this book will contribute to increased mutual under-standing on the part of both the clinical and legal disciplines, whose respective representatives differ from their counterparts only in having undergone a differ-ent kind of professional training. That understanding is indispensable to a rec-onciliation between the legal and mental health systems that would permit the realization of the legitimate goals of each without negating the ends of the other; it should be apparent that only a sympathetic understanding of both traditions of caring for and about people will lead to the attainment of this reconciliation.

THOMAS G. GUTHEIL, M.D.
PAUL S. APPELBAUM, M.D.

Introduction

When reading textbooks or articles that are really interesting, I am in the habit of underlining. In the case of this second edition, a thoroughly updated version of Appelbaum and Gutheil's, *Clinical Handbook of Psychiatry and the Law,* I found myself unable to put down my pen.

The curious and thoughtful reader of this invaluable book will, I believe, have an identical reaction to mine. The first edition of *Clinical Handbook of Psychiatry and the Law* won the Manfred S. Guttmacher Award of the American Psychiatric Association and the American Academy of Psychiatry and the Law as the outstanding contribution that year (1982) to the field of law and psychiatry. The first edition helped set the law/psychiatry agenda for the 1980s.

One might say that the first edition of this book was a "self-fulfilling prophesy." The book explained the law and its clinically relevant dimensions for the clinician, demystifying its possible negative impacts on doctor-patient relationships, thereby setting the stage for more extensive growth and understanding of this field. By identifying the structures and settings in which the law affects psychiatric practice and by preparing the clinician for intelligent responses to clinical/consultative opportunities, the format of the first edition served the field well. Happily this prize-winning format is again followed in this second edition.

This second edition offers even more than the first because, over the last decade, Appelbaum and Gutheil have persisted in the work and become identified as among the most outstanding practitioners and theoreticians in legal and forensic psychiatry. Each has also performed empirical research to sophisticate his views and advance the field. Therefore, this second edition reflects each author's clinical wisdom and vast experience involving the doctor-patient, doctor-client, and doctor-subject relationships. This clinical/consultative experience is reflected on every page. The many challenging case examples and illustrations demonstrate lessons learned and previously analyzed by Appelbaum and Gutheil in recent but now classic articles on law and psychiatry. For example, Appelbaum's previous work on the right to refuse treatment guides the reader toward improved understanding of how the procedural requirements of the law have come to pass, how meaningful consent can yet be obtained, as well as how to assess patient competency in many settings. Gutheil's dynamic expertise is reflected in the second edition's many discussions of countertransference and the dynamics of malpractice, how therapists' own perspectives or fears can get in the way of the their understanding of the law's requirements or the patient's dilemma.

There is even greater need for this book now than in 1982 because of the deplorable tendencies in the profession toward the practice of defensive medicine, the assault on professional values by third party payers and sometimes by the courts, the ever increasing regulation of psychiatry, the rising level of violence within our society, the fears of victims, but also, from a much more positive and hopeful perspective, the increasing sophistication of patients. Today's patients are better educated. They have more expectations and have learned to "talk back to their doctor." They have a better understanding of their rights and how to secure them. All of this requires flexibility of response from practitioners, as well as their ability to truly understand the patient's position. The reader's range of potential response is enhanced by the many sensitive discussions in this edition of the dilemmas of patients and their families.

Not to be lost, however, are the authors' point of view and values expressed throughout this book. The law's requirements and historical precedents are not as rigid as clinicians may imagine. Psychiatrists must ultimately adhere to their own professional values including, above all, commitment to their patients' therapeutic interests and dignity. It is the genius of this book to demonstrate how the historical, ethical, and case and statutory development of the law (and its variations within jurisdictions) need not detract from this perspective. Like a compass still pointing north, the authors sweep the horizon to demonstrate how the patient's best interests may be served in a variety of clinical situations.

Like its predecessor, this volume will be of considerable interest and use to a multidisciplinary audience including psychiatric clinicians, social workers, psychologists, and other mental health professionals. Trainees in the law and practicing attorneys will find much of value here. The point of view is that of well trained, experienced, and sophisticated clinicians who know law and its rationale and values, and, most importantly, how this affects psychiatric practice.

In my own experience, the most frequent consultative questions in today's complex environment relate to issues of confidentiality, the management of violent patients, the avoidance of malpractice and defensive medicine, and the demands of factual and expert witness testimony. Each of these areas is beautifully covered in this volume. Checklists included in the chapters in these areas, as well as in several other chapters, serve as a guide, not only to complete the task, but to open new vistas and ways of thinking for the clinician.

This second edition of *Clinical Handbook of Psychiatry and the Law* will be the place to begin for novice and expert alike who wish to treat their patients well and to evaluate their clients fairly and efficiently in the challenging professional environment of the 1990s.

Loren H. Roth, M.D., M.P.H.
Professor of Psychiatry
University of Pittsburgh
February 1991

Contents

1

Confidentiality and Privilege

I. CASE EXAMPLES

A. Case Example 1

A 27-year-old white man appears at a psychiatric hospital's emergency room looking dirty and disheveled, his communications impaired by marked loosening of associations. He is adjudged by the examining resident to require hospitalization, but because he has already included the doctor in his fluid paranoid system and has made a number of threatening remarks toward him, the resident requests that a security guard stand by in the room as the patient is processed for admission. During the course of eliciting the basic demographic data, the resident is stunned to hear the patient blurt out a confession to a murder. Expressing great remorse and desire for punishment, the patient recounts that he bludgeoned an elderly woman to death the previous night on the waterfront and then dumped the body into the harbor. The resident completes the admission, but is then uncertain how to proceed.

B. Case Example 2

For two years this 34-year-old white woman, diagnosed as a chronic paranoid schizophrenic, has been in intermittent supportive therapy with the same doctor. Several hospitalizations have taken place during this period. The patient has given birth to two children, but since one was given up for adoption several years previously and the second one is living with a foster family under the supervision of the Department of Welfare, they play little role in her life and are rarely mentioned. To the psychiatrist's surprise, she one day receives a subpoena to testify at a hearing concerning the younger child. Exploration with the patient reveals that the Welfare Department is now seeking permanent custody of the child. A call to that department uncovers the information that it is hoped that the psychiatrist's testimony will clinch the case for the unfitness of the child's mother. The psychiatrist's protestations that she knows nothing of the mother's capacity to raise children because they have never discussed it are dismissed. The patient firmly requests that the doctor not testify. In light of this, the doctor fears that any information that she gives will be perceived as a hostile act and will impair the fragile therapeutic alliance. She would like to avoid that outcome, but does not know how.

C. Case Example 3

A 28-year-old, newly married man is referred to a community mental health center from a nearby hospital. The social worker making the referral mysteriously refuses to say why it is being made. When the patient arrives, he is clearly distraught. After considerable discussion, he reveals that he has just received the results of an HIV (human immunodeficiency virus) antibody test, which was positive. He denies any history of homosexual activity or intravenous drug use, though he comes from a neighborhood in which experimentation with drugs is common among young men. The patient is uncertain whether he wants psychotherapy but agrees to a short-term contract to allow him to explore the issues surrounding his HIV status. During the second session, the patient mentions casually his intention to have a child with his new wife. When confronted, he says clearly that he does not intend to tell her about his HIV-positive status, because that would mean they could never have a child and he would not be a "real" husband. The therapist discusses over the next two sessions the risks posed to the patient's wife and to a child who may be conceived. However, the patient still refuses to discuss the issue with his wife or to permit her to be notified. Motivated by concern about his responsibility to the patient's wife, on the one hand, and about maintaining the patient's confidentiality on the other, the therapist ponders what to do.

II. LEGAL ISSUES

A. Confidentiality and privilege

Confidentiality refers to the right of an individual not to have communications that were imparted in confidence revealed to third parties. It is derivative of the broader right to privacy that guards against a variety of intrusions on an individual's freedom from unwanted attention.

Privilege, often called more accurately "testimonial privilege," can be viewed as a narrow offshoot of the right to confidentiality. An individual has a testimonial privilege when he has the right to bar another person from testifying based on information that person has gained from contacts with him. Privilege applies only in judicial or parajudicial settings and its extent is strictly limited by case law or statute.

B. The Concept of confidentiality

1. HISTORICAL EVOLUTION OF A RIGHT TO PRIVACY

In English common law, that corpus of court decisions reaching back to the Middle Ages that is the foundation of Anglo-American jurisprudence, no explicit formulation of a right to privacy exists. Here in the United States, it was not until 1890 that Warren and Brandeis' landmark article, "The Right to Privacy," offered the first theoretical construction of a general right to privacy, although before then a variety of doctrines had protected narrow interests in freedom from intrusion or in the confidentiality of particular communications (e.g., mail or telegraph messages). Individuals, however, had no remedies for invasions of privacy except in unusual cases in which a criminal statute was violated by the disclosure of personal communications, or the information revealed was untrue and thus constituted grounds for libel. The innovation in Warren and Brandeis' formulation was the idea that all citizens shared a general right to privacy which could be enforced by bringing suit for damages against those who violated it.

A right to privacy caught on slowly but ultimately became firmly ensconced in American common law. It is usually thought of as consisting of four separate components, guaranteeing freedom from intrusion on seclusion, appropriation of one's name or likeness for commercial purposes, publicity given to one's personal life, and publicity that places one in a false light. The area covered by the right to privacy has grown tremendously in recent years, as it has been declared by the U.S. Supreme Court to be inherent in the other rights granted by our Constitution; it has served as the basis for decisions at all levels of the judiciary, in such disparate areas as the right to use contraception, access to abortions, and the right to refuse psychopharmacologic agents.

The rights of patients in therapeutic relationships to protection of their confidentiality received little attention in the development of the law of privacy. None of the usual subcategories of a right to privacy are easily applied to therapists' breaches of patients' confidentiality. The one that comes closest, publicity given to one's personal life, has generally been held to require actual publication of the disclosure to a general audience. In contrast, those situations most disturbing to medical and psychiatric patients usually involve disclosures to a single person or a small number of persons, such as a spouse, an employer, or law enforcement authorities. Although the law was paying little attention to protecting patients' confidences, the helping professions themselves had not neglected the area.

2. ETHICAL BASES FOR PROTECTING CONFIDENTIALITY

Long before the development of a legal right to privacy, medicine had embraced an ethical proscription against the needless divulgence of patients' confidences. The Hippocratic Oath, as well as later codes, enjoined physicians from disclosing information they acquired from their patients: ". . . (W)hatsoever I shall see or hear in the course of my profession . . . if it be what should not be published abroad, I will never divulge, holding such things to be holy secrets."

The ethical foundations of confidentiality in medicine and the other helping professions are twofold. First, confidentiality is based on the belief that revelation of patients' confidences—communicated in the course of diagnosis and treatment—would discourage patients from seeking medical and mental health care. The resulting harm to society would exceed the benefits of disclosure. Thus, the greater good lies in shielding patients' communications. This form of argument, based on the principle that we should follow the rule that yields greatest good for the greatest number of people, is a form of utilitarianism. Note that it depends on empirically testable propositions, such as the assumption that incursions on confidentiality will affect patients' motivations to seek treatment.

Does such empirical support exist? Numerous surveys of therapists, patients, and non-patients support the importance of confidentiality in treatment settings. It has been harder to demonstrate that patients would be deterred from seeking treatment if confidentiality were not protected, although anecdotal evidence appears to be supportive, and many patients claim that this would be true. Most patients surveyed, however, are ignorant of legal protections of their confidentiality, or the lack thereof, instead trusting their therapists to protect their disclosures. Does this mean that legal protection is unimportant or only that patients believe they can take it for granted? The answer is unclear.

The second argument in favor of confidentiality, in contrast to the utilitarian approach, does not rely for its justification on the consequences of the rule chosen. Advocates of this approach argue that medical and mental health professionals induce their patients to reveal personal information by creating situations in which confidentiality is implicitly or explicitly promised. Having made such a promise, the clinician is obligated to keep it. An ethical argument of this sort falls into the category of a "deontologic" justification, dependent on an analysis of moral duties rather than on the consequences of the act. Even so considered, though, confidentiality is not an absolute principle. In the face of countervailing duties, as will be seen below, it may have to give way.

Most mental health professionals would probably offer both utilitarian and deontologic reasons for protecting patients' confidentiality, although it is the former that are most frequently discussed in the literature. Regardless of the ethical underpinning, every mental health discipline endorses the importance of confidentiality in its code of ethics.

3. CURRENT LEGAL BASES FOR CONFIDENTIALITY

The lack of clear-cut common-law doctrines for protecting confidentiality has not prevented the development of substantial legal protections for patients. Two mechanisms have been used to achieve this end, judicial and statutory. Courts have used traditional privacy doctrines to impose liability on physicians and psychotherapists who have disclosed information communicated to them in confidence by their patients. They have also begun crafting a new doctrine explicitly recognizing the right of persons in certain professional settings—including psychotherapy—to protection from disclosure. This new theory has generally gone under the term, "breach of confidence." One limit to this approach, of course, is that it provides a monetary remedy only after the damage has been done.

Simultaneous with this activity in the courts, legislatures have passed statutes attempting to prevent breaches of confidentiality in the first place. Prohibitions against disclosure may be found in physician or psychotherapist licensure statutes in some states, physician-patient or psychotherapist-patient privilege statutes (see Sec. II-C below), and in laws creating a "patient's bill of rights." All these sources of the doctrine of confidentiality prescribe a common standard governing the release of information: with rare exceptions, identifiable data can be transmitted to third parties only with patients' explicit consent.

4. RELEASE OF INFORMATION TO THIRD PARTIES

a. General principles

Although the principles of confidentiality require patients' consent prior to disclosure, the form of that consent varies. Oral consent may be adequate in some situations, particularly in emergencies or potential emergencies when the need to delay action until written consent can be obtained would place the health or safety of the patient or a third party in jeopardy. Other circumstances in which oral consent might be appropriate include situations in which consent is being obtained to intrainstitutional disclosure of information for therapeutic purposes; for example, a psychiatrist seeing a patient whose family is also being seen in family therapy might be satisfied with the patient's oral consent to discussion of the case with the family therapist.

In general, however, it is probably wise for therapists always to require the written consent of their patients before releasing information to third parties. Written consent is advisable for at least two reasons: (1) it makes clear to both parties involved that consent has, in fact, been given; (2) if the fact, nature, or timing of the consent should ever be challenged, a documentary record exists. The consent should be made a part of the patient's permanent chart. In order to maximize the understanding of both parties about the scope of the disclosure that has been authorized, and to protect the patient from future unauthorized disclosures, the consent should specify (if possible) the extent of the data to be revealed and should be considered valid only for one transmittal of data. Subsequent requests from insurance companies, governmental agencies, family members, and others should be filled only after the patient has consented anew. Some states have incorporated these procedures into their statutes.

b. "Special" third parties

Families.   Family members are not usually viewed as third parties by most therapists. In fact, those who take a family or systems approach to therapy consider the family to be as much a focus of the therapeutic effort as the identified patient. Families of the severely mentally ill, just now starting to play an active role in formulating mental health policy, often complain most bitterly of the failure of clinicians to discuss their relatives' conditions with them, even when they are the primary caretakers. Although there may be good reason to consider changing the usual rules concerning confidentiality in such cases, no state has yet taken a step in that direction. Thus, information concerning the patient's treatment and prognosis should, in most cases, be revealed to family members only with the patient's consent. Nonetheless, it may be possible for mental health professionals to be more helpful than they have been to family members, even within current constraints. Greater efforts can be made to obtain patients' consent for discussions; nonconfidential items can be revealed; and information relating generally to severely mentally ill persons (e.g., the side-effects of medication and how they can be treated) can be discussed without referring specifically to the situation of a patient who refuses to grant permission for disclosure. It may be the attitude of mental health professionals, which has often communicated the absence of an interest in collaboration, more than what is or is not disclosed, that has most upset family members.

Other physicians and therapists.   The casual exchange of information among professionals has long been a hallmark of cordial collegial relations. If the doctrine of confidentiality is to have real meaning, however, this practice must be superseded by a careful release of data only with the patient's consent, even to consultants. Exchange of detailed and identifiable information about patients with colleagues in casual conversation is unethical as well as potentially actionable.

The useful practice in many academic centers and group practices of obtaining informal consultations from colleagues and peers can, of course, continue, so long as the patient's privacy is protected by alteration of his or her name and other identifying data. Continuing case conferences and presentations in rounds and seminars should be governed by similar rules.

It is often particularly difficult to resist sharing information with clinicians who have previously had contact with the patient, but who are no longer actively involved. Having left the circle of those caring for the patient, however, these clinicians are no longer entitled to receive confidential information. Although this may require a good deal of tact to accomplish in practice, responding to such requests with a sincere apology, but a firm refusal, best protects the interests of the patient. Follow-up, to be sure, is an important element in the clinical growth of the therapist, but this is one occasion in which it must be sacrificed for a more important end.

Patients themselves.   Although patients themselves are technically not third parties, the question of patients' access to their own records is generally considered along with other confidentiality issues. Statutes in many states now grant patients the right to view and copy their own charts, though the records themselves are acknowledged to belong to the facility or clinician. Most such laws allow access to be restricted for psychiatric patients if, in the treating clinician's judgment, reading the records may harm the patient. Even in these cases, however, the patient can usually select a third party, often a clinician, to whom the records will be released. That person can then decide whether or not to allow the patient to view the material.

A growing number of studies have been performed to assess the effects of allowing psychiatric patients to see their records, in both inpatient and outpatient settings. Almost all studies suggest a positive effect from greater patient access, particularly when efforts are made to prepare patients for the session, and someone is on hand to explain material that may be unclear or confusing. In contrast, most studies of clinicians' perspectives on this process demonstrate their concern about the emotional impact on patients of reading progress notes and other materials. Clinicians are also troubled by the possibility that their charting practices may be distorted by the knowledge that patients will have access to records in the future. Detrimental impacts on the quality of charts that are made available to patients, though, have yet to be found.

An issue of special concern when patients receive information from their own charts is the possibility that the records will contain comments solicited from relatives or friends of the patient, based on assurances that patients would not learn of their role. Although ethical considerations similar to those involving patients apply to these other sources of information, the legal situation is not as clear-cut. In principle, data obtained from sources who have requested anonymity should be excised from records before they are released. Statutes, however, may not recognize the importance of this step, instead granting total access to patients. This is one area in which recording practices might need to change, with greater care taken to protect sources of information, or informants may need to be told frankly about patients' right of access to records. In fact, many clinicians who are reluctant to "keep secrets" from their patients already routinely tell informants that they will be disclosing the information communicated to patients. This practice obviously precludes later problems.

Insurers. Disclosure of information to third-party payers has become among the most problematic issues of confidentiality. Patients usually are required to sign blanket consents for release of all medical and psychiatric records as a condition of insurance coverage. Insurers have an unquestioned need to assess the basis for and progress of treatment. Recent pressures to contain health costs, though, have led insurers to demand increasing amounts of data, prior to, during, and after treatment. No longer satisfied with summaries of patients' care, perhaps because mental health professionals have been less than frank in the past about patients' diagnoses, insurers now demand actual records in many cases, sometimes in their entirety.

Professional organizations have been working with insurers to change these practices, but they are still widespread. It is difficult for clinicians to protect patients' confidentiality when insurers can compel patients to consent to release of all data or else bear the cost of their own treatment. Although some outpatients choose to pay the full cost of therapy to avoid passing records to their insurers, this is often not a practical option, especially for hospitalized patients. Threats to confidentiality are even greater when insurance forms are processed in-house by patients' employers, in an effort to hold down health-care costs. Insurers' dedication to confidentiality is suspect in the absence of state laws prohibiting redisclosure. The only reasonable approach at present is for clinicians to exercise great care in the information they include in patients' records in the first place, eliminating compromising information not essential to patients' care. Of course, this does not deal with the problem in its entirety, since even the fact of psychiatric diagnosis and treatment may be highly stigmatizing.

The federal and state-funded Medicaid program has given rise to numerous controversies over confidentiality of records. Aggressive fraud control units have demanded access to full patient records to determine if services billed for were actually provided. Therapists have argued, in opposition to such broad requests, that access should be restricted to billing records and appointment books, or that records should be redacted to eliminate personal information prior to inspection. The courts have split in their response to these cases, but at least several opinions have supported the importance of confidentiality and denied prosecutors blanket access. Legislative options to restrain overbroad prosecutorial initiatives have not been pursued, but would seem to be a promising approach in this area.

c. Release of information for research purposes

Protecting patients' confidentiality in research procedures. Gathering information for research purposes almost always creates risk that identifiable information about patients will become available to third parties. Federal regulations require that all limits on confidentiality be explained to research subjects, and their consent to participation be obtained. In addition, institutional review boards (IRBs), mandated to conduct prospective review of research protocols in institutions receiving federal research funds, have developed two strategies to minimize the risk of unnecessary disclosure: patient identifiers and confidential information are separated whenever possible, and the number of people with access to identifiable data is limited.

As a threshold matter, confidentiality is best protected if initial screening of patients for suitability for research is done, if at all possible, by their clinicians. This removes the specter of research assistants combing through the charts of dozens of patients to gather potential subjects. Once patients are identified as potential subjects, their clinicians can obtain consent for their being approached by researchers to discuss participation in the study. Alternatively, in institutions where a great deal of research activity occurs, patients' consent to have their charts screened or to allow their charts to be used for studies based solely on record reviews can be obtained prospectively. This is also helpful when it can be anticipated that patients may no longer be in treatment at the time of the screening. Though prospective consent of this sort is maximally protective of patients' rights to maintain confidentiality, the general practice of IRBs is to permit record screening and retrospective record reviews without patient consent.

Further protection to confidentiality is afforded if data forms contain codes, rather than patient names. If it is necessary to retain a record that links codes and names, for example to conduct a follow-up some months later, these forms can be kept separate from the data. Most IRBs require that research data be kept securely in locked files, and that identifiers be destroyed as soon as it is feasible to do so. The advantage to confidentiality in the last requirement is balanced by the loss of opportunity to use the same sample in subsequent studies not yet conceived. The possibility of future investigations must be considered carefully when confidentiality protections are being designed.

Publication of identifiable information. Not all research in psychiatry originates in formal protocols. Many important contributions have been made by clinicians who have reviewed and reported their clinical experiences with one or more patients.

Patients' privacy can be infringed by publication of data that are not sufficiently disguised to render them anonymous. The most famous case to reach the courts dealt with an analyst who published detailed transcripts of analytic sessions in a book. The courts held that despite the fact that the work was intended as a scientific demonstration for a professional audience, the patient's right to privacy had suffered. Obtaining the patient's consent to publication would have obviated the problem; however, the casual mention that the therapist is working on a book that might utilize case material of the patient, as occurred in the case noted here, was not sufficient. As the Group for the Advancement of Psychiatry noted, "Sometimes material may be so impossible to camouflage that it should not be published at all, in spite of its scientific value. Such ethical requirements take priority over research objectives." Of course, the same principles hold for videotapes and audiotapes of patients' sessions. (See also Chapter 4, Sec. II-C-2.)

d. Liability resulting from release of information to third parties

Patients whose confidential disclosures have been released without their consent can seek compensation from those responsible for harms they may have suffered, including emotional harms consequent on others knowing of their affairs. Courts have developed a variety of theories under which such claims are adjudicated, including actions in tort (the law of civil wrongs) for invasion of privacy, breach of confidentiality, and malpractice, and actions in contract for breach of an implied warranty that confidentiality will be maintained. (See Chapter 4, section II-C-2.) Several recent cases have indicated that those persons who induce a therapist to reveal confidential information (e.g., the patient's employer) may also be held liable for resulting harms.

Other options for the aggrieved patient include seeking punitive action against the clinician from the state's professional board of licensure. Theoretically, a complaint alleging breach of professional ethics can be brought before the therapist's professional association, although this is rarely done because of the limited sanctions available to such groups. If a "patients' bill of rights" exists in the jurisdiction, any penalties for violation that are provided for therein may also apply.

5. EXCEPTIONS

As important as confidentiality is to patients, from both utilitarian and deontologic perspectives, few people question that there are times when other interests must take priority.

Disclosure of information without patients' consent may be legally justified, or even required in such circumstances as:

a. During an emergency

Physicians, and probably other therapists, retain the obligations of a fiduciary relationship—to act in the best interests of the patient. When, in an emergency situation, a patient refuses to give consent or cannot be located for consent, a therapist may sometimes disclose appropriate data in the patient's interest. The situations in which this might be thought to be the case are so numerous—almost any refusal to grant consent can be construed as not in the patient's interest—that if the exception is not to swallow the rule, such action should be limited to situations in which the patient's immediate welfare is clearly at stake.

Some examples are fairly clear-cut. When the therapist is contacted by a hospital emergency room, where the patient, thought to be psychotic and unwilling to answer questions, is being evaluated, information concerning the patient's diagnosis, medications prescribed, pattern of illicit drug use, and the like may be essential to proper evaluation and treatment. It should be revealed, in the patient's interests, even without explicit consent, and if the patient's physical well-being is at stake, probably even over his explicit objections, with the justification for such action carefully documented.

When the patient's physical integrity is not at stake, the extent of an emergency exception becomes harder to define. A social service agency, for example, may contact a therapist asking for information that would establish the patient's continuing eligibility for subsidized housing. The patient has not been seen for some weeks, and consent for a disclosure of this sort was not previously obtained. Without the therapist's evidence, though, the patient will lose her apartment. Is this enough of an emergency to warrant a response in the absence of consent? In such circumstances, it may be best to rely on the assumption that a reasonable person would want a disclosure to be made, and to act accordingly. Some people who value confidentiality highly, however, may disagree with this approach. In any event, liability is extremely unlikely to be imposed if the therapist is acting in what he or she genuinely believes to be the patient's interest.

b. When the patient is incompetent

If the treating clinician believes that her patient is not legally competent to give or to withhold consent, for example, for release of information for disability benefits, she should attempt to obtain a substitute consent. If the patient has a guardian, that person is legally entitled to act on the patient's behalf. Many patients who are functionally incompetent, however, have never had a formal adjudication and lack guardians. In such cases, the consent of a close relative may be adequate. In situations in which a substitute for the patient's consent cannot be obtained (e.g., he has neither a guardian nor relatives available), the therapist can release information that she believes will serve her patient's best interest.

c. Acting to hospitalize or to commit the patient

When disclosure of information is required to effect the involuntary commitment of a patient (as by giving evidence of her inability to care for herself) or her voluntary hospitalization, such release is permitted in most states. Some jurisdictions, however, restrict therapists from releasing confidential information in commitment proceedings over patients' objections. In those states, special examiners conduct commitment evaluations without input from treating clinicians.

d. Acting to protect third parties

Prior to the mid-1970s, psychiatrists' obligations to protect third parties from their patients' violent acts were limited to situations in which psychiatrists took physical control of a potentially dangerous person, i.e., hospitalized that person. Their duties extended only to insuring that these patients did not escape or were not prematurely released due to the psychiatrist's negligence. There was no need to breach confidentiality to fulfill this duty.

Tarasoff v. Regents of the University of California, a case ultimately decided by the California Supreme Court in 1976, changed all that. *Tarasoff* recognized a duty of all mental health professionals, not just psychiatrists, to protect their patients' potential victims, even if the patient had never been hospitalized. Although the court required therapists to take "whatever steps are reasonably necessary" to discharge their duty, it especially emphasized the possibility that warnings may have to be issued to the victim and/or the police. Roughly 40% of the states now have similar judicial decisions, and about 25% of the states have adopted statutes defining some sort of obligation analogous to the one fashioned in *Tarasoff*. Most experts advise therapists in states without current law relating to a duty to protect to act as if some version of the obligation exists in their jurisdiction. (For a more complete discussion of potential liability resulting from a failure to fulfill the duty to protect, see Chapter 4, Sec. II-A-3-e).

As noted, the duty to protect is not synonymous with a duty to warn. Other measures can be taken without breaching confidentiality, and should ordinarily be considered first, including changing the nature of therapy to focus on the feared violence, adding or changing medications, expanding therapy to include a threatened intimate of the patient's, and hospitalizing the patient. There will be circumstances, however, in which disclosure will be necessary to protect potential victims. If the therapist fails to disclose and harm results, liability may be imposed. Conversely, disclosure made in a good faith belief that a third party is endangered will not result in liability for breach of confidence. Many states are now adopting statutes providing explicit immunity from suit in such circumstances.

The duty to protect was developed in the context of violent behavior by patients, but it has been extended by some courts to include property damage and harm caused by dangerous driving. Among the most problematic new areas to which a duty to protect may apply is the protection of sexual partners of persons infected with the human immunodeficiency virus (HIV). Laws in some states forbid disclosure of patients' HIV status to sexual partners, while others allow it. Suits against physicians for failure to inform a sexual partner have been rare, and there are substantial problems of proof (e.g., was the partner infected before or after the therapist learned of the patient's condition). But, whether or not required by law, many clinicians feel an ethical obligation to protect endangered sexual partners. It is generally agreed that efforts should first be made to get the HIV-infected patient to discuss the issue with his or her partner, and to bring that person in for counseling. Failing that, however, the American Medical Association and American Psychiatric Association have issued statements indicating their support for disclosure when necessary to protect a sexual partner. Public sentiment also appears to be swinging in this direction. No statutes yet mandate disclosure, but they may be on the horizon. An alternative approach for clinicians who are reluctant to contact sexual partners directly is to pass the information along to public health authorities, although the nature of their response will vary from state to state.

e. Acting in conformance with reporting requirements

States are imposing an ever-growing number of obligations on physicians, other mental health professionals, and other caregivers to report specified conditions and behavior. Although each reporting obligation that is adopted by the legislature represents a decision that public knowledge of the condition or behavior in question is more important than the maintenance of confidentiality, one must question the cumulative impact of these requirements.

Historically, all states have required the reporting of cases of specified communicable diseases to allow public health measures to be implemented. The range of conditions, symptomatic and asymptomatic, associated with infection with HIV is a controversial addition to this group. Similarly, all jurisdictions require professionals to notify authorities about cases of suspected child abuse, although the statutes vary considerably in their requirements. Some impose an obligation only if the professional has seen the child or if the abuse is recent and likely to continue; others require reporting even of abuse that has occurred in the distant past, whether or not the child has been seen in person.

New legislation is being enacted analogous to child abuse reporting statutes to cover other groups at risk of abuse. These include the elderly and the mentally and physically disabled. Some states are now attempting to enforce older requirements for reporting of persons who may be unsafe drivers, including but not limited to, the mentally ill, epileptics, and drug and alcohol abusers. Impaired health care professionals, especially physicians, who come to the attention of other providers must be reported in some jurisdictions. And there is a good deal of discussion about requiring mental health professionals to report instances of sexual contact between therapists and patients, when these are revealed by their patients.

Clinicians who fail to live up to their mandatory reporting obligations may be subject to the civil and criminal penalties that are part of many statutes. In addition, should harm later occur that would have been prevented had they reported the situation, potential civil liability may exist as well.

It should be noted that in almost every jurisdiction, and under federal law, previous crimes of a patient that come to the therapist's attention do not have to be reported. The common law doctrine of misprision, which required all citizens to report felonies of which they became aware, has been rejected repeatedly by courts in this country, although a few states retain misprision statutes. When evidence of a past crime raises the strong possibility of future crimes, however, as in the case of a repetitive sex offender, a clinician's duty to protect potential victims may require that some action (not necessarily reporting) be taken.

f. Supervisors and collaborators

It is not considered a breach of confidentiality to disclose information to those who are assisting the primary caregiver's efforts. This includes supervisors, members of a hospital's milieu staff, and colleagues who are involved directly in the patient's treatment. These individuals, once in possession of the data, are likewise under the same obligation to maintain confidentiality as the primary therapist. Inhouse quality assurance proceedings are undertaken under similar presumptions.

C. The concept of privilege

1. HISTORICAL EVOLUTION

Since Elizabethan times, when courts first assumed the power to coerce testimony from unwilling witnesses, there has been some sense that certain parties had a right—a privilege—to resist that coercion. Initially, it was the right of all gentlemen to refuse to divulge embarrassing confidences in court. As that privilege was abrogated, it was retained for a few groups. Clients were permitted to prevent their lawyers from testifying against them, on the grounds that to allow such testimony would so impair the lawyer-client relationship as to make it worthless. Husbands and wives were not permitted to testify against each other, although in part this privilege was motivated by the high risk of perjured testimony. These constituted the only protected relationships in English common law. Patients of physicians were never accorded a privilege comparable to that of clients of attorneys, despite arguments about the importance of protecting patients' disclosures.

It was in New York in 1828 that the first statute specifically granting doctors the right to refuse to testify was passed. Today, a majority of the states have some kind of medical privilege statute. Those statutes are generally under attack as unnecessary impediments to the discovery of truth in judicial proceedings. It is argued that the confidentiality they provide is not needed for the pursuit of good medical care.

Such arguments seem to carry less weight in the psychotherapeutic situation. Almost all states have provided some means of preventing compelled disclosure of communications by mental health professionals. Psychiatrists are covered by physician-patient privileges, where they exist, and by psychotherapist-patient privileges in most other jurisdictions. Ph.D. psychologists are included in the latter statutes, or may be covered by privileges specific to them alone. Other mental health professions, including clinical social work, marriage and family counseling, rape counseling, and school counseling are covered by privilege statutes in some states. Clergymen who conduct pastoral counseling may be granted privilege in those states that recognize a "priest-penitent" privilege. The trend is clearly toward broadening the classes of therapists covered by privilege statutes. Due to the patchwork of legislation, though, the actual terms of the privilege may vary substantially among professions even within the same state.

2. ETHICAL BASES FOR PRIVILEGE

As with confidentiality in general, two approaches can be taken to justifying a testimonial privilege, utilitarian and deontologic. Most discussions of privilege emphasize the former. Thus, the leading legal commentator on the rules of privilege, Wigmore, elaborated four rules governing when privileges should be recognized: when 1) the communication sought to be protected was made with an expectation of confidentiality; 2) confidentiality is essential to the relationship in which the disclosure took place; 3) the relationship is one that society should seek to foster; and 4) the harm to the relationship caused by disclosure is greater than the benefit to the litigation process. Mental health professionals have generally accepted this framework and argued that the psychotherapy relationship meets these criteria. When privileges have been applied to the mental health context, it has almost always been because this argument has been accepted.

In fact, though, as scholars have begun to point out, it is not easy to find empirical support for some of these propositions. Evidence exists, to be sure, about the importance that patients say they place on confidentiality, and there is a common-sense belief that widespread breaches would reduce patients' willingness to seek care. But the proposition that the absence of a privilege would impair psychotherapy is difficult to test. Would the small risk of disclosure in later court proceedings really deter patients who required mental health treatment from seeking it? The small number of jurisdictions without privileges do not, on first inspection, appear to have very different rates of patients seeking mental health care than do states with a privilege. Additionally, the fact that most privileges have many exceptions means that even where they exist patients still run substantial risks of courtroom disclosure. Is it only patients' unawareness of the risks, or their indifference to them, that keeps them coming to their therapy sessions?

The difficulty in validating the utilitarian requirements for a therapist-patient privilege (i.e., that there is a net gain to society) has led many people to turn to other ways of justifying it. They speak in deontologic terms of the value that privacy of the therapeutic relationship has in its own right. Such relationships should be protected from intrusion, they argue, even at some cost, because of the importance of providing a private sanctuary in which we can freely discuss our most personal thoughts. A society that encourages and protects such discussion and reflection, this approach maintains, is a morally better place to live.

3. CURRENT LEGAL BASES FOR PRIVILEGE

As noted, almost all privileges that affect the therapist-patient relationship have a statutory basis. A codified privilege represents the conclusion of the legislature that the sacrifice of evidence at trial is worth the benefits from protecting therapeutic confidentiality. Where a therapist-patient privilege is not explicitly provided for by statute it must be assumed not to exist. Courts still retain the power, however, to create privileges on a common-law basis, and may do so occasionally, using Wigmore's four requirements, listed above.

Federal courts, in cases in which they must apply federal law, constitute a somewhat different situation. The Federal Rules of Evidence do not contain an explicit psychotherapist-patient privilege—or any other kind of privilege—although one was included in the original draft. Rather, the Rules give the federal courts the power to create privileges on a case-by-case basis, "governed by the principles of the common law as they may be interpreted . . . in the light of reason and experience." The language, supported by the legislative history of the Rules, appears to allow judicial recognition of a psychotherapist-patient privilege in appropriate cases. Nonetheless, several federal courts have ruled that the absence of a psychotherapist-patient privilege at common law (i.e., in judicial decisions issued prior to the adoption of the Rules) precludes the courts from recognizing a privilege. Whether this will be the settled interpretation of the Federal Rules is unclear at this point.

Two federal statutory privileges should be noted. The first exists for records of patients in drug and alcohol treatment programs supported, even indirectly, by federal funds. Those records cannot be released without a specific determination by a judge that the public interest in disclosure outweighs negative effects on the patient and his treatment. Another privilege may be invoked for research records in projects for which the investigator has obtained a certificate of confidentiality from the appropriate federal agency. Certificates can only be issued under certain circumstances, but provide almost complete immunity from prosecutorial or judicial access to records.

4. EXERCISE OF PRIVILEGE

The right to bar testimony of a therapist belongs to the patient; that is, the privilege is his to exercise. If he chooses to waive his privilege and to permit testimony by his therapist, the latter has no basis on which to refuse to testify. In some cases the right to waiver may belong to the patient's guardian or heir. If the patient does exercise his privilege, the information that the therapist has obtained, though usually not the fact of treatment itself, may not be revealed in court in pretrial proceedings. If the patient is not present to claim his privilege, the therapist may be obligated to claim it for him, pending the patient's appearance. (See also Chap. 8, Sec. I.)

5. EXCEPTIONS TO PRIVILEGE

The situations in which a patient may not exercise testimonial privilege vary from state to state and in some cases may be interpreted so broadly by the courts as to almost negate the utility of the statutes. These exceptions include:

1. cases in which the patient has initiated litigation to which her mental status may be relevant (the so-called patient-litigant exception).
2. if the examination has been ordered by the court for purposes of determining competency to stand trial or criminal responsibility.
3. if the therapist was asked to aid in the commission of or avoidance of punishment for a crime or tort.
4. after the patient's death (some jurisdictions limit this exception to issues concerning the disposition of the deceased's property).
5. when the patient represents a danger to herself or others.
6. if the patient has initiated a malpractice suit against the therapist.
7. when a patient fails to pay her bill and the therapist undertakes court proceedings.
8. in criminal cases (though some jurisdictions explicitly permit privilege to be exercised even in criminal actions).
9. in child custody cases, where on balance the good to be gained for the child outweighs the negative effects of disclosure (some states extend this standard to all court proceedings).
10. in investigations of billing fraud by the therapist. Federal rules governing access to therapists' records may be deemed to override state privilege statutes in such cases.

It should be emphasized that the extent of exceptions differs from state to state, and a careful reading of local law is essential before testimony is undertaken. In all jurisdictions if the patient herself testifies about some aspect of the privileged relationship, she is considered to have effectively waived all future claims of privilege.

6. SUBPOENAS

Any litigant can obtain a subpoena to compel the appearance of a witness and/or the production of relevant documents in court or at deposition for the purpose of examination. The mere fact that a subpoena has been issued does not compel a therapist to testify, only to appear. At that point, it is for the judge to decide whether the testimony or records in question are subject to a claim of privilege. Receipt of a subpoena should be a stimulus for the therapist to contact the lawyers involved to determine the information sought. If the right of a patient to claim privilege may be at issue, the patient or his lawyer should be notified too. Finally, this may be a good time for the therapist to contact his own attorney to clarify his rights and responsibilities in the case at hand. Under no circumstances should records be altered or destroyed when a subpoena is received.

7. COMMUNICATIONS MADE IN THE PRESENCE OF THIRD PARTIES

Traditionally, statements made in the presence of third parties were held not to be susceptible to a claim of privilege. Court opinions in recent years have differed as to this, however; some states may void privilege if any third party is present, others only if that party is not involved collaboratively in the patient's care (e.g., as a social worker or a nurse would be), while other states continue to permit privilege to be claimed. In such cases, the therapist may be exempt from testifying but the third party may still be obligated to testify. The most difficult cases of this sort are divorce proceedings, in which one spouse may attempt to force the therapist to testify about statements made by the other spouse during marital therapy. The success of a claim of privilege here will vary with the jurisdiction.

8. GROUP THERAPY

Revelations made before groups represent a special instance of communications in the presence of third parties. Unless the privilege statute explicitly grants privilege to the group situation, as suggested in the American Psychiatric Association's Model Law on Confidentiality, it should be assumed that testimony about any material revealed in the group can be compelled from any member of the group.

D. Confidentiality and informed consent

As exceptions to confidentiality in mental health treatment have multiplied, questions naturally have arisen as to how much patients should be told about the risks of disclosure. Some clinicians have argued that all possible threats to confidentiality should be revealed to patients at the start of therapy, so that they can decide whether they are willing to run the risk that confidential information may leave the consulting room. At least one state recently has adopted a statute requiring psychologists to disclose this information.

This approach, while affording patients maximal information prior to entering into therapy, is not without costs. Patients may interpret the unfortunately lengthy list of circumstances under which disclosure may take place as meaning that their confidences will almost certainly be revealed. At the point where their own ambivalence about entering treatment is at its height, the perception that they are about to embark on a venture that is likely to end with embarrassing information becoming public or being used to their disadvantage may well lead them to reject the idea of treatment altogether. A more reasonable approach can certainly be outlined.

1. PROVIDING INFORMATION AT THE START OF THERAPY

For most patients, the risk that information discussed in therapy will be revealed is small. Most risks, in fact, have such a low likelihood of materializing that a reasonable patient would not take them into account in making a decision about entering treatment. Even under the most rigorous views of informed consent, (see Chap. 4, Sec. II-B-2-a) discussion of such information with patients is not required. That conclusion is reinforced by the likelihood of patients being frightened away from therapy at its inception.

On the other hand, for some patients it may be possible to identify risks of disclosure that are more than minimal. A patient with a long history of violent or self-destructive behavior, for example, might well create a situation in which the clinician felt compelled to breach confidentiality to protect a third party or the patient herself. It may well be appropriate to inform these patients at the initiation of therapy, or when the potential for breach of confidentiality becomes apparent, what the therapist intends to do. This ensures that even if the patient's confidentiality must at some point be violated without her consent, she will not have consented to participate in therapy without an understanding of the possible consequences.

2. PROVIDING INFORMATION PRIOR TO DISCLOSURE

Even if the precautions described above are taken at the initiation of therapy, there inevitably will be situations in which the therapist unexpectedly learns in the course of treatment of information that must be revealed. If at all possible, disclosure of confidential information should be discussed with the patient before it takes place. The reason for disclosure can be discussed and the patient asked to consent to the therapist's action, or to suggest some alternative. This process changes non-consensual disclosure into a more collaborative decision.

Patients, of course, may not consent to the disclosure. Even so, studies suggest that patients are less likely to leave treatment if clinicians make an effort to inform them of the reasons confidentiality is being broken. Such discussion allows the therapist to explore the patient's responsibility for creating the situation that warrants breach of confidentiality in the first place. In cases in which the therapist may wish not to disclose, but be compelled to do so by existing law, that too can be made clear.

III. CLINICAL ISSUES

A. Trust as the basis for the therapeutic alliance

The alliance in therapy is based on a collaboration between the therapist and the nonpathologic (or "healthy") aspects of the patient's personality. To attain this collaborative stance, the therapist attempts to "see the world through the patient's eyes," striving for a state of empathic rapport. At the same time, in tension with this collaborative approach, the therapist must inevitably work in opposition to the pathologic (or "sick") aspects of the patient's psyche (e.g., a tendency toward harshly punitive self-appraisal), in effect acting as an advocate for the healthy side of the patient.

The foregoing requires from the patient an openness of self-disclosure and comfort with candor, in respect to which the physician owes the protection of confidentiality.

1. CONFIDENTIALITY AND THE QUESTION OF AGENCY

The term "agency" describes for whom one is working, who as employer has hired the therapist. The agency is thus the operational basis for the therapeutic alliance. There are several varieties of agency.

a. Individual patient agency

This is the outpatient adult model. In this model, the consenting adult hires the therapist as a consultant specialist; therefore, the therapist is considered to be working for that patient only. The individual patient's material is kept confidential from all other parties, in the absence of consent.

b. Couples, group, or family agency

In these models, the therapist works for the good of the couple, group, or family as a unit; this may mean at times contravening the wishes of one member, even the "designated patient." In any case, confidentiality is kept within the couple, group, or family.

One potential problem with this matter should be noted. It is a well-known fact in family therapy that families may keep secrets as part of their normal or pathologic functioning. The danger is that the treatment team may fall into this pattern and perpetuate secrets in treatment through avoidance or other defense mechanisms. This may represent an exaggeration of a right to confidentiality to nonconstructive degrees. For example, a family may maintain that their psychotic son would "go crazy or kill himself" if he finds out that he is adopted. The treatment team may fall into the trap by viewing the son as too fragile to be told this information. Both groups (the family and the treatment team) may fail in this manner to recognize the fact that the perceived fragility of the son is, in and of itself, a symptom and product of the adoption secret.

In this example, the therapist is being asked to divide agency "within his patient" (the family). Approaches to this problem demand treating this wish to keep a secret as resistance to the process of therapy. The therapist should explore the family's fantasies as to the results of "telling" and reaffirm that the contract with the family is to explore areas that may be causing family distress. Finally, the therapist should urge family members to consider revealing the secret themselves, within the family therapy session, if possible, to permit maximum utilization.

c. Institutional agency and "split" agency

In the United States (as opposed to the Soviet Union, for example), pure institutional agency in treatment situations is rare; rather, the clinician's agency is usually split in varying proportions between the individual and the institution. Examples of a split therapeutic agency might occur in military, court, school, or industrial mental health work. Although the clinician in those settings owes some loyalty to the institution, the well-being of the patient is not usually completely ignored.

In some cases, confidentiality may also be split between the individual and the institution in varying degrees. A court psychiatrist, for example, may owe disclosure to the court concerning material relevant to the purpose for which the evaluation is being performed; in some jurisdictions the extent of the disclosure may be limited by statute. A military psychiatrist may be obliged to report on whether a soldier is a security risk, for example, but may keep other material confidential, subject to the absence of formal privilege in military law. (See also Chap. 6 concerning forensic evaluations.)

d. Confusion of agency

It is important to realize that confidentiality should work only one way; that is to say, nothing should be told about the patient (or family or group) to the outside world. Relevant outside information, however, should (and in some cases must) be reported "in"; that is, phone calls, letters, and other kinds of information that come to the therapist from outside ethically belong to the treatment process and should be reported to the patient. Failure to follow this guideline, especially with paranoid patients, may result in their flight from treatment or other unfortunate results. For example, the mother of a paranoid schizophrenic patient may call with certain information and may urge the therapist not to tell the patient that she called. There are some approaches found useful in such situations. Some therapists attempt to state, as early as possible in the conversation (interrupting if necessary), that information will be shared with the patient; this approach mitigates possible feelings of betrayal in the caller that might arise from being told, after having revealed a confidence, that it will be shared. The therapist might tell the mother that he must tell the son about their conversation by virtue of the contract, but the therapist should encourage the mother to tell the patient first. Failing that, the therapist must tell the patient about the call *at the earliest opportunity.* Delay in reporting this call may leave the patient unclear as to whether the therapist would have told him without the matter coming up in the process of treatment. Thus, the therapist must, as it were, remain above suspicion in his willingness to report material from the outside into the treatment. Such doubts can be severely problematic in work with paranoid patients.

A second example might be when the parents of an adolescent girl demand to know from the therapist about the patient's sexual or drug-related activities. The family may argue, "After all, we are paying the bill." The approach here requires clarification with the parents about the differences between the therapeutic contract and the contractual arrangements concerning payment for the sessions. Again, as in the above example, the therapist should urge discussion with the patient herself. If no resolution is possible, the therapist must refer to the original confidentiality or agency agreements that, ideally, are made at the outset of the treatment of either a minor patient or an incompetent patient. Clearly, when the payment will be coming from a source other than from the patient, identification of the arrangements concerning confidentiality should be made before treatment begins. Thus, the therapist might say at the outset: "I will be seeing Johnny in treatment and you will be receiving the bills. I will rely on Johnny to tell you as much as he wishes about the therapy. If you want to talk to me about something, I will get Johnny's permission and we will meet with him present. Is that acceptable?"

Such an agreement, negotiated during what may be a period of calm at the very start of treatment, goes a long way toward averting misunderstandings and antagonisms that may flow from feelings stirred up by crises in the treatment or in the patient's evolving relationship with the family. Under certain circumstances, should all of the above measures fail, treatment may have to be stopped by the therapist, since his alliance with the patient is shattered (but see Chap. 4, Sec. II-A-3-h regarding abandonment).

2. The ethical issue in agency

Split agency is not necessarily a problem; ethically, however, candor is required to delineate the nature of the agency *before* material is explored in any situation where agency is not limited only to the patient. Thus: "I am evaluating you for the court (school, company, battalion), Mr. Jones; what you tell me will be (may be, may in part be) shared with the court (etc.), so please keep that in mind. Within that limitation, however, I would like to be as helpful to you as I can." Obtaining the patient's informed consent to the split in agency is essential to prevent the patient from being, or feeling, victimized by the situation. (See also Chap. 6, on forensic evaluations.)

B. Release of information to third parties with consent

It must be kept in mind that the patient's signed consent overcomes only the *legal* barrier to release of information. Clinical standards require a separate scrutiny.

1. How much to tell

The best rule to follow in deciding how much to tell third parties about confidential material must be designated the "rule of austerity"; to wit, the minimal necessary data to answer the question posed by the third party is the preferred amount. In selecting data, one must keep in mind that facts are more useful than speculations and that direct observations and personal assessments are more useful than reports or hearsay data.

Certain information can be conveyed with minimal disclosure by the use of negatives in writing an opinion; for example, "There are *no* psychiatric *contra*indications at this time to (driving a car, getting a job, moving into special housing)." The use of this double negative format may avoid the necessity of extensive supporting data.

In general, unconscious material, fantasies, and psychodynamic formulations have no place outside the immediate clinical sphere and should be excluded from communications to third parties. Some exceptions to this approach should be noted. Under some statutes patients may have the right to authorize release of their entire record. Even without an explicit statute, patients generally have the right to release complete records to attorneys, third-party payers, administrative agencies, and subsequent treaters.

2. HANDLING THE PATIENT'S WISH FOR ALTERED CLINICAL DATA

On occasion, a patient may directly or indirectly request altered data for either social, monetary, narcissistic or legal gain. For example, for social gain, the dangerous alcoholic may request a letter supporting the return of his driver's license to allow greater convenience in using his car. In the monetary realm, the patient may request a reimbursible diagnosis on an insurance form or may request a statement of (nonexistent) disability in order to permit collection of benefit payments. In the narcissistic realm, the patient with a grandiose paranoid illness may request statements addressed to various places that "nothing is wrong," in order to perpetuate her denial of the illness. In the legal realm a patient who is in therapy as a condition of parole from a criminal sentence may request that the therapist "not tell them anything," despite agreement from the outset on regular reporting to the parole officer; similar requests may be made in those circumstances where treatment is an element of probation.

(1) The therapist may be fallible, but should not be corruptible; that is, although he may make mistakes or miss something relevant, he should not knowingly falsify, misrepresent, or ignore factual data.

(2) The therapist must represent reality or the viewpoint of realistic observation.

(3) All the issues above can and should be discussed at length to extract the maximum data about the patient's ego functioning and world view that can subsequently be utilized in therapy.

3. REVIEWING THE INFORMATION WITH THE PATIENT

As a rule, whenever it is possible, the therapeutic course is advanced when doctor and patient have the opportunity to review together any material that is going to third parties; this may include forms, letters, and discharge summaries. As a general rule, a joint review tends to support the alliance position. Indeed, the majority of difficulties that arise around confidentiality do so, not because confidentiality is breached per se, but because the patient is surprised by finding out that some unexpected person or agency knows something about her that she did not anticipate. This "surprise factor" appears to be the major trigger for litigation in this area (see Chap. 4, Sec. III-A). Reviewing with the patient everything that leaves the office is thus the best liability preventive measure, as well as a means of conveying respect for the patient.

In handling the release of sensitive information, one issue that frequently arises is the question of the patient's or a third party's judgmental interpretation of certain technical and descriptive terms. Such terms might include "latent homosexuality," "incestuous wishes," and the like. Although these terms have specific meanings to the therapist in relation to the patient's unconscious dynamics, they are often experienced by laypersons (who may include third parties) as critical or pejorative. More importantly, third parties, including legal authorities, tend to see these terms as literal, conscious, and action-related rather than symbolic, unconscious, and fantasy-oriented. The distinction between these two categorizations may be unclear to the uninitiated.

The following approaches are suggested: First, the use of judicious euphemism is indicated in writing the report. The word "oedipal" or "developmental" rather than "incestuous" would be a preferable way of stating this issue; in a similar manner, "identity concerns" would be preferable to "fear of homosexuality."

Another valuable approach involves blending candor in the written discussion with an eye to maintaining a perspective on human experience. This would mean indicating to patients or third parties that these seemingly deviant feelings are common to all human beings and are part of the normal human experience.

A third approach embodies the diplomatic choice of expressions. One resourceful clinician, working in a clinic where all patients read all notes, wrote the following self-explanatory entry: "This woman seemed so suspicious, I wonder if she is paranoid, though she says she is not." This manner of describing the episode clearly communicates to clinicians who might read the record in the future the important clinical data that it was intended to communicate.

C. Release of information to third parties without consent

1. EMERGENCIES

Emergencies in general constitute exceptions to the usual rules governing confidentiality. Under certain emergency conditions involving danger (risk of suicide, impending assault, etc.), confidentiality may (and in certain circumstances, must) be breached without consent as noted in Sec. II-B-5-a above. For example, the therapist may tell the patient's spouse that the patient is suicidal and may urge that the police be called, thus breaking the confidentiality of the therapist-patient relationship. In such situations the alliance has been temporarily abandoned. The therapist is forced into the position of social agent, both by law, and more importantly, by the overriding concern for the safety of the patient and others (See Chapter 2.)

Such breach, needless to say, has effects on the alliance itself. The patient may feel abandoned or betrayed during the emergency and may feel herself in opposition to (rather than allied with) the therapist. During the emergency, the therapist should candidly describe what is happening: "I am breaking our agreed-on confidentiality because in my judgment we face an emergency situation (explain), and I must act in your interest, even against our agreement."

After the emergency is resolved, attention should be paid to the repair of the transiently broken alliance. In this approach, the therapist invites the patient to join with him in a study of how the loss of alliance occurred and why it was necessary temporarily to abandon the agency of the individual patient.

2. IN COURT

Under certain circumstances, testimony may be compelled from the therapist with privilege absent or waived as described above (see Sec. II-C-5). The effects of such forced testimony may be similar to those of other instances of disclosure without the patient's consent. The therapist should personally explain to the patient the circumstances of this disclosure and should pledge to divulge the minimum necessary information. Under specific circumstances, and preferably with the advice of counsel, the therapist may choose to refuse to testify on certain points, even at risk of contempt charges, if he feels such testimony will harm the patient in some way and he is willing to face the consequences.

3. Obtaining a History

On occasion, an evaluating clinician in an emergency setting will be unable to obtain sufficient data from the patient alone and is forced to turn to third parties, even without the patient's consent. At this point, a tension develops between (1) the patient's right to privacy and confidentiality concerning the emergency and (2) the evaluator's need to get information to treat the patient appropriately, since it is difficult to gather data without revealing some aspect of the patient's situation. The evaluator must decide on clinical grounds how much information must be revealed to third parties in order to elicit necessary treatment-related information.

> *Example 1:* An evaluator calls the parents of a floridly psychotic teen-ager, despite his objections, to obtain a possible history of drug inges-tion that would directly affect the decision to use neuroleptics. He does this even though the call betrays to the parents, against the pa-tient's will, the fact of the patient's illness, evaluation, and possible hospitalization.

Many informants (e.g., family and friends) are extremely concerned about, and interested in, the patient and may press the evaluator for information, statements, and prognoses. Here again, the evaluator must reconcile the patient's right to confidentiality with the often-pressing need to enlist and recruit family, friends, etc., for future work with the patient.

> *Example 2:* After their son was admitted in an acutely psychotic state, the parents pressed the ward social worker for quotations from the patient, especially what he was saying about them. The son adamantly refused permission to talk to the parents. The social worker compro-mised by telling the family: "I am legally forbidden to talk to you, but I can listen to what you tell me that may help your son. When he's better, he may well give permission and we can talk then; meanwhile, let's meet regularly."

4. Acting as Informant

At times the evaluator is on the other side of the fence, as informant in an emergency situation. Here, too, trade-offs similar to the foregoing may be called for, as well as some use of discretion and ingenuity.

> *Example 3:* The lawyer for a patient newly admitted in an emergency telephoned the psychiatrist to ask if the patient was in that hospital, since he had to meet with him to discuss charges arising out of the

patient's actions during the current psychosis. The psychiatrist explained that acknowledging without permission any patient's presence in the hospital was a breach of confidentiality. The lawyer nevertheless reiterated his demand. Realizing that the patient's interests were at stake, the psychiatrist acknowledged the patient's presence at the hospital. The lawyer arrived at the hospital to meet his client shortly afterward.

Example 4: A psychotic inpatient had adamantly refused permission for the staff to talk to her parents. The patient's mother visited while the patient was still acutely ill and, shortly after seeing her daughter, sought out the psychiatrist on the case. Tearful, frightened, and desperate, she besought, "What's wrong with her? She doesn't even recognize me! Will she ever know me again?" The psychiatrist realized that a dry recitation of the rules of confidentiality would have alienated the mother as a potential ally for the treatment and further would be nonresponsive to her human distress. He elected to use the "generalized third person," thus, "Sometimes when people are very ill they can't recognize their loved ones for a time; when we get the illness under control, they usually know them again." In addition to relieving the mother, the psychiatrist's comments, generalized to "patients," betrayed nothing confidential to the patient in question.

In bona fide emergencies, the patient's welfare must predominate over other considerations. The evaluator should attempt to convey to other institutions or providers the nature of the emergency to obtain needed data; such steps, of course, require careful documentation at both ends of the conversation. At a later point, the evaluator should explain to the patient in retrospect the reasoning behind any such interventions, especially those that took place against the patient's will. The goal is not only reestablishment of the alliance as founded on the patient's best interests, but modeling of a realistic assessment of a situation.

5. PRESERVING THE ALLIANCE WHILE BREACHING CONFIDENTIALITY

In addition to the patient's review of materials that leave the office described above (see Sec. III-B-3), other techniques can preserve the working alliance with the patient even when confidentiality must be breached. These include:

a. Advance notice

Whenever possible, clinicians should alert the patient to possible need for a breach in anticipation of its being required. Examples include patients involved in child abuse, reportable diseases, AIDS, histories of violence, and the like. Such anticipatory discussion permits the subject to be broached at a calmer time than when an acute crisis makes sound judgment more difficult.

b. Use of a hierarchy of interventions

When, for example, a patient is persisting in driving in dangerous or potentially destructive ways, the clinician should not "blow the whistle" as the first intervention. Rather, the clinician should first counsel the patient about driving, exploring the matter therapeutically; then, recommend some alteration in driving behavior; that failing, strongly urge the patient to change his ways; then, threaten to intervene; finally, tell the patient that the patient must cease driving or report the matter to the Bureau of Motor Vehicles, or the therapist will. The speed with which the steps of this hierarchy are accomplished depends on the situation. Careful documentation of this process (and consultation if needed) have become particularly important in the wake of the driving cases that have sprung up in the courts recently. (See Chap. 4, Secs. II-A-3-e and III-A-2-g-i.)

Finally, even when confidentiality must be breached without the patient's permission, the patient, again, should be told of the breach as a courtesy, and the matter therapeutically explored.

c. Remembering the nature of the alliance

The clinician should bear in mind that her alliance is with the healthy side of the patient against the illness. Thus the clinician is not working against the patient or turning into an agent for social control merely by opposing certain destructive behaviors or honoring reporting requirements. Even child abuse/ neglect reporting (See suggested readings—Harper et al.) or management of the violent patient can be managed in a tactful, supportive, and ultimately more useful way by attending to the alliance with that part of the parent that wishes not to abuse the child, that part of the violent patient that wants to keep control, that part of the self-destructive patient that wants to survive, and the like.

D. The "circle" of confidentiality

As a summary, note Figure One. Within the circle, patient information may be shared; those outside the circle require the patient's permission to receive such information.

The patient's family or attorney are "outside" the circle; being a relative or one's legal representative does not consititute entitlement to obtain clinical information. For a patient in the hospital the outside therapist is also excluded from the circle of confidentiality, although, as a matter of clinical wisdom, permission should be obtained as early as possible to obtain essential historical material and to discuss the case, for the patient's benefit. Indeed, experienced clinicians believe that data gained during hospitalization of a patient who is in therapy can often serve a valuable consultative function to the ongoing treatment.

The police, too, are outside the circle. If the police call a hospital or mental health center and ask if a certain individual is there, the only proper response is, "We cannot give out that information. However, we will make inquiries and, if anyone by that name is here, we will encourage him to call you." Note that this response is appropriate regardless of whether or not the sought individual is, in fact, there as a patient.

Within the circle, information may, and perhaps should, be shared. Staff supervisors in teaching settings are considered to be within the line of responsibility and thus part of the treatment team. The same would be said for treatment staff of all disciplines.

In a similar fashion, those consultants who actually see the patient (as, for example, a gynecology consultant for a patient in a psychiatric hospital) clearly must be informed about the clinical situation to be of any value.

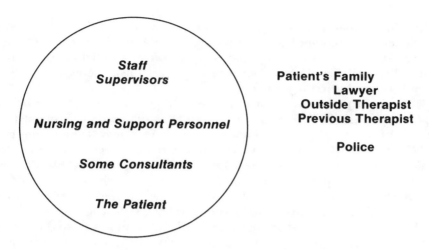

Figure 1.1.   The "circle" of Confidentiality.

Finally, the patient herself is inside the circle–a point perhaps so obvious as to be overlooked. Since the patient has no professional obligations to anyone, the patient might, theoretically, appear on national television and reveal the secrets of her life story to the entire country. In more practical terms, clinicians should recall that the patient, if able, may pass along information in those ambiguous situations where the requirements of confidentiality are uncertain. The patient can inform family, agencies, other caregivers, and so on. The more tricky and complex the situation, the more valuable this patient's role.

Having the patient convey important information has a particular value in a most counterintuitive context, having the patient himself warn a putative victim of his own dangerousness to the latter. Empirical experience suggests that while such communication cannot always be achieved, direct conversation by supervised phone call or monitored visit may defuse the actual danger potential in the relationship, a result far more desirable than merely meeting some legalistic "duty to warn." When patient and victim are talking to each other, they are not shooting at each other; paranoid fears and fantasies can be tested under clinical supervision, misunderstandings corrected, spleen safely vented, and tension eased. Having the patient "do the warning," then, in those rare instances where this is indicated, avoids the ethical tension caused by the clinician's unilateral breach of confidentiality, no matter how justified.

E. Patient's request to see own records

At certain junctures in the treatment process, the patient may request to see her own records. In the usual situation, this is an expression of certain fantasies about the state of the treatment and requires, among other things, exploration in the therapy as well as a reality response. In general, exploring the reason for the request implies identifying fantasies that are frequently related to the patient's questions "How am I doing?" or "What do you think of me?" One attempts in managing this to deal with these concerns and questions in the usual exploratory manner.

In certain situations, the wish to see a record may have a basically paranoid core with delusional components; for example, the patient may believe that some of her secret thoughts are being read or that accusing indictments are being leveled at her in the content of the record and that this is being revealed or is potentially revealable to third parties.

The request to see the record may be used constructively to advance the therapeutic process, both because of the fantasies that may be brought to the surface and because distinct advantage to the therapy may accrue from going over the actual chart material under certain circumstances. The patient and therapist might, for example, review together certain nursing observations made during the time the patient was psychotic. When properly handled and with proper preparation within the therapy, this review may aid integration of the patient's psychotic experiences into her nonpsychotic self-image.

All the difficulties cited above (see Sec. III-B-3) with regard to the patient's potential misinterpretation of technical terms in disclosed information are equally applicable to the patient's review of the record. The goal of all clinicians should be to avoid such difficulties by eschewing the use of misinterpretable technical terms in the patient's record (see Sec. III-G-2 below), that is, by writing the record in anticipation of the patient's reading it.

F. Confidentiality in group therapy

Group therapy poses special problems with regard to confidentiality, which experienced group therapists attempt to minimize by using the following approaches: (1) use of only first names of members in conducting the group and in keeping charts on group members; (2) urging group members to see themselves as *cotherapists* together with the group leader and thus subject to the same moral obligation to keep group material within the group (in this way, one appeals to the group's conscience and the conscience of individual members to encourage confidential behavior); (3) discouraging members from meeting or socializing, etc., outside the group; (4) analyzing breaches of confidence, if they occur, as part of the normal group process; and finally, (5) terminating treatment with members who breach the group's confidentiality to outside parties.

G. Informed record keeping that protects confidentiality

1. CLARITY OF SOURCES

In keeping records, it cannot be overemphasized how important it is to distinguish clearly data known by observation to be fact from speculation, report, and allegation. It is also important to note both the source of any data not obtained by observation and that source's reliability. For example, one might note, "The arresting officer reports..." or "The parent, known to be a good historian, reports . . . ," and so forth. For potentially or ostensibly criminal matters, the word "alleged" is proper usage, as in: "the alleged theft, assault, rape, felony, etc." (See Chap. 4, Sec. III-A-3, for extensive discussion of this topic in terms of malpractice prevention.)

2. THE CONCEPT OF "TWO SETS OF BOOKS"

A useful approach is to distinguish between *process* notes (which are a record of the patient's (or even the therapist's) fantasies, feelings, and experiences, intended for the therapist's use in treatment) and *progress* notes (objective records of facts, observations, and treatments for use in communications to other parties and in utilization review of care given). The latter should theoretically be open to the patient and third parties following the provision of consent as earlier described, and should be written from a perspective that anticipates such release. The former are totally private, although still recoverable by subpoena, of course.

For clinicians working in institutional settings, the process notes remain their property, even after they leave the facility. Therapists who intend to write papers based on data collected from their clinical work can use process notes for this purpose, since they will ordinarily be denied access to patient's records (the official progress notes) at a facility at which they no longer work (but see Chap. 4, Sec. II-C-2). Once active work with a patient is terminated, it is advisable for the therapist to remove identifying marks from the process notes, so that their later use for didactic or academic purposes will not jeopardize the patient's confidentiality. This can be done by removing the patient's last name or by using a numbering system for coding the records and keeping a copy of the code elsewhere. In most circumstances, the progress notes, which are the property of the facility, should not be photocopied for these purposes. Many facilities have rules explicitly forbidding such copying for personal use, a situation again underscoring the utility of keeping process notes.

OUTLINE OF PROGRESS VERSUS PROCESS NOTES:

	Progress notes	Process notes
LOCATION	"Front," "ward," "clinic," or "public" chart	Therapist's private notes
CONTENT	Facts, observations, tests, procedures, treatments, services, lab results, medications *only*	"Anything that comes to mind," conscious or unconscious, fact or fantasy
VIEWPOINT	Operational/Descriptive	Therapeutic/Investigative
PURPOSE	Treatment planning, recording, documentation, and utilization review	Understanding total patient for treatment
LANGUAGE	Austere, factual, descriptive, clear and legible, showing follow-up of problems, may be problem-oriented format	May be quotations from doctor or patient, may use private shorthand or abbreviations, etc.

3. AIDS AND RELATED MATTERS

Since our society at large is still undecided as to how to view AIDS, HIV seropositivity, and the presence of risk factors for infection, it is not surprising that considerable confusion and inconsistency prevail around record-keeping on this topic. Some jurisdictions require separate consent and/or separate charting (or use of a designated section of a chart) for HIV-related material.

In the present state of flux, clinicians must familiarize themselves with relevant local regulations and statutes. A potentially useful rule of thumb, in novel or ambiguous situations like this one where local regulations have not yet addressed the matter or do not offer guidance, may be to treat HIV-infection as though it were syphilis and invoke public-health-based principles of reporting and intervention. Expert consultation is particularly valuable here.

IV. PITFALLS

A. Inappropriate secrecy

Appropriate attention to confidentiality may be confused with a patient's countertherapeutic demand for secrecy; inappropriate secrets in the milieu of the inpatient ward, however, can be very destructive. For example, the patient may ask a new staff member not to reveal her plan for suicide or escape because that would violate the patient's "trust and confidentiality." This loaded secret leaves the staff member in an impossible and no-win position. Either the staff member loses the alliance and trust of the patient or, on the other hand, may lose the patient herself. This approach by the patient usually reflects covert hostility toward the staff member. A second example might be a case in which a male patient's homosexual concerns make the resident so anxious that, in the name of confidentiality, he does not pass them on to the staff. The staff, not being warned about this, may inadvertently provoke a panic by allowing male staff members to come too close to the patient, rather than preferentially utilizing female staff members, as is ordinarily done in such clinical states.

B. Confusion of agency in informing

Most clinicians are alert to the importance of not discussing a patient with, say, the patient's family member without permission. However, a family's urgent request not to tell a patient about a phone call, ostensibly to avoid needless upset, may be very forceful and persuasive, leading the clinician to omit telling it to the patient. Here the clinician may be influenced by overidentification with the parent's protective impulse. Other seemingly trivial information coming in about the patient from various sources may similarly, but inappropriately, be dismissed as irrelevant to the patient's care and thus undeserving of being passed on to the patient.

Here, wishes to spare the patient distress may fuse with considerations of convenience, expediency, and the wish not to be the bearer of bad tidings to the patient. The pitfall here is clear: a patient who learns from other sources that the clinician knew something (no matter how trivial) and did not pass it on may not easily recover trust for the clinician. The wish of outside sources to "sneak" information past the patient to the clinician can be explored with the various parties as a legitimate therapeutic issue.

V. CASE EXAMPLE EPILOGUES

A. Case Example 1

Because the hospital and the resident are not obligated to report the patient's confession to the police, and since a confidentiality statute in the state where this occurred bars such disclosure even in criminal cases, it would appear that the resident has no further legal obligation. He is concerned, however, that the patient's story, if true, might shed light on his future dangerousness and on the need for involuntary commitment, both estimations which he is legally obligated to perform. The need to confirm the patient's story appears to conflict with the principle of confidentiality.

Fortunately, a means is available of verifying the patient's account without breaching confidentiality. The resident calls the police and, without informing them of the patient's identity, reveals the nature of his confession. The police officer reports that the site of the alleged crime was used for a massive fireworks display the previous night and, given the tight security precautions, it is highly unlikely that the patient could commit such an act undetected. In addition, no body was found in the harbor that morning. The resident takes no further action. action.

One week later, after medication has rendered the patient much less psychotic, he admits that his confession was a fabrication.

B. Case Example 2

In this case, the doctor could be the beneficiary of the state's privilege statute, which bars disclosure of material gathered in therapy. Unfortunately, the statute specifically exempts child custody hearings from a claim of privilege when the presiding judge determines that disclosure of the information in question is more valuable than maintaining the confidential doctor-patient relationship.

The doctor, prior to her appearance in court, discusses her dilemma with the patient and explains that, though she does not want to testify, she may be compelled to do so. When she arrives in court, prepared to ask the judge to receive her data *in camera* in order to rule on its applicability, she discovers that the judge disavows any knowledge of the privilege statute. As she has not brought a copy of the two-page statute along with her, she can not refer him to its specific provisions and, faced with a direct order to testify or to face contempt proceedings, she acquiesces.

The resulting breach of confidence provokes the expected difficulties in her relationship with her patient, who is much more reticent about talking with her thereafter.

C. Case Example 3

This jurisdiction has no statute regarding the disclosure of information about patients' HIV status, although it does require patients' written consent for the disclosure of information from mental health facilities, except in emergencies. The therapist must therefore judge whether the threat to the patient's wife is serious enough to warrant being called an emergency. He is also concerned that if word gets out that the mental health center is contacting sexual partners of

HIV-positive patients, such people will stop coming in, despite their need for care.

   After considerable thought, he decides he must contact the patient's wife, unless the patient does so first, and so informs the patient. At this point, the patient says he has already told his wife, and that she has agreed with his plan to try to have a child. The therapist doubts the accuracy of the patient's report. In order to forestall the patient's intercepting his communication, he sends a registered letter to the patient's wife, asking her to come in to discuss an important issue with him and the patient. When she arrives, she discloses that the patient has told her about his HIV-status, but only after the letter was received. She is confused about the meaning of the test result, and simultaneously angry at her husband and fearful of losing him. The therapist supports an airing of the issues by both husband and wife, then arranges for them to meet with a counselor specializing in AIDS-related issues to discuss the implications of the patient's status. Although angry at the therapist for forcing him to tell his wife, the patient agrees to counseling and to continue in therapy.

VI. ACTION GUIDE

A. Checklist for Release of Information to Third Parties

   1. *Explore* reason for request.
   2. *Determine* extent of disclosure required.
   3. *Be certain* patient understands potential implications of data release.
   4. *Obtain written* consent for disclosure
      a. Should specify the content of the material to be disclosed (e.g., history of outpatient treatment since 1985, or lifetime medication history)
      b. Should be renewed for each subsequent disclosure.
   5. *Organize* material to be released.
      a. Whenever possible *communicate* in writing, not on phone.
      b. *Reveal* minimum necessary data.
      c. *Stick* to facts and firsthand knowledge.
      d. *Avoid* psychodynamic material.
      e. *Write* letter as if patient will read it—patients often will.
   6. Whenever possible, *review* letter with patient before it is sent.
   7. When patient requests falsification or omission
      a. Stance should derive from incorruptibility.
      b. Therapist sides with healthier part of patient's ego.
      c. *Discuss* issues thoroughly with patient.

B. Checklist for Release of Information Without Patient's Consent

   1. *Determine* if one of usual exceptions apply:
      a. Clearly acting in emergency situations and in patient's best interest;
      b. Patient incompetent and substitute consent not available;
      c. Patient incompetent and substitute consent obtained;
      d. Acting to hospitalize or commit patient;
      e. Acting to protect third parties;
      f. Required to report data by state law;

g. Sharing data with collaborative caregivers or supervisors.
2. *Document* efforts to obtain patient's consent and existence of exception.
3. *Alert* patient that information is to be released.
    a. Discuss basis for decision.
    b. Discuss impact on therapeutic alliance.
4. *Reveal* minimum necessary data, in writing if possible.
5. *Repair* alliance afterwards, focusing on how situation evolved and patient's feelings about it.

C. Checklist for Release of Information from Patient's Record to the Patient

1. *Explore* reasons for request.
    a. *Identify* fantasies.
    b. *Be alert* for delusional basis.
2. *Determine* laws governing patients' access to records in your locale.
    a. If release required, *skip* to #3 below.
    b. If release required except when not in patient's interest, *make* determination and *document* basis for decision in patient's record.
    c. If release not required, *determine* if in patient's interest to release and *act* accordingly.
3. *Prepare* patient for impact of disclosure.
    a. *Discuss* confusing, technical, or seemingly pejorative terms.
    b. *Discuss* possible impact on ongoing therapy.
4. Whenever possible, *go over* record together with patient.
5. *Use* material revealed to advance therapy.
    a. *Use* as means of integrating past experience.
    b. *Explore* effect of fantasies confirmed or denied.
6. *Do not release* material obtained from other sources (e.g., hospital records, former therapists, family members)—patient must obtain that information directly from those sources.
7. *Do not alter or destroy* records before patient sees them—potential legal liability.

D. Checklist for Revelation of Information in Court Proceedings

1. If request is from patient, no privilege applies—*handle* as in C above.
2. If request is from party opposing patient, *determine* laws governing privilege in your locale.
    a. If no patient-doctor or patient-psychotherapist privilege, *handle* as in B-3, 4, 5 above.
    b. If privilege exists, *determine* if this case constitutes an exception or not.
3. When subpoena arrives, *remember* that it only mandates your appearance—judge must still decide if privilege exists.
4. *Consult* with lawyer requesting subpoena to see what information is desired.
5. *Notify* patient and patient's lawyer of arrival of subpoena, giving them a chance to challenge it.
6. Consultation with your own lawyer may be useful.
7. If your testimony is inevitable, *follow* C-3 to C-7 above.

VII. SUGGESTED READINGS

A. CONFIDENTIALITY AND PRIVILEGE

1. Appelbaum, P.S.: Confidentiality in psychiatric treatment, in L. Grinspoon (ed.), *Psychiatry 1982: The American Psychiatric Annual Review.* Washington, DC, American Psychiatric Press, 1982.

2. Knapp S. & VandeCreek L.: *Privileged Communications in the Mental Health Professions.* New York, Van Nostrand Reinhold, 1987.

3. Shuman D.W. & Weiner M.E.: *The Psychotherapist-Patient Privilege: A Critical Examination.* Springfield, IL, Charles C Thomas, 1987.

4. American Psychiatric Association: *Guidelines on Confidentiality.* Washington, DC, APA, 1987.

5. Group for the Advancement of Psychiatry: *Report No. 45—Confidentiality and Privileged Communication in the Practice of Psychiatry.* New York, 1960.

6. Model law on confidentiality of health and social service records. *Am. J. Psychiatry* 136:137–147, 1979.

7. Roth, L. & Meisel, A.: Dangerousness, confidentiality, and the duty to warn. *Am. J. Psychiatry* 134:508–511, 1977.

8. Cross, W.: Privileged communication between participants in group therapy, in Kittrie, N., Hirsch, H., Wegner, G. (eds.), *Medicine, Law, and Public Policy.* New York, AMS Press, 1975.

9. Huber, G. A., & Roth, L. H.: Preserving the confidentiality of medical record information regarding nonpatients. *Virginia Law Review* 66:583–596, 1980.

10. Note: Breach of confidence: an emerging tort. *Harvard Law Review* 82:1426–1468, 1982.

B. THERAPEUTIC ALLIANCE

1. Gutheil, T. G., & Havens, L. L.: The therapeutic alliance: contemporary meanings and confusions. *Int. Rev. Psycho-Anal.* 6:467–481, 1979.

2. Dickes, R.: Technical considerations of the therapeutic and working alliances. *Int. J. Psychoanal. Psychother.* 4:1–24, 1975.

3. Friedman, L.: The therapeutic alliance. *Int. J. Psychoanal.* 50:139–153, 1969.

4. Greenson, R. R.: The working alliance and the transference neurosis. *Psychoanal. Q.* 34:155–181, 1965.

5. Harper, G. & Irvin, E.: Alliance formation with parents: limit setting and the effect of mandated reporting. *Am. J. Orthopsychiatry* 55: 50–60, 1985.

C. RECORD KEEPING

1. Gutheil, T. G.: Paranoia and progress notes: a guide to forensically informed psychiatric record keeping. *Hosp. Community Psychiatry* 31:479–482, 1980.

2. Slovenko, R.: On the need for record-keeping in the practice of psychiatry. *J. Psychiatry Law* 7:399–440, 1979.

3. Rappaport, R. G.: The psychiatrist on trial. *J. Psychiatry Law* 7:463–469, 1979.

4. Roth, L. H., Wolford, J. & Meisel A.: Patient access to records: tonic or toxin? *Am. J. Psychiatry* 137:592–596, 1980.

5. Short, D.: Some consequences of granting patients access to consultants' records. *Lancet* I:1316–1318, 1986.

6. Kinzie, J.D., Holmes, J.L. & Arent, J.: Patients' release of medical records: involuntary, uninformed consent? Hosp. Community Psychiatry 36:843–847, 1985.

2

Legal Issues in Emergency Psychiatry

I. CASE EXAMPLES
II. LEGAL ISSUES
    A. The psychiatric emergency
    B. Legal responsibilities of the clinician in the emergency setting
        1. WHEN A DUTY OF CARE EXISTS
        2. CLINICIANS' DUTIES IN THE EMERGENCY SETTING
          a. Evaluation
          b. Disposition
             i. No further treatment
             ii. Outpatient treatment
             iii. Hospitalization
    C. Voluntary hospitalization
        1. HISTORY OF THE CONCEPT
        2. TYPES OF VOLUNTARY ADMISSION
          a. "Pure" voluntary admission
          b. "Conditional" voluntary admission
         3. THE QUESTION OF COMPETENCE
    D. Involuntary hospitalization
        1. HISTORY OF THE CONCEPT
          a. Confinement of the mentally ill in the colonies and the young republic
          b. Involuntary commitment in the nineteenth century
          c. Involuntary commitment in the twentieth century
        2. LEGAL RATIONALES FOR INVOLUNTARY COMMITMENT
          a. Police powers
          b. *Parens patriae*
          c. An alternative perspective: the survival of *parens patriae* justification for commitment
        3. CURRENT STANDARDS OF INVOLUNTARY HOSPITALIZATION
          a. Emergency commitments
          b. Court-ordered commitments
              i. Danger to others
              ii. Danger to self
              iii. Unable to care for self
              iv. Danger to property
              v. In need of treatment
              vi. At risk of deterioration
              vii. Miscellaneous criteria
         4. PROCEDURAL ISSUES

      a. Standards of proof

      b. Other procedural requirements

E. Assessing the current system of involuntary commitment

    1. EXCLUSION OF THE NONDANGEROUS PATIENT IN NEED OF HOSPITALIZATION

    2. DIFFICULTIES PREDICTING DANGEROUS BEHAVIOR

      a. Theoretical considerations

      b. The empirical data

    3. DISTORTION OF THE ROLE OF THE MENTAL HEALTH SYSTEM

F. Alternatives to the current commitment system

    1. INTRODUCTION OF MODIFIED NEED FOR TREATMENT CRITERIA

      a. The American Psychiatric Association model law

      b. More limited efforts

    2. RELAXATION OF DANGEROUSNESS CRITERIA

    3. RELAXATION OF PROCEDURAL REQUIREMENTS

    4. OUTPATIENT COMMITMENT

    5. NON-STATUTORY APPROACHES

III. CLINICAL ISSUES

A. Performing the emergency assessment

    1. THE HISTORY AND THE RECORD IN THE EMERGENCY ASSESSMENT

      a. Obtaining the history from the patient and others

      b. The evaluator as user of informants

      c. Informant reliability

      d. Ulterior motives

      e. Solicitation of information as an alliance threat

      f. Documentation

    2. ASSESSING THE PATIENT AND THE ENVIRONMENT IN EVALUATING AN EMERGENCY

      a. Risk factors

        i. External risk factors

        ii. Internal risk factors

      b. Resource factors

        i. External resource factors

        ii. Internal resource factors

B. Assessment of suicidality

    1. DIAGNOSTIC CONSIDERATIONS AND HISTORY

      a. The personal context

      b. Previous history and background

      c. Current stressors

      d. Personality disorder factors

      e. Psychiatric illness

      f. Symptomatology

      g. Context of the suicidal act

      h. Clinical wisdom concerning suicide

    2. ASSESSMENT OF SUICIDE ATTEMPTS

    3. MANIPULATIVE SUICIDE AND THE PROBLEM OF REGRESSION

C. Assessment of dangerousness to others

    1. DIAGNOSTIC CONSIDERATIONS AND HISTORY

      a. Past violence

      b. Age

      c. Gender

      d. Race

      e. Socioeconomic status and stability of employment situation

      f. Substance abuse

      g. Clinical wisdom concerning dangerousness to others

      h. Predictions in the presence and absence of past violence

I. CASE EXAMPLES

A. Case Example I

A middle-aged man shuffles into the office of the resident psychiatrist on duty in the emergency room and slumps into the chair; his deep sigh releases a whiff of alcohol, and he remarks, "Perhaps I shouldn't have come." He is graying, unshaven, and his somewhat disheveled clothes fit him loosely.

Empathic questioning reveals that two months ago he lost his job because of alcohol-related absenteeism. This event proved to be the last straw for his wife, who took the children and decamped to her parents' home. He is sleeping little;

his appetite is gone. His drinking buddies no longer find him "fun to be with"; his parents are not interested in hearing from him; he has no relatives or close friends in town. He has been thinking seriously of suicide.

The doctor on call recommends hospitalization. The patient demurs at first, then argues, then threatens. The doctor is firm. The patient looks searchingly at the doctor for a long moment, sighs quietly, and says, "OK, Doc, you've convinced me. I'll go pack some things and meet you here in an hour." Rising, he turns toward the door.

B. Case Example 2

A middle-of-the-night call to an emergency service of a community mental health center announces the imminent arrival of a transfer from a nearby general hospital. The patient in question, age 28 and mildly intoxicated, had just received extensive stitching for two self-inflicted superficial lacerations running the length of each arm. After the lacerations were sutured, the patient went into the bathroom of the emergency ward and removed each stitch. He was resutured and is now being transferred for hospitalization.

On his arrival, it is apparent that he is not psychotic, but is furiously angry with his stepbrother, with whom he has been staying since his arrival in the city three weeks ago. When his stepbrother ordered him to leave the house after an altercation, the patient procured a razor blade from the bathroom and, in front of his stepbrother's little daughter, carved up his arms. He will not say whether he intended to kill himself or if he is still bent on self-destruction. He does give a history of previous hospitalizations after other self-destructive acts, all of which ended with his angrily signing himself out of the hospital within a few days. After eliciting this story, the resident pauses to consider his options for handling the case.

C. Case Example 3

Nearly frantic with concern, the mother of a 23-year-old woman calls a psychiatric center to ask for help. Her daughter, who until last month had held a responsible secretarial job, has, since then, been acting rather strangely. She has withdrawn large amounts of money from her bank account to buy flashy clothes, has begun to drink a good deal, and has left her boyfriend of two years to begin a series of wild one-night stands with men she meets in bars. In addition, she is now extremely suspicious of her mother, with whom she formerly had a very close relationship.

On the previous night the daughter had gone with her boyfriend to a disco, but soon left the establishment somewhat intoxicated in the company of another man. Her boyfriend discovered that she had taken his car and not far from the disco had smashed it into a guardrail on the highway, causing extensive damage, but no injuries. He does not wish to press charges, but would like to see her get psychiatric care. She was last seen leaving the scene of the accident in the company of a cabdriver who had stopped to help. A friend reported that she had called to say that she was spending the night with the cabdriver. The mother pleads that something be done to give her daughter the care she needs.

II. LEGAL ISSUES

A. The psychiatric emergency

The clinician who sees patients with presenting complaints of an emergent nature, whether in the office or in the psychiatric emergency room, is faced, as the examination proceeds, with two critical clinical-legal decisions: (1) does this patient require hospitalization or is some less drastic form of intervention preferable; and (2) if hospitalization is required and the patient refuses to consent to admission, does the patient meet those criteria that would permit hospitalization against his or her will? Clinicians are concerned, as well, with the impact of both of these decisions on their potential liability should something untoward occur. Although most of the court cases arising from emergency treatment settings have involved physicians, the principles elaborated are applicable in most circumstances to other clinicians as well.

B. Legal responsibilities of the clinician in the emergency setting

1. WHEN A DUTY OF CARE EXISTS

A clinician becomes responsible for a patient's care only when a treatment relationship is established between them. Thus, a clinician accosted in the street by someone whom she has never previously met and who threatens suicide is, moral considerations aside, not legally obligated to undertake an evaluation or to arrange a disposition. When a patient is seen in a treatment setting, however, such as a private office or a walk-in clinic, and it becomes apparent even during the initial assessment that an immediate intervention is required, a therapeutic relationship is assumed to exist despite the absence of a formal contract. Facilities advertising emergency services have a duty to provide urgent care to all comers. Failure to provide for proper care (which may consist merely of referral to another, more appropriate facility) leaves the clinician open to a charge of abandonment. Before a patient is permitted to leave, an assessment ought to be made sufficient to rule out the possibility that further immediate steps are required.

The determination of whether the care-giver has assumed a duty of care toward the patient is not always clear-cut. Phone calls from people who have not previously been in treatment but who are seeking aid or the casual inquiries of friends that reveal emergent issues leave the clinician in an ambiguous position. Though no definite pronouncement is possible, courts have frequently held that where a physician has responded to the inquirer as a physician—not merely as a friend—a therapeutic relationship has been established and a duty of care exists.

2. CLINICIAN'S DUTIES IN THE EMERGENCY SETTING

Clinicians have two general obligations toward patients once a duty of care is established in an emergency setting: evaluation and proper disposition.

a. Evaluation

The nature of the duty to evaluate the patient differs somewhat in the emergency context. Mental health evaluation in office, clinic, or hospital-based practice can be a deliberate process. Information is gleaned from patients over a protracted period. Many practitioners make little attempt to structure interviews, in the belief that, with time, the most important material will rise to the surface. Records of previous mental health contacts are requested by mail. Once the therapist has a reasonably firm relationship with the patient, family members or other informants may be invited to join the patient for a session at which their perspectives can be explored. As long as no symptoms require urgent attention, the completion of the evaluation, along with formulation of a working diagnosis and initiation of definitive treatment, can all be postponed.

Emergency evaluations have quite a different character. In a brief period of time, the clinician must gather sufficient information about the patient to assess her current condition and to formulate plans for immediate intervention. This data-gathering process, in contrast to the one described above, is focused and rapid. Interviews are highly structured. Information from other care-givers is obtained by telephone, rather than by mail. Informants who have accompanied the patient to the evaluation are interviewed on the spot. Laboratory tests may be performed, with results returned before the evaluation is completed (e.g., serum lithium level, blood alcohol level, toxic screen). If a definitive diagnosis cannot be established, at least a differential diagnosis is formulated, with the most likely possibilities identified.

There are several important legal implications that flow from the unique nature of the emergency assessment. First, the standard of thoroughness to which the clinician will be held is not the same as in a nonemergent context. The law will recognize, should legal proceedings ensue as a result of the evaluation, that the resources (including information and time) available to the emergency evaluator are restricted. Although resources that are at hand should be utilized, decisions may need to be made before all the information that one would desire is available. For example, the patient's therapist may be unreachable during the evaluation, and critical data concerning the patient's functioning may have to be foregone. Thus, the questions asked to evaluate the clinician's performance will be: did he make reasonable efforts to obtain the necessary information; and, given the constraints on available data, was the assessment performed as well as could be expected?

An important corollary to this limitation on the degree of expected completeness of the evaluation is that a decision about the nature of the patient's condition—at least sufficient to make disposition plans—cannot be deferred simply because not all the information is in. Clinicians dealing with emergencies have to tolerate a fair degree of uncertainty, but must make their best judgments. A decision to defer intervention pending further data is equivalent to a judgment that the situation is not emergent enough to require intervention. When some intervention is clearly required, the law will shield the mental health professional who acts despite gaps in the data base but may hold culpable the clinician who cannot make up his or her mind.

b. Disposition

Three options are available to the emergency evaluator: no further treatment, outpatient treatment, and inpatient hospitalization.

No further treatment.   The clinician in an emergency setting is not obliged to recommend further psychiatric treatment. Psychiatric emergency rooms are frequently visited by persons who may neither need nor desire psychiatric care. These include homeless people hoping for bed and board in a psychiatric hospital; persons brought by family members or friends because the latter perceive a problem (e.g., premarital sexual activity) that on evaluation turns out not to be indicative of psychopathology; persons brought by the police because of bizarre or violent behavior, but who are personality disordered, unreceptive to treatment, and therefore essentially untreatable. Once an appropriate evaluation has been performed and both its conclusions and the recommendations given to the patient carefully documented, the clinician may well decide that the "emergency" does not represent a situation that requires further involvement from the mental health system.

Outpatient treatment. Even the presence of a genuine emergency does not mandate hospitalization. Most patients who come to psychiatric emergency rooms or walk-in clinics are referred for outpatient follow-up. To recommend outpatient treatment, the emergency evaluator does not have to reach conclusions concerning the patient's definitive diagnosis or ultimate treatment plan. She need only determine that the patient can be safely maintained in the community until the follow-up visit is scheduled, at which time reevaluation of the patient's status can take place.

Ordinarily, the degree of anticipated cooperation by the patient and the availability of supports in the community are important determinants of whether an outpatient option is feasible. If the patient resists the referral, or it appears clear that he will not follow through, consideration must be given to whether the patient meets the criteria for involuntary treatment—on an outpatient basis in some states (see Sec. F-4 below) or on an inpatient basis. If the patient is not committable, and all efforts to negotiate an acceptable treatment plan with the patient have failed, there may be no alternative but to allow the patient to leave. For patients whose competence to make decisions about treatment may be in question, family members can be advised to seek an adjudication of incompetence. This may allow the appointment of a substitute decisionmaker to consent to treatment on the patient's behalf. (See Chap. 5, Sec. II-C-1.)

It is important to note that the outpatient option remains available even if the patient qualifies for involuntary hospitalization under applicable state laws (see Sec. D below.) These laws are permissive, not mandatory. That is, they define circumstances in which commitment may occur, not conditions under which it must. In fact, many statutes now incorporate a "least restrictive alternative" criterion, permitting commitment only when no outpatient option is feasible. Recent studies showing that only a minority of "committable" patients are hospitalized involuntarily may help ease the fears of clinicians about treating such patients in the community.

Hospitalization. Often the only reasonable option for dealing with a psychiatric emergency is to seek the patient's hospitalization. This may occur on a voluntary basis (see Sec. C below) or involuntarily (see Sec. D below). When the patient is amenable to the recommendation, voluntary hospitalization is often the most desirable course of action. If the patient resists hospitalization, however, the clinician must determine whether he meets the criteria for involuntary commitment, and if so, begin that process.

Confusion often exists as to whether patients who desire voluntary hospitalization may be committed anyway. Some states limit this practice, but the majority erect no barriers to it. Involuntary hospitalization may be preferable when the patient has a history of signing out of the hospital soon after admission; in these circumstances it simplifies the task of treating the patient, and it provides a message to the patient about the seriousness with which the staff view his situation. Commitment may also be the best choice when state laws would make it difficult to hold the patient if he later elected to sign himself out of the hospital but would probably allow commitment in the emergency context.

As if the clinician did not face sufficient difficulties in considering whether or not to hospitalize a patient, there is an additional worry. Common law rules, codified in some places, have held those who unjustly deprive a person of his freedom to be liable for suit in tort for false imprisonment. While any patient can claim that she has been unjustifiably committed, the key point here is that the courts are unlikely to hold liable a clinician who acts in good faith, in accordance with the laws of the state, to hospitalize a mentally ill person. Many state commitment statutes have provisions that grant immunity to clinicians who act in compliance with statutory mandates. Liability is limited to those cases in which the clinician has acted willfully and maliciously to deprive a person of his or her freedom, knowing that the patient did not meet the required criteria. Good record keeping, with a clear recitation of the basis for the decision, should effectively foreclose liability.

C. Voluntary hospitalization

1. HISTORY OF THE CONCEPT

Ironically, the idea that the mentally ill might be able to sign themselves voluntarily into psychiatric hospitals is a relatively new one. Although the first statute allowing a mental patient to enter voluntarily was enacted in Massachusetts in 1881, by 1949 only 10% of patients were voluntarily admitted. It was not until 1972, following two decades of widespread revision of commitment laws to encourage voluntary status, that the majority of admissions were accomplished in a voluntary manner.

The reasons voluntary admissions took so long to become common fall into two categories. First was the issue of administrative convenience; it was feared for many years that permitting a patient to leave a psychiatric facility at will, as the concept of voluntary admission seemed to allow, would paralyze the treatment program and overwhelm the paper-processing apparatus. Secondly, many felt that the presence of mental illness per se rendered a person incompetent to consent to hospitalization and required the intervention of a court.

Psychiatrists were the strongest advocates of voluntary hospitalization, particularly after the psychoanalytic movement made its mark on the country. They felt that a patient's cooperation was essential for effective treatment and that such collaboration in treatment should begin at the time of admission. Advocates of patients' rights for many years had also favored voluntary status as less restrictive of patients' freedom.

Today, the debate over voluntary hospitalization has changed somewhat. Many advocates of patients' rights oppose any admission without court review, holding that the mentally ill are often subject to unwarranted coercion at the time that the admission decision is made. These proposals, if adopted, would represent a return to the situation as it existed in most jurisdictions in the 1940s, and they evoke the arguments that were then urged in favor of removing the admission process from the courts: a lessening of the stigma of admission to a mental hospital, which resulted in part from the quasi-criminal procedure; a greater sense of autonomous functioning on the part of the patient who has chosen to sign himself into the hospital; an explicit contract for treatment between the patient and the hospital. In addition, there are substantial practical problems with requiring scarce psychiatric resources to be spent in hours of court hearings, not to mention the burden on the courts themselves. For all of these reasons, almost all mental health professionals, and probably a majority of the mental health bar, favor the retention of voluntary admissions as the most frequently used means of ingress to a psychiatric hospital.

A final irony should be noted. The percentage of voluntary patients in state hospital systems has been falling in recent years as the policy of deinstitutionalization has drastically reduced the number of available beds. Some public mental health systems now restrict hospitalization only to involuntary patients in an effort to hold down inpatient censuses. Others will accept only patients who meet commitment criteria, though they may allow them to sign in voluntarily. Voluntary, but noncommittable patients will be sent to the private sector or, if they lack insurance coverage, simply turned away. Voluntary hospitalization, once encouraged as a means of enlisting patients in their treatment, has become a victim of widespread retrenchment in mental health services.

2. TYPES OF VOLUNTARY ADMISSION

All states today permit patients voluntarily to enter psychiatric hospitals with some statutes additionally requiring that the patient be in need of care and that the facility be capable of providing such care. The age at which adolescents can consent to their own care ranges from 12 to 18. The different types of voluntary status vary as to the procedure for ultimate egress.

a. "Pure" voluntary admission

Under this status, sometimes called "informal" admission, the patient is free to leave the hospital whenever he chooses. Because of the potential for manipulation by patients of the therapeutic situation with such leeway, some states limit, by law or policy, the scope of pure voluntary admissions.

b. "Conditional" voluntary admission

A modification of the pure form, this status allows the facility to detain a patient for a certain period of time, usually several days, after notice is given of a desire to leave. This interval is designed to be used for the evaluation of the patient with respect to the possibility of instituting proceedings for involuntary commitment, and for preparing discharge plans if the patient must be released. If the facility decides to seek commitment, the patient can continue to be held until the commitment hearing takes place. Otherwise the patient is free to go. This period is frequently used in practice as an interval during which an angry, impulsive, or manipulative patient can reconsider her decision to leave.

3. THE QUESTION OF COMPETENCE

If one were to analogize the act of voluntarily entering a mental hospital to other acts of great importance to the individual, such as making a will, one would assume that the person would need to be legally competent to be able to do so. Early statutes authorizing voluntary admissions, indeed, made this requirement explicit. More recent laws, however, designed to encourage voluntary admission on the theory that it aids treatment, omit such requirements in all but a handful of states.

The dilemma is that requiring competence to consent to hospitalization would probably deprive many patients of the benefits of such admission; some experimental data exist to support this conclusion, though the strictness of the definition of competence will have an obvious impact on the proportion of patients found to be incompetent. On the other hand, ignoring the question of competence leaves psychiatrists and facilities open to charges of improperly manipulating clearly incompetent patients (for example, severely demented patients). Some legal experts argue, in addition, that the benefits of voluntary status are illusory and are easily outweighed by the lack of automatic judicial review and the potential deprivation of freedom that follows from it. At present the issue is unresolved, although in practice the question of competence is usually ignored.

A recent U.S. Supreme Court decision (*Zinermon v. Burch*) may draw increased attention to this issue. The court held that in those states, such as Florida, that require a patient to be competent before signing in voluntarily, the failure to screen out incompetent patients violates those patients' constitutional rights. It is unclear whether the Court would actually restrict voluntary hospitalization only to those patients found competent, assuming a state's statute is silent on the issue. The decision itself did not address this question, but some of its wording suggested that the Court may be leaning in this direction. Clearly, there are legitimate interests on both sides.

Any resolution of this dilemma would require an accommodation between two conflicting societal values: on the one hand, a desire for consistency in the law, which generally requires that a person who takes a major step (e.g., making a will, signing a contract, accepting or refusing treatment) be competent to do so, and on the other the recognition that to insist that psychiatric patients meet this standard is unrealistic and may substantially interfere with their treatment. The deeper values underlying these positions are a desire to maximize individual autonomy, as opposed to a benevolent interest in treating incompetent mentally ill patients for their own benefit. It seems likely that some sacrifice of the autonomy interest is warranted in the best interests of the patient as an individual in need of care. Should the law choose to move in this direction without invoking the full panoply of judicial procedures, options that have been suggested include: the use of criteria of the "peer-review" type for given diagnoses within which treatment could be undertaken for a limited period; the use of in-hospital review committees to oversee treatment of assenting incompetents; and the provision of a substitute decisionmaker for incompetents, empowered to consent to a limited course of treatment on their behalf. The alternative of judicial review of each admission in which a question of competence is raised, either prospectively or retrospectively, would face severe practical problems of implementation, delaying treatment and overburdening the resources of both the courts and the treatment system.

D. Involuntary hospitalization

While the power to hospitalize a psychiatric patient against his will is often taken for granted by many caregivers, it actually represents a marked deviation from the traditional tendency in Anglo-American jurisprudence to maximize individual autonomy. To understand the unique position of the mental patient—for example, no competent medical patient can be "signed in" against his will—one needs to examine the evolution of the concept and the underlying rationales.

1. HISTORY OF THE CONCEPT

a. Confinement of the mentally ill in the colonies and the young republic

In the earliest years of the settlement of North America, no facilities for the specialized care of the mentally ill were created. Indigent persons with mental illness who did not present a threat of violence were cared for by their own communities in poor houses. Here they were mixed with the physically ill, widows and their children, and the unlucky destitute. All of these groups could be detained against their will at the order of the overseers of the poor. Occasionally, towns made provision for harmless mentally ill persons to be boarded out to local families at town expense.

Separate provisions were made for violent mentally ill persons, sometimes called the "furiously mad." They might be detained in jail until it was thought safe to release them. At that point, if they were not residents of the town, they would be transported to the borders of the community and "warned out," responsibility for their care falling to the next town along their path. A similar fate befell nonresident, harmless mentally ill persons who wandered into a community.

As the colonies matured, hospitals began to be established, the first in Philadelphia in 1751. These institutions treated both physically and mentally ill persons, with similar procedures for admission used in each case. Ordinarily, family members brought prospective patients to the hospital, where admission was determined by two factors: a doctor's judgment as to the need for hospitalization and the family's ability to pay for a period of care in advance. Patients played little or no role in negotiating these admissions, or in deciding when they might leave.

b. Involuntary commitment in the nineteenth century

This informal system of hospitalization, free of statutory control, began to change in the second quarter of the nineteenth century, as the first great wave of building state hospitals got underway. With the states taking responsibility for care of the mentally ill, a statutory framework was required. The earliest statutes, though, did little more than formalize the existing system. Families and hospital superintendents dominated the admission process, with overseers of the poor standing in for families in the case of indigents. The only criterion applied to determine the appropriateness of commitment was whether the patient was in need of treatment. Patients' sole recourse if they felt unjustly confined was to seek a writ of habeas corpus from the courts, which precipitated a hearing on the issue. It appears from the extant records that relatively few cases went that route.

In the 1860s and 1870s, allegations of abuse began to rise, probably in connection with a decline in the quality of institutional care. Included among these were legendary stories of wives "put away" by their malevolent husbands, with the connivance of psychiatrists. These protests led to the introduction of criminal-style procedures, designed to insure that deprivation of liberty was not arbitrarily undertaken. Judicial hearings were required, representation by counsel allowed, free communication with the outside world guaranteed, and in some states, even trial by jury on the issue of mental illness was afforded. Although some states clung to a family- and physician-dominated model for several more decades, by the end of the nineteenth century most jurisdictions had adopted judicial review of commitment.

c. Involuntary commitment in the twentieth century

With a single exception, all of the major changes in commitment law after 1900 were prefigured before that time. The first two-thirds of the twentieth century saw an alternation between periods in which the primary concern was that criminalized commitment procedures made it too difficult to hospitalize those in need of care, and in which worries about protecting patients from unjust confinement predominated. Marked relaxation of procedures occurred during the Progressive Era (1900–1920) when short-term, emergency commitment on physician certification was introduced. A similar period followed World War II, with psychiatry's prestige at its peak, when statutes were widely revised and judicial procedures relaxed. Every period of procedural relaxation was followed by an era of tightened procedures, as no permanent accommodation between the conflicting interests could be achieved.

The most recent period of widespread reform, however, beginning in the early 1970s, differs from all that preceded it. To be sure, the usual, periodic recriminalization of commitment procedures took place. In addition, an assault was made on the standards for involuntary hospitalization for the first time in American history. Standards based on need for treatment were rejected by many courts (the leading case was *Lessard v. Schmidt,* a 1972 federal court decision in Wisconsin) as unconstitutionally vague and overbroad. Such courts ruled that only standards based on clear evidence of patients' likelihood of endangering themselves or others were permissible. Meanwhile, legislatures had been coming to similar conclusions, albeit generally for a different set of reasons. They saw narrowed commitment criteria as an easy mechanism for trimming the size of state hospitals, encouraging deinstitutionalization, and saving money. By the end of the 1970s, almost every state in the nation had shifted to commitment criteria based on dangerousness.

2. LEGAL RATIONALES FOR INVOLUNTARY COMMITMENT

Contemporary common wisdom holds that two separate bases exist for involuntary hospitalization of the mentally ill.

a. Police powers

The government has always had the power, reserved in this country by the U.S. Constitution to the individual states, to take those actions necessary to maintain the safety of society. These are broadly referred to as the "police powers." The extent to which each state can go to protect the public is limited by the state's constitution and by the Fourteenth Amendment of the U.S. Constitution, which guarantees all citizens "due process" and "equal protection" of the laws.

Use of the police powers to confine the mentally ill dates back to colonial times, when the "furiously mad" were incarcerated in local jails. These days some theorists would argue that all dangerousness-based commitment laws rely for their validity on the state's police powers. The legitimacy of confinement, in this view, is based on the state's power to prevent mentally ill persons from hurting others or themselves. Police powers are also exercised in so-called "criminal commitments," including hospitalization of prisoners whose competence to stand trial is in question, or (at least for the period immediately following trial) who have been found not guilty by reason of insanity.

b. *Parens patriae*

The concept expressed by the Latin phrase *parens patriae* denotes the state as acting in place of the parent. It derives in Anglo-American law from the power of the English kings, who were viewed as the "fathers" of their subjects, to act in their subjects' presumed interests when the subjects were not capable of protecting themselves. Historically, this meant that the king might appoint a representative to oversee the castle and estate of a nobleman gone mad. *Parens patriae* justifications for involuntary confinement of the mentally ill in this country date back to colonial confinement of the insane in poor houses to allow the community to provide them effective support. As statutes began to be passed establishing need for treatment as the main criterion for commitment, *parens patriae* became the theoretical linchpin of commitment law. The state was acting, in theory at least, from purely beneficent motives in hospitalizing the mentally ill. Many observers believe that the shift to dangerousness-oriented statutes in the 1970s rendered *parens patriae* justifications irrelevant to American commitment law.

c. An alternative perspective: the survival of *parens patriae* justification for commitment

The widespread belief that current commitment laws are based solely on the state's police powers is almost certainly mistaken. Although the state may have a substantial interest in protecting the public order, by itself that interest is insufficient to justify commitment of the mentally ill. Persons who are likely to harm others, but who are not mentally ill, cannot be detained against their will until they have committed a crime. This is true even for criminal recidivists with long histories of violent behavior. Similarly, persons who behave in ways likely to cause themselves injury—rock-climbers who fail to use safety equipment, for example—cannot be confined unless they too are mentally ill.

If the state's police powers are at issue here, why should the presence of mental illness make a difference? Why is the presence of dangerous behavior by itself not sufficient to justify state intervention? The only reasonable conclusion is that actions to protect society's interests—standing by themselves—are insufficient bases for state action when significant deprivation of liberty is the cost. The difference between a dangerous psychotic person and a dangerous non-mentally ill criminal is that hospitalization of the former is likely to benefit him, and not incidentally, allow ultimate return to society in a more functional state. Confinement of the latter would be solely for preventive purposes, and might have to be indefinite to achieve that end. In short, it is the availability of care and effective treatment that justifies dealing differently with the mentally ill. *Parens patriae* rationales are therefore inherent in any system of commitment, even one limited to dangerous persons. The commonly accepted dichotomy is false. (See also Chap. 5, Sec. II-E-1.)

3. CURRENT STANDARDS OF INVOLUNTARY HOSPITALIZATION

Standards for involuntary commitment vary greatly from state to state, even under prevailing dangerousness-based approaches, and are frequently subject to revision by courts and legislatures. Here we shall attempt to outline the principles underlying the various criteria. It is the obligation of every clinician to remain informed about the most recent developments in his or her jurisdiction. Professional societies can often supply copies of current statutes, and will keep members up to date on changes as they occur. Every clinician should take the time to read the state's commitment statute, and other legislation relevant to mental health practice.

a. Emergency commitments

Most jurisdictions provide for the short-term hospitalization of patients in emergency situations until a court hearing can be held. The period of time before the hearing may vary from as little as two days to as long as three weeks. Usually a physician or psychologist must sign the commitment certificate, but some states require more than one professional to sign, and some allow agencies, such as the police or the courts, to initiate commitments when no mental health professional is available. Some states have screening requirements of varying degrees of rigor. At the lower end of the spectrum, states mandate that the committing clinician call in to a central screening officer to obtain permission for commitment, at least when the patient's bill will be paid by a public mental health agency. More significantly, other states require a full investigation by an independent agency of the need for hospitalization and the availability of alternative placements in the community.

Most often the criteria that must be met are identical to those required for court-ordered commitment. Facilities must decide at the end of periods of emergency commitment whether to release the patient or to petition for court-ordered hospitalization. The strict time limits on the duration of an emergency commitment are sometimes subverted in practice by the long periods of time required for the court to schedule a hearing. Thus patients may be involuntarily detained for many weeks or months before a hearing. The power to commit represents such a significant limitation on the freedom of the individual that those who hold it should exercise it only with extreme care.

b. Court-ordered commitments

After the expiration of an emergency commitment, or if dangerousness is not an issue at the time the decision to hospitalize is made, the court of appropriate jurisdiction can be petitioned for an order of commitment. The hearing that follows may take place, depending on the state, in a district, superior, family, or probate court. A small minority of states substitute an appearance before an administrative board or hearing officer in lieu of a formal judicial hearing. Some states guarantee the patient the right to have a jury decide on the question of commitment, but the vast majority of cases are heard by judges. In some states the duration of the commitment is explicitly limited to six months or one year; recommitment following that period requires a rehearing. Other states specify no period for commitment or allow an indefinite period, depending on the patient's condition. Recent court decisions suggest that even in this latter group of states a periodic review of the patient's status is constitutionally required to determine if the criteria for involuntary commitment continue to be met. The standards that the patient must meet to be committable include, as a result of being mentally ill:

Danger to others. Many states require this danger to be imminent, and some require proof of a threat, attempt, or occurrence of harm (often called an "overt act"). These demands for concrete evidence of dangerousness reflect society's trade-off of some measure of protection of the public at large in favor of a more stringent limitation on the number of those who face involuntary commitment. While these requirements appear to objectify the decision-making process, in fact a great deal of discretion remains in the hands of the committing physician, who now must judge the dangerousness of a person's threats or acts, rather than the degree of danger represented by his mental state.

Danger to self. This criterion addresses suicidal or severely self-destructive behavior (e.g., self-mutilation). Criteria tend to be less strict here than for dangerousness to others, but even so there are states that do not allow long-term commitment of suicidal patients (California, for example). Immediacy of harm and direct evidence of threat or attempt are other frequently included requirements.

Unable to care for self. Usually limited to an inability to provide for the essentials of food, clothing, and shelter such that the patient is at risk of serious physical harm, this standard can be subsumed under a broad definition of dangerousness to self. The ability of care need not meet middle-class levels; many chronic patients who live on the streets have developed remarkable talents for meeting their basic needs. In some areas this standard is known as "gravely disabled." Even if the patient cannot care for himself, hospitalization may not be permitted if alternative provision is available in the community.

Danger to property. This is an infrequently used criterion. Court decisions have indicated that involuntary commitment on the basis of danger to property in general is unconstitutional, but statutes requiring that the danger be one of substantial property loss or damage may pass constitutional muster.

In need of treatment. This is the old pure *parens patriae* standard but no longer stands on its own. It is frequently used in combination with the criteria above; patients not in need of treatment, despite dangerousness to self or others, may not be committable in these states.

At risk of deterioration. A few states, beginning with Washington state in 1979, have permitted involuntary hospitalization if a severe deterioration in the patient's condition is likely. This represents an effort to reinject something of a need-for-treatment approach in commitment law. (See Sec. F-1 below.)

Miscellaneous criteria. A small number of jurisdictions require that patients be incompetent to make treatment decisions (see Sec. F-1-a below), at least under certain of their commitment criteria (e.g., grave disability in Texas). An increasing number of states, spurred by court decisions, require that the option of commitment be the "least restrictive alternative" that will meet the patient's needs. This generally means excluding nursing home and group home placements, day hospitalization, and outpatient care as options before hospitalization is pursued. There are a number of practical difficulties in utilizing a "least restrictive alternative" analysis. While legal thought has always assumed that a lesser degree of governmental intervention is inherently less restrictive, that assumption may not always hold true in psychiatric settings. Critics of the concept have pointed to the difficulty in determining whether it is truly "less restrictive" for a psychotic patient to wander the streets uncared for or for him to be involuntarily hospitalized in a safe, clean, therapeutic milieu where not only his physical needs can be met, but the grip of the psychosis on his mind can be broken. Some clinicians and researchers have advocated a substitution of "most therapeutic alternative" in place of the "least restrictive" test. The courts, however, who will be the final arbiters of any such change, have not yet shown themselves inclined to accept it. (This question is also addressed in Chap. 3, Sec. II-B-1.)

4. PROCEDURAL ISSUES

a. Standards of proof

The degree of legal certainty required before commitment can ensue was the object of a 1979 U.S. Supreme Court decision (*Addington v. Texas*). The possible standards include: (1) a preponderance of the evidence—the standard in civil cases and generally conceived of as "more likely than not" or 51 chances out of 100; (2) clear and convincing evidence—roughly 75 chances out of 100; and (3) beyond a reasonable doubt—the standard in criminal cases, approximately 90–95 chances out of 100. Deciding amongst these, the Court ruled that the preponderance standard was insufficient when liberty was at stake, but, given the difficulty psychiatry would have in meeting the most stringent standard (of beyond a reasonable doubt), clear and convincing evidence was all that was constitutionally required. Nonetheless, some states, either by statute (e.g., Hawaii) or by state court decision (e.g., Massachusetts) continue to require proof beyond a reasonable doubt. Given the inherent difficulties psychiatrists have in the prediction of future behavior, this is a difficult standard to meet. But it should be kept in mind that what must be proven is *not* that it is beyond a reasonable doubt that dangerous behavior will occur. Rather, since almost all states specify that a "likelihood," "significant risk," or "imminent risk" of dangerous behavior is required, it is only the existence of that risk that must be proven beyond a reasonable doubt. It is a good deal easier to be certain that someone is at risk than to be certain that the risk will materialize.

b. Other procedural requirements

The trend toward criminal-style procedures in civil commitment cases reached its apogee in *Lessard v. Schmidt,* the 1972 Wisconsin case. There the court required: comprehensible and timely notice to the subject of the hearing of the allegations on which the request for commitment was based; similar notice of all rights, including the right to trial by jury; no detention longer than 48 hours without a hearing on probable cause; no detention longer than two weeks without a full hearing on the grounds for commitment; and the right to representation by adversary counsel, to exclusion of hearsay evidence, and to remain silent when examined by a psychiatrist or at trial. Some states, in addition, consider information revealed by patients to treating clinicians as privileged (see Chap. 1), and—regardless of relevance--exclude it from evidence at the hearing.

Not all courts, and certainly not most legislatures, have gone this far. The rights to notice, timely hearing, and assistance of counsel have been widely accepted. States vary considerably, though, in rules governing the need for and timing of a probable cause hearing, the use of hearsay evidence, and the right against self-incrimination. There may be considerable differences governing probable cause hearings, usually conducted a few days after detention, often by nonjudges, and full-fledged commitment hearings. In general, though, the latter are required to stick fairly closely to the kinds of procedures seen in criminal cases.

How closely do the courts adhere to procedural requirements? Studies prior to the reforms of the 1970s showed hearings in many jurisdictions to be *pro forma*, with little effort made to investigate the patient's status. Post-reform studies show many jurisdictions still having difficulty adhering to a full adversarial model, but in many others procedural requirements are rigorously observed.

E. Assessing the current system of involuntary commitment

Current approaches to civil commitment, which link dangerousness-based standards with criminalized procedures, are usually critiqued on three grounds.

1. EXCLUSION OF THE NON-DANGEROUS PATIENT IN NEED OF HOSPITALIZATION

Many, perhaps most, clinicians believe that existing commitment criteria and procedures make it too difficult to commit patients who are desperately in need of inpatient care. These patients are not dangerous to others, and may at this point represent no immediate threat to their own physical safety. Yet, they are suffering great emotional distress and run the risk of severe deterioration. Included in this group are: manic patients in the early stage of an episode, whose poor judgment is threatening their own well-being and that of their family; disorganized schizophrenic patients, roaming the streets, but able to beg or find enough food to sustain themselves; and depressed patients in considerable anguish, but so pessimistic about the possibility of improvement that they reject care.

There are numerous papers in the professional literature reporting anecdotes of patients not qualifying for commitment under current standards, who later came to harm. Most clinicians can offer examples from their own experience. Surprisingly, though, it has been difficult to demonstrate the existence of such a group in the few empirical studies that have addressed the question. Those patients most in need of treatment seem to get admitted. The "unable to care for self" criteria apparently absorb most of them. Few are released.

Needless to say, the research to date is not without flaws; noncommittable patients may not make their way to the emergency room, as those who would ordinarily bring them have learned of the futility of the effort. But the failure so far to identify significant numbers of such patients is provocative. It suggests that, in most cases, dangerousness-based criteria, including inability to care for self, may not significantly restrict hospitalization of patients truly in need of care. Rather, it may be the sustained policy of reducing inpatient beds, followed in most states for more than two decades, that accounts for the largest part of the difficulty in hospitalizing mentally ill persons.

2. DIFFICULTIES PREDICTING DANGEROUS BEHAVIOR

Most mentally ill persons are not dangerous, either to themselves or others. In fact, existing research suggests that mentally ill persons are only marginally more likely to be dangerous to others than the non-mentally ill. As in the general population, therefore, prediction of future dangerousness requires identification of a small fraction of problematic people from a much larger group. A common objection to the prevalent dangerousness-based commitment criteria is that they require mental health professionals to perform a task that simply cannot be accomplished, the prediction of future behavior dangerous to self or others.

a. Theoretical considerations

Some authors have pointed to the statistical impossibility of accurately predicting a low-frequency event (e.g., violence or suicide) without accruing a large number of false positive findings (e.g., nonviolent individuals incorrectly classified as violent). These authors cite examples similar to the following; assuming 100,000 mentally ill individuals are screened each year, of whom 1% are potentially violent, with a test that is 95% accurate in predicting violence, then 950 of the 1000 violent patients would be detained. However, given the 5% inaccuracy, 4950 of the 99,000 nonviolent patients would also be detained. The use of a less accurate screening test, which is probably closer to the actual situation, gives even poorer results.

Other factors have been cited as contributing to this tendency toward over-prediction. These include the fear of the clinician that if even one violent or suicidal individual is mistakenly discharged, the clinician will be subject to public castigation and to damage suits in the courts; the desire of the clinician to treat illness wherever possible, leading him or her to err in favor of committing potentially treatable patients; and the apprehensions of violence that many psychiatric patients evoke, even in the professionals who deal with them daily. It is difficult to imagine measures that might be effective in reversing these biases. Many question whether the benefits of detaining a small number of potentially violent or suicidal individuals are worth the costs of violating the rights of a large number of nondangerous patients.

b. The empirical data

The often-cited studies on the predictability of dangerousness towards others typically involved the follow-up of patients released against a psychiatrist's advice from a prison or a court setting. These studies show that psychiatrists tend to over-predict by factors of two to five in deciding who is potentially violent. The difficulty with these studies is that they do not disprove the ability of psychiatrists to predict violence in certain acute situations (as where recent acts of violence have taken place) or among specific subpopulations of patients (e.g., manics or excited catatonics). In fact, a generation of more recent studies, based on short-term predictions made in hospital emergency rooms about violent behavior following hospitalization, reveal much better results, with predictive accuracy in the range of 40–60% and considerable consistency among clinicians in judgments of dangerousness. Even these studies may underestimate the rate of correct predictions, since the institutional setting in which patients are placed may preclude the predicted dangerousness from becoming overt. Despite the methodologic difficulties that affect these studies, they do suggest that predictions of dangerousness by mental health professionals—with an accuracy, at their best, in the range of 50%—are problematic bases on which to rest a deprivation of patients' liberty.

Another set of studies have taken an actuarial approach to prediction. Using large populations and many variables thought likely to correlate with violence, they have tried to come up with formulae that would separate patients who will later be violent from those who will not. These efforts have been even less successful than clinicians' attempts at prediction. Whatever the limits of clinicians' abilities, they are identifying variables that appear to be difficult to specify or quantify for actuarial purposes.

Oddly, many fewer studies have examined the prediction of suicidal behavior than violent behavior, although a large number of correlates of suicide have been identified. Actuarial-type studies have been no more successful in predicting which patients will attempt to harm themselves than in identifying those who may harm others. Self-harm resulting from grave disability has, to our knowledge, not been studied in the same way. Most clinicians feel more comfortable with predictions of this sort, but whether that comfort is justified remains to be established.

3. DISTORTION OF THE ROLE OF THE MENTAL HEALTH SYSTEM

Even assuming the problems with prediction could be managed, many mental health professionals object to dangerousness-based approaches because of the effect they have on the functioning of the mental health system. By emphasizing the need to identify and treat dangerous persons—especially those dangerous to others—current statutes force clinicians into quasi-police roles. This may lead patients to identify the mental health system with the criminal justice system, making it more difficult to encourage them to come for needed care and to confide in their treaters.

Further, as state hospitals continue to dwindle in size, the emphasis on dangerousness had led to high concentrations of violent patients, making them difficult places to work and making it hard to treat other types of problems. Ironically, the effect may be to force out those patients with the most easily treatable problems (e.g., depression, acute psychosis) in favor of patients who are most resistant to current approaches (e.g., patients for whom dangerous behavior is the target symptom, especially those with personality disorders). A few efforts have been made to document these effects. Although the increasing percentage of patients who are dangerous to others has been confirmed in a number of studies, it is unclear if the rate of in-hospital violence has risen. Almost all studies agree that patients committed solely because of dangerousness to others represent a small fraction of committed populations.

F. Alternatives to the current commitment system

Given the level of dissatisfaction suggested by the previous section, it should come as no surprise that many proposals have been offered to alter the dominant approaches to civil commitment.

1. INTRODUCTION OF MODIFIED NEED FOR TREATMENT CRITERIA

If the emphasis on dangerousness is the cause of many current problems in civil commitment, a logical response would be to move away from exclusive use of that standard. Several proposals have been offered to supplement or replace dangerousness criteria with need-for-treatment based standards, modified to respond to the objections of civil libertarians that the old standards were too vague and overbroad.

a. The American Psychiatric Association model law

The most ambitious of reform proposals was offered by the American Psychiatric Association in 1983. Based on the work of psychiatrist Alan Stone, the model law would establish the following commitment criteria:

 i) presence of a severe mental disorder;
 ii) a reasonable prospect that the disorder will be treatable at the facility to which the patient will be committed, and that this is the least restrictive alternative for treatment;
 iii) refusal or inability of the patient to consent to treatment;
 iv) lack of capacity of the patient to make an informed decision regarding treatment; and
 v) likelihood that the patient, as a result of the severe mental disorder, will cause harm to self or others, or will suffer substantial mental or physical deterioration.

The effects of the APA proposal would be to limit commitment to patients who, though dangerous to self or others, also lacked the capacity to make their own decisions about treatment of their severe mental disorder. This emphasizes the *parens patriae* basis for commitment, since many commentators argue that this doctrine can only be applied when the person is incompetent to make her own decisions.

Another important change would be the hospitalization of patients who were not dangerous, but were likely to suffer deterioration associated with significant distress. This is a group that, though its size is unclear, attracts a great deal of attention from those unhappy with the present system.

No state has adopted the APA model in its entirety, although as will be noted below, several states have borrowed pieces of the model. States' reluctance may be based on their fear that the APA approach would increase the number of committable patients, flooding the public mental health system. Recent data suggest, however, that requirements similar to the APA's, especially severe mental illness and lack of capacity, actually restrict the number of committable patients when compared with straightforward dangerousness standards. Thus, the APA model might effect a true reorientation of the commitment system toward more severe, and perhaps more treatable, types of psychopathology.

Additional reasons for reluctance, however, are less easily dealt with. Civil libertarians are, in many cases, unalterably opposed to any effort to move away from dangerousness criteria. Further, the APA model would exclude from hospitalization persons dangerous to self or others, yet competent to make treatment decisions or not seriously mentally ill. That would limit commitment of many personality-disordered patients now apparently absorbed by the system. Legislatures may be leery of giving up the idea of the state hospital as a dumping ground for persons that no other system has the ability to deal with.

b. More limited efforts

A number of states have adopted one or another of the kind of proposals embodied in the APA model. Several have followed the lead of Washington state in adding commitment of patients likely to suffer substantial deterioration to their dangerousness-based criteria. These statutes may require significant functional impairment to be associated with deterioration, or evidence of previous deterioration in similar circumstances. They open the commitment net for an important population but do not otherwise address the problems associated with dangerousness criteria.

2. RELAXATION OF DANGEROUSNESS CRITERIA

The original dangerousness-based statutes of the 1970s frequently were framed in highly restrictive language. They required an overt act indicating dangerousness prior to commitment, sometimes within a specified period of time, or they mandated that the threat of dangerous behavior be "imminent and substantial." A number of states have modified these requirements in light of concerns over the rigor of their statutes, deleting the overt act requirement or allowing a verbal threat to serve in its place, and abandoning the language defining the degree of risk. Other states have added inability to care for self criteria to statutes that were previously limited to danger to self or others.

3. RELAXATION OF PROCEDURAL REQUIREMENTS

Procedures for involuntary commitment are always susceptible to modification when reform appears called for. There is, after all, a century-and-a-quarter's tradition of such moves. Yet there has been surprisingly little activity on this front since the statutory efforts of the 1970s. Criminalized procedures have come to be taken for granted by most participants in the commitment process, and there are few serious proposals for change. Perhaps the debates over substantive commitment criteria have diverted attention from the procedural aspects.

4. OUTPATIENT COMMITMENT

Easier access to inpatient hospitalization is not the only possible answer to current problems with civil commitment. A particularly frustrating group of patients are those who stop their medications shortly after discharge, rapidly deteriorating and soon requiring rehospitalization. Although statutes with deterioration criteria for commitment might allow that trajectory to be interrupted, they would not help to stabilize the patient in the community. This is where proposals for outpatient commitment come in.

In some respects, outpatient commitment is an old idea, related to the practice of "paroling" mental patients from state hospitals or giving them trial discharges. Patients who failed to adapt to the community could then be recalled to the hospital without further legal proceedings. In its new guise, however, it is not limited to former inpatients but can serve as a disposition of choice at a commitment hearing. Courts can order patients "committed" to a course of outpatient treatment specified by their clinicians. Even some civil libertarians endorse outpatient commitment (albeit in a limited fashion) as an alternative to more restrictive inpatient settings.

Almost every state has implicit or explicit provisions authorizing outpatient commitment in its statutes, but only in relatively few states are they used with any frequency. This is due, in part, to the lack of clinical and administrative structures to carry out court-ordered outpatient treatment. Other problems include judicial unfamiliarity with the concept, the absence of discrete criteria for outpatient commitment, and the absence of enforcement mechanisms.

The states that have taken outpatient commitment seriously, including North Carolina, Hawaii, Arizona, and Tennessee, have created different criteria for outpatient than for inpatient commitment. The criteria focus on the likelihood of relapse that would eventuate in future dangerousness, and in some cases require that a pattern of dangerous behavior when unmedicated be evident. Enforcement of judicial orders is a major problem, with most statutes silent on how this is to occur. Even statutes that make provisions for patients to be brought before a judge if they fail to comply usually limit the judge's power to admonishment; inpatient hospitalization is only possible if patients are found to meet the usual commitment criteria.

A small number of empirical studies have demonstrated varying results with outpatient committed patients. Much of the variance may be due to the different capacities and interest of mental health systems in undertaking involuntary outpatient treatment. There is also the long-range question of whether some enforcement mechanism (perhaps short-term detention and involuntary administration of medication) will be needed when patients discover that they can often avoid current orders with impunity. Outpatient commitment is an interesting approach that bears careful study as different models are tried out in a number of jurisdictions.

5. Non-statutory approaches

Not everyone believes that changing commitment statutes is the best way— or even a very good way—to reform commitment practices. Some experts in the area hold the opinion that commitment law changes, especially changes in substantive criteria, make relatively little difference in who gets committed. They see decisionmakers as operating independently, within broad bounds of statutory criteria, guided by their innate sense of who belongs in a hospital and who does not. As noted above, the state of empirical research on effects of commitment law changes does not allow us to comment definitively on this contention.

There is evidence, however, of a great deal of discretion embedded in the current system. Witness the frequent phenomenon of sharp rises in local commitment rates following well-publicized acts of violence by mentally ill persons. Some people argue that the best way to affect commitment decisions is to educate gatekeepers about the consequences of severe mental illness, thereby leading them to broaden the scope of cases they will define as commitable.

Nonstatutory approaches may also be of use in amending commitment procedures. Much of what takes place in the commitment process is determined not by statutes, but by administrative rules, judicial practices, or simple custom. The National Center for State Courts has issued guidelines for reforming the less functional elements of the commitment process, and suggests that groups of concerned participants from the mental health and legal systems meet regularly to discuss problems and implement these local-level reforms.

III. CLINICAL ISSUES

A. Performing the emergency assessment

The emergency evaluation is often a precipitous, stressful, unprepared-for encounter between strangers, both caught up in the tensions of the moment. Moreover, patients, families, and members of the community may turn to the hospital, sometimes quite unrealistically, as a panacea for personal, familial, or social dysphoria. These conditions may give rise to an oppositional posture of clinician and patient operating at cross purposes or seeking different goals. To the clinician belongs the challenge of "reaching for the alliance" despite the circumstances; her basic wish to help must lead her to reach out empathically to make contact with the distress in the patient. This process holds true even if the evaluator must finally disappoint, refuse, or turn away the patient on clinical grounds.

Specifically, the evaluator seeks the patient's best side, the resources and strengths, and attempts to recruit these traits to the tasks of data gathering and intervention. Without this fundamental rapport, the emergency encounter is more a collision than a collaboration.

In practice the decisions that must be made at the point of a psychiatric emergency address the issues of treatment versus no treatment; hospitalization versus no hospitalization; and psychiatric versus nonpsychiatric intervention (e.g., an apparent psychiatric emergency may in reality be a matter for neurology, internal medicine, or surgery, or for the criminal justice system).

In relation to these considerations, the emergency assessment may involve legally significant compromises, procedures, and trade-offs rarely employed in nonemergent settings or situations. One implication of this situation is that emergencies in general are considered exceptions to many well established rules. For example, breaches of confidentiality and many treatment interventions, even if involuntary, are understood to be permitted in the context of a bona fide emergency. Predictably such an extension of the clinician's license to act mandates well documented assessment and identification of the factors which make the present situation a true emergency.

1. THE HISTORY AND THE RECORD IN THE EMERGENCY ASSESSMENT

a. Obtaining the history from the patient and others

Significant data that need to be obtained from the patient include the details of previous episodes of the current illness or problem, previous successful interventions, and previous attempted solutions. When the patient cannot provide historical data, the evaluator is forced to turn elsewhere for the information, even without the patient's consent, under color of the emergency.

When obtaining information from informants requires revealing information that may prove embarrassing to the patient (e.g., that he is mentally ill and in need of hospitalization), the harm done to the patient's right to confidentiality must be carefully weighed against the expected benefits. But the immediate clinical needs of the patient should always be the primary determinant of the course chosen. (See Chap. 1, Secs. II-B-5-a and III-C-3.)

This illustrates another important clinical/legal difficulty of emergency assessment. In general, certain steps taken under color of the emergency may involve acting *on* the patient (e.g., involuntary hospitalization or emergency breach of confidentiality), which may pose future difficulties for the therapeutic alliance when the issue is working *with* the patient in a trust-based collaboration.

b. The evaluator as user of informants

The evaluator is frequently in the position of structuring the inquiry to elicit usable data from random and unsystematic observations and perceptions of family, friends, school personnel, police, passers-by, and so on. While to the lawyer these may represent "hearsay" evidence, such observations may be the only sources of information for the front-line clinician. The optimal approach to gathering data focuses on previous psychiatric history; recent behavior or behavioral change; significant alteration of circumstances (e.g., loss of job); bizarreness of ideation or action; threats to self or others, or related behavior such as the purchase of poison, rope, or a gun; history of substance abuse, and the like. By concentrating on factual elements in the informants' presentations, rather than on their subjective evaluation of the situation, one minimizes the possibility that a patient will face a major, potentially liberty-depriving intervention without adequate justification. Of course, the responses that the patient elicits in others may be useful data in themselves, but they should be viewed merely as another element in the picture, not as a necessarily accurate appraisal of the patient's mental state.

One practical tip of inestimable value is often overlooked in the rush and confusion of many emergency settings: obtaining names and telephone numbers from anyone who has accompanied the patient, including family, police officers, and individuals from other agencies. If the patient is admitted and a more exhaustive workup can be undertaken, these numbers prove enormously useful for following up on clinical issues raised during the emergency evaluation. Obtaining this information from all accompanying individuals should become a reflex for emergency room clinicians.

c. Informant reliability

The variation in reliability of informants represents one of the complexities of the emergency evaluation. The evaluator is charged with assigning a weight of apparent veracity to each informant's data based on a necessarily brief, ad hoc assessment of that informant in a situation lacking both leisure and a contract for an intimate evaluation of the informant (i.e., one cannot easily, or at least overtly, administer a mental status examination to the informant). Such factors as apparent prejudice toward the patient, anger at the patient, fear of the patient, or wishes to shield, blame, or deny must enter into this determination. Certain types of professionals (e.g., police officers) may be by training more skilled in observation and more objective than family members, especially under conditions of stress.

d. Ulterior motives

Under certain circumstances informants may reveal data that is distorted, selective, or even fabricated for ulterior motives.

Example 1: A family wishes to be at least temporarily rid of a patient whose chronic psychosis has exhausted them for days; they exaggerate the patient's distress, dangerousness, suicidality, or symptomatology in the hope of having the patient admitted.

Example 2: A medical doctor, wishing not to take care of an alcoholic patient, refers the patient to an emergency psychiatrist without mentioning the obvious odor of alcohol as a possible causative factor in the stated symptoms of confusion and hallucination.

Example 3: The husband whose wife has just, in hysterics, declared her intention to leave him, presses for her admission on fabricated grounds, out of the magical wish that the hospitalization will "cure her" of her wish to leave.

It should be emphasized that admission *may* in fact be indicated or contra-indicated in any of these examples; the point at issue is the contamination of informant reliability by ulterior motives.

e. Solicitation of information as an alliance threat

In many cases, the very act of solicitation of information may provoke violent objections that threaten the alliance with the patient. The evaluator attempts to keep the assessment as the task before them, a task to which all parties must address themselves and in which all parties have a common interest; thus this community of interest serves as an initial framework for alliance formation in the emergency setting.

Example 4: As the evaluator turns to the psychotic teenager's mother, the patient screams furiously, "Who are you gonna believe, me or her? *I'm* the one who needs help!" The evaluator responds: "Look, we have a real crisis here and we'd be unwise to pass up hearing anything from anyone that might help us to figure out what's going on. I'm not here to believe her or you, just to understand what's happening."

The use of "we" in the example enlists all parties present into the evaluative effort, while the shift of emphasis from "belief" to "understanding" paves the way toward the nonjudgmental exploration of future issues.

f. Documentation

It should be underscored that the assessment process described in the foregoing sections must be documented explicitly in the record; the documentation should include (but should clearly distinguish among) observations, allegations, and direct examinations. The differential weighting and the inclusion or exclusion of data should be described together with the evaluator's rationale. Such documentation alone may prove the decisive preventive against a claim of negligence in regard to the evaluation.

The clinician is well advised to document more extensively the decision to take the less conservative approach. That is, the decision to release or send out a patient in an ambiguous situation should require a far more careful risk-benefit analysis than when the patient is being definitively hospitalized or treated. (See Chap. 4, Sec. III-A-3.)

2. ASSESSING THE PATIENT AND THE ENVIRONMENT IN EVALUATING AN EMERGENCY

In addition to the more traditional historic and diagnostic elements of the evaluation, the evaluator must clarify those factors that influence the urgency of the current situation. These factors extend beyond the concept of "precipitants," and may be grouped into risk factors and resource factors, external and internal. Careful determination of these factors provides the legal justification for clinical interventions.

a. Risk factors

Factors under this heading tend either to increase the urgency of the current situation or to decrease the supportive or coping mechanisms available to the patient. The patient's past behavior, given a set of risk factors similar to the current ones, is often the most useful prognostic guide.

External risk factors.   External risk factors include:

- Loss, alienation, or absence of significant objects (family, therapist, lover, etc.) or circumstances (job, residence, school, etc.)
- Hostile environmental factors (family wants patient dead, patient only black in racially troubled neighborhood, etc.)
- Acuteness of and/or lack of preparedness for emergency situation

Internal risk factors.   Internal risk factors include:

- Lack of ability to use available resources (severity of disturbance in cognition or behavior—all toxic states, retardation or other organic impairment, language barrier, etc.)
- History of marginal intellectual or interpersonal adaptation, poor achievement or level of functioning (never employed, high school dropout, lives on streets, cannot make friends)
- History of impulsivity, substance abuse, criminal record, violence or suicidality
- Intolerably dysphoric feeling state (rage, panic, agitated depression, etc.)
- Preoccupations, obsessive thoughts or fantasies with destructive content (constant thoughts of revenge, "resting in peace," etc.)

b. Resource factors

Factors under this heading tend either to decrease the urgency of the current situation or to increase the supportive or coping mechanisms available to the patient.

External resource factors.   External resource factors include:

- Availability of family, spouse, friends, therapist, protective setting (group home, halfway house, commune)

- Preservation of supportive circumstances (boss will give back job, school open for reapplication, etc.)
- Availability of specialized resources (VA benefits, medical treatments for disabling conditions, financial supports, social agencies, etc.)

Internal resource factors.   Internal resource factors include:

- History of impulse control, obsessional defenses, intellectual and social achievement, high functioning, "rootedness" (home and work stability)
- Absence of history of substance abuse, toxic or organic states
- Presence of a number of personally acceptable options or choices at point of crisis
- Durable religious faith or ethical convictions with low conflict about them
- "Marketable" vocational or professional skills
- Social skills, ability to enlist and relate to others

B. Assessment of suicidality

This assessment represents, among other things, a special case of the risk/resource evaluation described in general terms above. The central clinical and legal concerns involve negligence in evaluation and in involuntary interventions (usually hospitalization). While this topic might well occupy a book in itself, we here outline general principles in review, drawing on both empirical data and "received wisdom."

1. DIAGNOSTIC CONSIDERATIONS AND HISTORY

While many scholars in the area of suicide assessment and prediction have considered the epidemiology of suicide in subject populations, our focus here will be primarily on the individual and his assessment, whether in an emergency room or office—an assessment that should be performed routinely on intake of individuals seeking psychiatric treatment, whether or not overtly depressive features dominate the presentation. We present an outline of factors demonstrated in suicide research (see, for example, Suggested Readings—Roy) that appear to have empirically validated utility.

a. The personal context

Research suggests that men are more at risk than women and that the years after reaching middle-age are the riskier ones for suicide. Despite the rise in suicide rates among young people, this finding remains significant. The divorced and the widowed are at higher risk, closely followed by the separated. Perhaps the most important variable is that of psychological isolation. This can derive from a number of sources. For example, immigrants who have failed to find a local community, those who are retired or unemployed, those living alone, even those living in transient or disorganized areas such as resort towns whose populations fluctuate wildly on a seasonal basis. Finally, Catholic faith appears to pose some barriers to suicide; of the three major American faiths, Protestant faith appears the most vulnerable to it.

b. Previous history and background

Important variables appear to be family history of affective disorder, suicide, or alcoholism. Previous suicide attempts themselves are complex predictors, in that frequent suicide attempts may paradoxically decrease the likelihood of serious intent.

c. Current stressors

Important stressors likely to be associated with suicide are acute bereavement or separation from loved ones; recent geographic move, especially to a more isolated situation; loss of job; complications of alcoholism; physical illness; and, with the elderly, terminal illness.

d. Personality disorder factors

Issues most relevant here appear to be cyclothymic personality and sociopathy (antisocial personality), intensified by substance abuse of any kind.

e. Psychiatric illness

Depression predictably leads the list of illnesses correlated with suicide, especially in the context of recurring depression or full-fledged bipolar disorder. Substance abuse is highly represented, as are various forms of organic conditions and impairments in the elderly. Recent data suggest that panic disorder significantly increases suicide risk, and that as many as 10% of schizophrenics ultimately kill themselves.

f. Symptomatology

Again leading the list are depressive symptoms or a recent history of the same (the patient at the time of presentation may be less acutely depressed than before, having made the decision to die) and communicated suicidal intent in both verbal form and in suicide notes. Particularly serious are states of agitation and dysphoria in the depression that convey an "excruciating" quality. Patients in this condition are subjectively extremely difficult to sit with; indeed, the examiner's countertransference impulse to retreat from the patient may have diagnostic force. Other significant ominous feelings are pessimism, hopelessness, and, in particular, ideas of reunion with the lost loved one.

g. Context of the suicidal act

Suicidal acts of a high risk, low rescue sort (see Sec. B-2) are particularly ominous, as are suicide attempts accompanied by certain preparatory actions (suicide notes, giving away possessions, etc.). Lethal and violent methods should alert clinicians to particular risk.

h. Clinical wisdom concerning suicide

In addition to the above empirically validated elements of the assessment, some useful lore in the form of "clinical received wisdom" may stand a practitioner in good stead. One finding is that individuals attempting suicide through what might be styled "respiratory" means—hanging, drowning, gas, various forms of asphyxiation or strangulation—may represent a somewhat more lethal sub-population of suicide attempters. The one exception to this rule is individuals, usually male, who are attempting a strangulation experience to intensify masturbatory excitement in the form of auto-erotic self hangings. This paraphiliac activity may trigger social responses as though it represented attempted suicide, whereas it is really a variant of erotic activity.

The second point important in the assessment of the suicidal patient is the understanding that one of the clinician's most essential tools, empathy, may mislead or misguide the evaluator. The reasoning here, though subtle, is clinically very important. Individuals on the brink of suicide may be cut off from their own despair. Thus, the evaluator attempting empathic linkage with the patient may perceive someone who "seems to feel OK." In this context, the examiner may have to exercise humility and augment the empathic assessment with what might be termed "cerebration," in which careful attention is paid to the actuarial risk factors earlier delineated. The individual who appears to have a serious loading of risk factors but who "feels OK" in the immediate evaluation may require use of more active safeguards until the entire situation is better understood than may be possible in the brief emergency context. Further investigation and use of ancillary sources may clarify the situation either way.

Other elements of the clinical picture that appear to increase the risk of suicide are the presence of psychosis, especially with command suicidal hallucinations; a history of suicide attempts, successful suicides, or psychosis in either the patient or family; and the presence of specific anniversaries.

Religion may operate to increase risk through fomenting guilt but may decrease risk through prohibition of suicide; as a rule of thumb, patients who state that their religion forbids suicide should have this resource taken seriously, absent strong evidence to the contrary. A common omission for clinicians in dealing with suicidal patients is failure to explore the patient's religious history. This information helps to identify risks *and* resources and to capture a picture of the afterlife to which the patient is considering sending himself.

Finally, some experienced evaluators note that as part of the normal response to the depressed patient, the evaluator feels somewhat depressed. Confronted with the suicidal patient, however, the examiner may feel an inexplicable fear. Careful introspection and attention to this diagnostically useful countertransference response may be extremely illuminating and helpful.

A series of factors validated by experience define a continuum of increasing suicidal risk, which may aid the clinician in assessing the urgency of the situation.

Suicidal ideation. Nearly a universal experience under certain circumstances.

Suicidal intent.   The decision to die; may be accompanied by an ominous *decrease* in tension or dysphoria and *increase* in calm or an elevation of mood.

Presence of specific plan.   Gives increasing focus and affective intensity to fantasy around intent; may channel energy toward goal.

Availability of means.   The pills, gun, rope, specific bridge, etc., are immediately accessible.

Attempt.   The patient has actually taken action against himself.

2. ASSESSMENT OF SUICIDE ATTEMPTS

Patients may present to the emergency setting at the last stage of urgency, i.e., after having already attempted suicide and survived; referral may come from general medical physicians or from the police. A useful guideline for assessing such attempts is the risk/rescue rating popularized by Weisman and others (see Suggested Readings—Weisman & Worden). The evaluator must bear in mind throughout this determination, however, that the population of suicide attempters (regardless of low risk, high rescue circumstances) is at greater risk for suicide than other populations. In increasing order of lethality, typical examples are:

- Low risk, high rescue: patient takes a small number of aspirins and immediately tells friend.
- Low risk, low rescue: patient attempts to slash wrists with piece of glass while alone.
- High risk, high rescue: patient shouts "I'm going to jump!" and lunges for distant window of crowded room.
- High risk, low rescue: patient buys gun and rents motel room under false name.

It is important that, when the evaluator makes a determination that serious suicidal risk exists, she act decisively and without permitting delay, postponement, or an unobserved or unprotected interval during which the patient "gets some things." Patients at the crisis point may attempt suicide in the emergency room itself, in rest rooms, while going for a cigarette, etc. When significant suicidal risk is present, the approach must be guided by a consistent, serious, and unambiguous assumption of responsibility for the patient by the clinician.

This authoritarian "taking over" is guided by the truism that depression is usually temporary and treatable; suicide is permanent. The evaluator aims at a realistic moratorium on action, not an ominipotent interdiction against death. A very experienced clinician used to say to patients at the brink: "It would be a pity if you killed yourself while depression clouded your judgment. Let's get you undepressed; then, if you still want to kill yourself, I know I can't stop you." This posture conveys the locus of eventual responsibility, the indirect optimism for treatment, and the realistic limitation of the evaluator's power.

3. MANIPULATIVE SUICIDE AND THE PROBLEM OF REGRESSION

Although the idea is confusing to the layperson, a number of people "attempt suicide" without a wish or intention to die; rather, their goal is to change or to improve their manner of living. Not all such patients require hospitalization or even intervention.

Example 5: When her boyfriend breaks up with her, a high school girl slashes her wrist superficially and blames her guilt-stricken boyfriend when he meets her in the hospital emergency room. The boyfriend begs her to make up and swears eternal fidelity. Suicidality in the patient disappears, at least temporarily.

Example 6: A woman in her twenties arrives at the admission office with two paper bags, ostensibly containing clothes and possessions, sits down and glares at the admitting doctor. Asked, "Can I help you?"

she barks, "I'm here to be admitted!" Asked to say more, she retorts, "There's nothing to say, I'm here to be admitted." When told she must give a reason, she states, "Admit me or I'll kill myself." Many minutes of questioning reveal that the woman is enraged at her live-in boy-friend and had hoped to be admitted to "show him."

Other examples of the threat of suicide with nonlethal intent include the destitute patient seeking a roof for the night and the felon wishing to escape detection by the police. These clinical situations must be distinguished from true suicidality.

A specific population requiring consideration is the group of chronically, as opposed to acutely, suicidal patients. This type of patient offers a unique challenge to the diagnostician in the emergency setting, since actual suicide is a perpetual risk, yet hospitalization tends to promote regression and should often be actively resisted. This poses a legal dilemma as well as a clinical one, since the clinician faces the constant fear of a jury finding her negligent because "that one time" the patient's usually half-hearted attempt succeeded. Furthermore, laypersons tend to view hospitalization as a panacea and rarely grasp that hospitalization may be *harmful* to such patients.

The clinician must place the best interests of the patient first and act accordingly; however, careful attention to documentation of the clinical rationale is mandatory when the calculated risk (not admitting the self-confessedly suicidal patient) is taken.

A useful guideline in this difficult situation may be to assess the patient's capacity (or competence) to follow through on treatment planning or, more particularly, to weigh the risks and benefits of giving or withholding information from clinicians about suicidal impulses. Essentially, this assessment helps distinguish the patient who *can* report to the clinician about her condition—but chooses to withhold this information—from the patient too ill, sick, hopeless. depressed, or regressed to do so. This may have some implications for future liability assessment.

The essence here is that the clinician make (and document) an assessment of the patient's ability to be a reporter on his own internal state of risk. This permits the clinician to draw useful conclusions about the state of the alliance with the patient, which may be itself a significant suicide preventive.

C. Assessment of dangerousness to others

Dangerousness to others is in certain ways more complex and more emotionally charged than suicidality, since the danger threatens to involve innocent bystanders—a situation exerting significant influence on the degree of risk the clinician can accept. Nevertheless, prediction of dangerousness is a fundamentally unreliable endeavor (see Sec. II-E-2 above.) The diagnostician is constantly challenged to balance the individual patient's rights and freedoms against the safety of society.

The situation is profoundly complicated by the fact that threats against others (including, of course, the therapist) are an extremely common event, a result in part of the mobilization of powerful feelings that often occurs in psychiatric treatment. It would be unreasonable, unethical, and surely impossible to respond to every one of such threats as though it represented an acute and present danger to others; yet legal decisions like the *Tarasoff* ruling (see Chap. 4, Sec. II-A-3-e) intensify the pressure on the diagnostician to winnow the chaff of idle threats from the wheat of serious intent to harm, since different courses of action must follow, and a different tack must be taken in regard to an alliance-threatening breach of confidentiality. The "duty to protect" must be weighed against the possible risk to the therapeutic relationship.

In light of the evidence presented earlier that strongly suggests that psychiatrists are poor predictors of dangerousness (see Sec. II-E-2), it may seem paradoxical to outline herein a framework within which that determination can be made. Several arguments, however, can be offered in support of such an attempt to clarify the bases of psychiatric prediction of dangerousness: (1) it may be that psychiatrists (and other clinicians) predict poorly because they do not utilize the criteria that have been offered in the literature to aid the process; (2) there may be subpopulations of violent patients (e.g., acutely manic patients) in whom the determination of dangerousness is more reliable; (3) the courts have not yet recognized that psychiatry's predictive powers are limited, and they continue to hold clinicians responsible for the failure to predict their patients' violent acts (while often simultaneously refusing to accept such predictions in commitment cases); (4) given all the imperfections in the prediction process, it remains the only means in many states by which patients in desperate need of treatment can receive it without their consent; (5) despite what seem to be inherent limitations on the accuracy of the prediction of dangerousness, if any progress is to be made in the field, the development of valid guidelines will continue to require the thoughtful attention of the mental health professions.

1. DIAGNOSTIC CONSIDERATIONS AND HISTORY

As in the assessment of suicide, the data used in this prediction consist of both statistically validated findings (see Suggested Readings—Monahan) and received wisdom derived from practice in the field.

The following include elements repeatedly found in empirical studies to correlate with future dangerousness to others:

a. Past violence.

This factor repeatedly appears as the strongest correlate in actuarial studies of violence and related phenomena. Clinicians must overcome their denial, based on discomfort with the issue of violence, in order to make a specific inquiry about this subject. A particularly useful question is: "Have you ever, for any reason, accidentally or otherwise, caused death or severe injury to another human being?" This may elicit unexpected but highly relevant data, including incidents involving police, negligent homicide through vehicles, military combat experience, and the like.

b. Age.

This represents another familiar variable in violence assessment. Violence peaks in the teenage years, declines slowly through the 30s, then drops precipitously after age 40.

c. Gender.

Males overwhelmingly predominate as agents of violence. The ratio in many studies is 9:1.

d. Race.

Even corrected actuarial data that attempt to filter out differential selection due to preferential arrest of racial groups conclude that non-white individuals have significantly higher rates for violent crimes.

e. Socioeconomic status and stability of employment situation.

Multiple studies suggest that economic stability and employment are inversely correlated with recidivism for violence.

f. Substance abuse.

Use of many psychoactive substances, particularly alcohol, clearly correlates with increased violence. Phencyclidine ("PCP") and cocaine—two currently popular drugs of abuse—are believed by many clinicians to be major triggers of violent behavior.

g. Clinical wisdom concerning dangerousness to others.

Moving to the "received wisdom" in the field, clinicians note that patients with a tendency to externalize are more likely to see the locus of their problems as residing in the outside world and to seek solutions by acting on it there. This category would of course include the host of paranoid conditions, the "impulse disorders," and substance abuse as earlier mentioned.

Other features historically considered important include:

— history of dangerous intentions or thoughts (lasting grudges, obsessive thoughts of revenge or retribution, persecutory delusions fixed on specific persons, and some forms of the delusion known as erotomania: the belief that a person, usually someone of higher perceived status, is secretly in love with oneself).
— membership in violence-oriented ethnic or cultural groups (e.g., street gangs) may militate in favor of increased dangerousness.
— history of victimization (recipient of child abuse; of adult violence; public shame, humiliation, or loss of face; rejections, provocations, and related narcissistic injuries, particularly in significant relationships such as loved ones).
— ownership of weapons and related items (gun collection, knife collection, martial arts degrees, membership in mercenary groups).
— tendency by history to make lists (mental or written) of people who have wronged one and whom one would like to "pay back," kill, see dead or eliminated; diaries or journals with similar content.

Clinicians should forthrightly explore these areas since, although commonly omitted in the casual assessment, they are of significant value in rounding out a picture of the patient's potential for danger.

h. Predictions in the presence and absence of past violence.

When a patient has no history of previous violence, a judgment must be made as to the relative balance of inhibitory versus instigative factors. In close decisions, the longer the period of time that the present balance has existed, the stronger the possibility that it represents a stable equilibrium. When the situation is rapidly changing, in contrast, there may be some value in erring on the side of safety.

In the presence of a previous history of violence, the assessment becomes somewhat easier. The clinician must ascertain those factors that appeared to contribute to the previous violent act and determine the degree of amelioration. The greater the change, the lower the likelihood of recurrence.

2. RELATIONSHIP OF DANGEROUSNESS TO MENTAL ILLNESS

After a crime of violence, the assailant who has been examined by a psychiatrist at some point may be seen in hindsight by a jury as clearly mentally ill and the crime, as clearly the product of that illness. For the diagnostician the problem prospectively is far more difficult to clarify. The diagnostic listings offer "explosive disorder"; but does this really include the alcoholic who is belligerent when drunk, or the street-corner pugilist whose multiple fights ("assaults") are more the products of deliberation than explosiveness? Empirical research repeatedly demonstrates, moreover, that previous criminality determines future criminality; mental illness independent of this consideration "drops out" as a variable. Such findings tend to refute the popular fusion of mental illness and crime.

The situation is further complicated by the fact that the violent psychopath who is not psychotic has found a nosologic home in neither the psychiatric nor the criminal justice systems. Again, in retrospect, a jury may have difficulty seeing that a patient who has "traveled through life on his fists" may have "no mental illness"; yet only in the presence of "real mental illness"—i.e., a disorder likely to benefit from available psychiatric interventions—may the clinician lawfully intervene with such sanctions as involuntary hospitalization. Theoretically, all other situations are matters for the police.

3. CLINICAL ASSESSMENT OF DANGEROUSNESS

a. Appearance: clues to dangerousness include physical tension (grimacing, clenching fists or jaw, etc.), preoccupation, pacing, presence of real or possible weapons (knife, length of pipe, etc).

b. Mood and speech: angry; threatening; glaring or hostile looks, words, or threats.

c. Thought content: persecutory delusions, command hallucinations directing violent acts; the obsessive thoughts, fantasies, and ruminations of assault, loss of control, revenge, and the like.

d. Circumstances: patient brought in, in handcuffs, by four policemen after assault; patient seen raving in restraints, etc.

e. State of controls: The clinician must assess the "impulse versus controls" balance in a manner similar to the "risk versus rescue" balance in suicide.

External: A number of concerned, strong family members may be able to sit with the patient until alcohol wears off and transient dangerousness passes, whereas a lone patient just arrived in town may have no such resources.

Internal: An obsessional patient terrified of losing control is more likely to maintain it than an impulsive, amphetamine-abusing street fighter.

D. Assessment of ability to care for self

This category reflects the awareness by lawmakers that not all psychiatric emergencies are characterized by a clearly definable "active risk" of dangerousness to self or others. A significant category of patients who need immediate care includes those who are so psychotic, hallucinated, demented, etc., that they represent a "passive risk" to themselves: being run over in traffic, being mugged, raped, or assaulted, dying of pneumonia from exposure to cold, or starving to death.

By its very ambiguity, this category is the most ethically, as well as diagnostically, challenging, since its breadth of scope creates—depending on one's viewpoint—the greatest flexibility to bend the law to help the patient or, contrariwise, the greatest potential for paternalistic abuse. To aid clinicians in thinking rigorously about this issue, structured scales have been developed for the assessment of ability to care for self. (See Suggested Readings—Grisso.)

1. THE "ILLNESS VERSUS FUNCTIONING" DILEMMA

Assessment of the ability to care for self depends far more on the history and observed evidence of functioning than on any diagnostic category or even the severity or chronicity of illness. An example would be the so-called "street schizophrenic" who is able to exist (though perhaps not thrive) by means of a practical knowledge of sources of food, clothing, and shelter unknown to the average urban dweller.

Example 7: One such man lived for seven months in this manner, seeing his father only to pick up a social security check, otherwise living on the streets. He was hospitalized only when a combination of unusually cold weather and purulent leg ulcers made this way of life untenable.

2. THE ISSUE OF AVAILABLE RESOURCES

Patients may be rendered unable to function only when certain resources break down or become unavailable. Being evicted from a halfway house or a nursing home may snap the thread that makes extrainstitutional living possible; a similar "last straw" may be the patient's alienating a supportive family member or a trusted therapist, nurse, or aide, or even the temporary absence of a nursing home dietician on vacation. These and similar seemingly minor events may threaten the balance of resources so as to render a previously equilibrated patient unable to continue self-care. The clinician must seek for problems remediable by direct interventions, short or long term, to return to the patient the capacity for self-care or to provide the necessary caretaking environment.

E. Clinical aspects of emergency assessment

1. DOCUMENTATION

Interventions made in the emergency setting should reflect a well-thought-out formulation of the problem that generates a rationale for the type of intervention used; meticulous documentation and record keeping should demonstrate not only careful efforts at data gathering and at assessment of the patient, but also the steps of reasoning followed to arrive at the treatment plan.

> *Example 8:* A forensically unsound emergency room note found in a patient's chart read, in its entirety: "Chief complaint—can't sleep. Rx Elavil 25 mg qid. # 50, see Tues." The author of the note omitted documenting several forensically crucial steps including the fact that:

(1) the assessment of the patient revealed depression at the cause for insomnia;
(2) the assessment revealed no acute suicidality, implying, first, that the patient would probably *live* until Tuesday and, second, that a potentially lethal amount of antidepressant could be prescribed safely at one time.

2. CONSULTATION TO EXISTING RELATIONSHIPS

The emergency room serves as the arena where difficulties in relationships (including therapeutic relationships) may be played out:

> *Example 9:* A patient, refused minor tranquilizing medications by his doctor, continued to obtain them from an emergency room psychiatrist who did not inquire about current treatment.

> *Example 10:* A patient whose husband minimized her anxieties convinced him to bring her to the emergency room with an unconscious intention of proving she was "that upset."

The evaluator is often challenged to perform what is essentially a consultation to an official or unofficial therapeutic relationship; the consultative effort may be obvious or subtle.

> *Example 11:* A patient in therapy came to the emergency room with an anxiety attack, feeling he could not "bother his doctor with these trifling concerns." The emergency room evaluator merely pointed out that the patient was self-defeatingly undermining his psychiatrist's taking him seriously and that something serious enough for the emergency room was serious enough to call the doctor about. The patient agreed and called.

> *Example 12:* A couple with two teenagers came to the psychiatric emergency room demanding commitment of the younger child as a result of a tremendous family fracas just before a long trip; the parents were furious, the children upset but clearly not in need of hospitalization. Careful exploration and considerable time spent interviewing

the whole family revealed that the trip in question would have been, in all probability, the last time the family would have seen the seriously ill grandparents alive, though the family had kept this fact from conscious awareness. The upset had resulted from submerged tensions about this, and the visit to the emergency room had aborted the conflicted trip. The family was encouraged toward psychological termination with the grandparents.

Although the issue is generally not considered in these terms, an intervention with the patient threatening harm to another party could also be looked at as having consultative force, since the relationship—now potentially violent or homicidal—is badly in need of external modification. One device may prove beneficial, not only in diminishing the actual dangerousness of the situation but subsequently in diminishing liability in the event of a bad outcome: have the dangerous patient actually contact the putative victim (for example, by making a phone call from the evaluator's office) and share her grudge verbally. This verbal contact, in addition to being superior to physical ones, may permit the reality testing of paranoid fantasies, the ventilation and catharsis of unmanageable rage, and other salutary processes which may defuse the dangerous situation (see Suggested Readings—Wulsin et al.).

3. Environmental Manipulation

In broadest terms, this intervention usually boils down to removing a patient from a noxious situation and/or placing the patient in a more protected environment. The former action may involve, e.g., finding an emergency shelter for a battered wife; the latter may involve hospitalization in a psychiatric facility.

a. Voluntary hospitalization

Hospitalization is offered to decrease the pressures of external responsibility when the patient is overwhelmed by them and to provide structure, a supportive milieu, protection, "intensive care," closely supervised pharmacotherapy, electroconvulsive therapy, or other forms of treatment. A voluntary patient by definition accepts the treatment recommendations of hospitalization.

b. Involuntary hospitalization

The legal indications and standards for involuntary hospitalization have been well delineated in Section II of this chapter. The clinical problems require a different perspective, directed to preservation of the alliance despite an involuntary (i.e., by definition, oppositional) position due to circumstances. Since involuntary commitment is sought not only during emergency circumstances but also as a response to the wish of the voluntary inpatient to leave, we will address both circumstances here.

Some jurisdictions appropriately indicate a preference for voluntary hospitalization over involuntary. On occasion this leads to a form of emergency room "blackmail" of the committable patient: "If you do not sign in voluntarily, I will commit you." The voluntarity of such a signature, of course, is highly suspect.

Both clinical and ethical good practice enjoin clear separation of the two issues. If the patient *is* committable, the clinician should express this unambiguously: "I plan to bring you into the hospital; if you wish to sign in, you may do so. However, your condition requires admission regardless of whether you sign in."

Wishes versus interest.   The patient's *wishes* determine most of the treatment except when the patient's *interests* (survival, preventing harm to others) take primary priority; the evaluator may make this quite explicit: "Though you feel everything is hopeless, Mr. Jones, I am obliged to act on your behalf to hospitalize you until we get your depression under control."

The conflicted wish for hospitalization.   Most clinicians are familiar with the paranoid position, in which a patient may wish for some response, but is prohibited from asking for it by the need to project (externalize the issue); in certain circumstances, then, the wish *not* to be hospitalized or the wish to leave the hospital may be a highly ambivalent one, so much so that the conflicted wish to *stay* is actually the stronger. The overt expression of a wish to avoid hospitalization or to leave the hospital may be intended *by the patient* as a test of the therapist's caring.

An interesting ethical dilemma here arises in relation to cases of questionable dangerousness. In most jurisdictions dangerousness alone constitutes the grounds for commitment; this criterion is the judge's concern, separate from issues of the patient's need for, or likelihood of benefiting from, treatment. If the physician were the final arbiter of the commitment decision, it would be inappropriate to petition on grounds other than clearcut dangerousness; however, the judge is the final arbiter, through a due process to protect adequately the patient's rights.

Because of this automatic judicial review process, the physician need not feel totally constrained to use a rigid and clinically narrow dangerousness standard, especially when the dangerousness is unclear, unpredictable, or labile; since due process protects the patient, the physician may freely petition in doubtful cases and leave the outcome to the legal process, even though actual commitment may be uncertain.

This petition has clinical advantages. As experienced by the patient, the act of petitioning may convey that the clinician takes the patient's problem or illness seriously and wants to take care of him. Thus, even if the judge releases the patient, a strong statement of seriousness of intent (another form of "commitment") has been made by the clinician that may form the nucleus of the outpatient treatment alliance.

To put it another way, the clinician need not feel required to anticipate or to second-guess the judge's ruling, especially since judges (or even the same judge at different times) are notoriously unpredictable in this regard.

Judicial unpredictability and the alliance.   In a paradoxical way, the very unpredictability of judges may serve to support the therapeutic alliance. Patient and therapist can see the situation as one in which they are in opposition around the question of hospitalization, and are placing their disagreement in the hands of an authorized "referee." Both parties are in ignorance of what the judicial ruling will be and are thus united in uncertainty, which may serve as the nucleus of a bond: patient and therapist jointly discuss the question of what will happen and the possible consequences, in a state of equal perplexity. This alliance posture of joint discussion may pave the way for future collaborative efforts after the issue of commitment is resolved. (See Chap. 3, Sec. III-F-3.)

4. CONTRAINDICATIONS TO HOSPITALIZATION

A number of clinical situations pose relative contraindications to hospitalization. The clinician is reminded that, given the layperson's view of hospitalization as a panacea, the decision *not* to admit a patient who wants to be admitted or who seems to need hospitalization requires fully as much documentation as the decision to admit. It may perhaps require even more, since not admitting a patient who is threatening suicide, even if the threat is considered specious, involves a calculated clinical and forensic risk. The clinician is well advised to "think out loud" for the record, carefully noting the evidence on which the decision is based. (See Suggested Readings for Chap. 1—Gutheil; and see Chap. 4, Sec. III-A-3-c.)

Typical situations include:

1. The patient without psychotic or suicidal symptomatology feels anxious and overwhelmed by reality factors (e.g., final exams coming up) and wants to get away from them. Here, the patient is discouraged from using the hospital in this way and encouraged to make reality decisions instead.
2. The patient has no place to go. This factor should very rarely be the *sole* reason for admission; the patient is better directed to a shelter, "crash pad," Salvation Army station, or the like. Exceptions may, of course, be made.

   > *Example 13:* A geriatric patient who is found to be unsuitable for psychiatric admission is sent from a nursing home that then refuses to take him back after the assessment. Admission may be the only humane alternative to the patient's being sent back and forth numerous times between the two institutions; placement can then be attempted anew.

3. The chronically suicidal patient. As earlier noted (see Sec. III-B-3), such patients must sometimes be actively denied admission to forestall serious regression and fostering of disabling hospital-centered chronicity.

These considerations clearly do not apply to those hospitals that uncritically offer admission to anyone having adequate insurance, even for "a rest"; this approach, though sometimes defensible, is often inappropriate from both a clinical and forensic perspective and raises serious questions of resource allocation.

5. "INVOLUNTARY NON-ADMISSION": SENDING THE PATIENT OUT

For completeness in this section we may consider involuntary or "administrative" non-admission. This term defines the situation when a patient is refused admission against her will for reasons not purely clinical; these include (1) lack of insurance, (2) treatment refusal, (3) infraction of rules (e.g., assaultiveness, theft, sexual acting out).

Each of these situations, though not defined in strictly clinical terms, nevertheless requires the hospital to maintain a clinical perspective. If a patient's coverage has lapsed and that patient clinically needs the hospital, the hospital is obliged to arrange transfer to a free facility. The patient refusing treatment for whom it *is* safe to leave may be sent out, but alternative care (e.g., outpatient appointments, referral) must be offered. Even the noncommittable patient abruptly sent out for rule infractions must be offered at least a list of possible places to stay (e.g., shelters) if no residence exists already (of course, the patient too ill to be discharged safely may not ethically be discharged; other approaches must be invoked.) This issue is further explored for inpatients in Chap. 3, Sec. III-G.

IV. PITFALLS

A. Denial and underreaction

The anxiety of dealing with life and death emergency situations may mobilize in the evaluator a number of defensive operations including denial of acuteness, seriousness, urgency, and dangerousness. In the first case example at the beginning of the chapter the evaluator might well have been influenced by the patient's apparent acquiescence to the plan of hospitalization so as to permit the patient to "visit home briefly" despite the danger of this move. Evaluators must be cognizant of both their own defenses and statistical and epidemiologic trends in emergency populations. Often, underreaction takes the form of a focus on detail at the cost of the total picture.

> ***Example 14:*** A psychotic woman, before witnesses, energetically stabbed herself with a knife. The evaluating resident fixed on the fact that the knife was somewhat dull and did not inflict too deep a wound. This minimizing perspective missed the severity of the psychotic disturbance and the resultant dangerousness of the total clinical state.

B. Contagion and overreaction

At the opposite extreme, the evaluator who attempts an appropriately empathic assessment may be swept out of a position of perspective and into the contagious urgency of the patient or others. A panic-stricken family, frenziedly demanding the admission of one of their number, may interfere with dispassionate assessment of the actual need for hospitalization on patient-centered clinical grounds; in addition, the alternative—refusing to admit the patient—may be rendered difficult by the family's belligerent, threatening, or litigious demeanor.

The patient's own anxiety and urgency may impair the calm thoughtfulness of the emergency evaluation and create the pressure within the evaluator (like that within the patient) to "do something immediately"—a pressure that may promote precipitous, ill-thought-out action before the clinical situation is sufficiently clear.

In a related manner, the empathic assessment of severe depression may breed specious hopelessness and helplessness in the evaluator that belie the actual likelihood of a favorable response to treatment of this illness.

C. Failure to act or to confront

This pitfall stands in relation to denial as action is to perception; that is, even if the danger is acknowledged, decisive action may be blocked by counter-transference-based conflicts around aggression, sadism, and authoritarianism.

Involuntary commitment, for example, represents the very opposite of the desirable alliance posture of amicable collaboration; instead, the evaluator directly opposes the patient's intention, risking the latter's anger, enmity, or accusation. These fears work against the clinician's natural wish to be liked by patients or, at least, to be seen as a helper or a benevolent ally. From this viewpoint the position of opponent or enemy represents a narcissistic injury for the clinician.

Similarly, though acting within well-defined legal sanctions, the evaluator who participates in involuntarily hospitalizing the patient may feel himself to be in the position of "pushing the patient around," "controlling" or "punishing" him as well as behaving like a jailor or a tyrant. Sadistic and aggressive feelings evoked by these fantasied roles may generate conflicts in the evaluator.

Such conflicts impair the evaluator's ability to overrule and override the patient's stated wishes, threats, or demands when the clinical situation calls for such a decisive response.

Confrontation of the patient, moreover, is often rendered difficult by the patient's own unflinching denial; manic euphoria, elation, and grandiosity; or relentless paranoid projection of responsibility or blame. The unassailable conviction and energy with which such patients can maintain delusional views may well make an evaluator quail at the thought of opposing the patient's forcefully stated wish or intent.

V. CASE EXAMPLE EPILOGUES

A. Case Example 1

The resident is momentarily nonplussed, but manages to get the patient to wait. Summoning additional personnel, the doctor explains forcefully that he is taking over responsibility for the patient since his depression is clearly impairing his judgment, at least temporarily. The patient threatens a lawsuit, but grudgingly complies.

Three days after admission, he confesses that he had bought a gun on the day of presenting to the emergency room, and—had he been allowed to go home "to pack some things"—would have used it on his wife and then on himself. Six months later, when his vocational and alcohol rehabilitation are well on their way, he expresses gratitude for having his momentary wish overridden.

B. Case Example 2

It seems likely that this nonpsychotic but impulsive patient, with a borderline personality organization, would not benefit a great deal from hospitalization. His previous history suggests that his despondency over the rejection by his stepbrother would soon be externalized and transformed into anger against the hospital staff, a process facilitated by the regressive hospital environment. The only indication for hospitalization is the threat of further self-injury in the immediate future, which might justify a brief inpatient stay.

After an initial assessment, the resident elects to let the patient sit in a supervised area for several hours to think about his situation, while the resident explores alternatives to hospitalization. In repeated interviews during this period, the resident insistently tries to shift responsibility for the patient's care back to the patient himself. As his demands to be cared for are met with offers to help him plan his own care, the predicted externalization takes place. Becoming angry at the resident, the patient reveals that in three days he has a court hearing scheduled on a rape charge and that he had hoped that hospitalization would help him avoid the hearing. He is furious that the hospital has not cooperated in this plan. Nonetheless, he is no longer despondent and now convincingly denies self-destructive intent. Consequently, he is permitted to leave the facility with the strong recommendation that he return when the outpatient clinic opens in the morning to begin a long-term course of outpatient treatment.

C. Case Example 3

The evaluator feels moved to help the obviously distressed mother, but recalls that signing a commitment petition on an unexamined patient is both clinically and legally unsound. The evaluator empathizes with the mother's concern about her daughter, but stresses that unless the latter is willing to come to the hospital or to a private psychiatrist's office for an evaluation, there is, regrettably, little that can be done. This is followed by an explanation of the laws governing involuntary commitment and of the criteria that must be met. It is carefully explained that the determination of dangerousness to oneself or to others that was required for hospitalization can, despite the genuine nature of the mother's story, be made only after an examination of the patient herself. The distraught mother is advised as to the means that could legitimately be used to persuade the daughter to come for evaluation, as well as the possibility of the family's involving the police or the courts if the patient's behavior seems acutely dangerous. Finally, an attempt is made to stress the systemic nature of the difficulty, particularly with hypomanic patients, whose judgment, though poor and often resulting in acts deleterious to themselves, is not always clearly *dangerous* to themselves. The mother is enlisted to work within the confines of the system to help the daughter to receive an evaluation. Later that day, having been persuaded by her boyfriend and mother, the patient appears at the center for assessment. She is found to be imminently dangerous to herself and is committed on an emergency basis.

VI. ACTION GUIDE

A. General Principles

1. *Document* data, source, reliability, reasoning, and rationale in developing plan, interventions.
2. *Decide* recommendations explicitly and record them, together with availability of resources.
3. *Obtain* consultations freely as needed to determine course of action.
4. *Determine* whether specific intervention is necessary.

B. Dangerousness to Others

1. *Overcome* denial about violence potential of individuals being interviewed.
2. *Look for* past violence, including encounters with police, vehicular homicide, military combat experience and the like.
3. *Note* age, gender, race, socioeconomic status and stability of employment situation.
4. *Consider* substance abuse, especially disinhibiting materials such as cocaine, PCP, and alcohol.
5. *Weigh* patient's tendency to externalize, presence of paranoid conditions and impulse disorders.
6. *Determine* history of dangerous intentions or thoughts, fixed persecutory delusions, grudge lists.
7. *Determine* membership in violence-oriented ethnic or psycho-cultural groups.
8. *Obtain* history of victimization, narcissistic injury.
9. *Inquire* concerning ownership of weapons, especially collections, and related factors.

C. Dangerousness to Self

1. Suicidality
    a. *Evaluate*
        i. the personal context: stages of life, psychological isolation, religious faith;
        ii. previous history and background: family history of affective disorder, suicide or alcoholism; suicide attempts (remember variability);
        iii. current stressors: acute bereavement/separation, recent geographic move, job loss, alcoholism, physical or terminal illness;
        iv. personality disorder factors: cyclothymic personality and sociopathy;
        v. psychiatric illness: depression, especially recurring depression or bipolar disorder, panic disorder, schizophrenia;
        vi. symptomatology: depressive symptoms, communicated suicidal intent, states of agitation and dysphoria, hopelessness and ideas of reunion with loved one;
        vii. context of suicidal act: high-risk/low-rescue attempts, preparatory actions, recent violent methods.
    b. *Consider* "received wisdom" issues:
        i. "respiratory" suicide, pitfalls of empathy,
        ii. command hallucinations,
        iii. history of suicide attempts, successful suicides, or psychosis in patient or family,
        iv. anniversary phenomena,
        v. mixed role of religion,
        vi. depressive countertransference response in observer.
2. Inability to care for self
    a. *Check for* degree of illness versus degree of functioning by history, availability of resources (residence, family, others).

      b. *Assess* present functioning, remediable problems.

      c. *Attempt* return to self-care state or *provide* caretaking environment.

D. Therapeutic Interventions

1. Crisis intervention
   a. Verbal: *allow* abreaction, ventilation; *define* problem; *validate* difficulty; *attempt* to reestablish perspective.
   b. Chemical: *treat* acute states with appropriate psychopharmacologic agents; *begin* long-term antidepressants if safe and indicated.
2. Consultation to existing relationships
   a. *Assess* point or issue of breakdown of preexisting relationship.
   b. *Attempt* to restore relationship, recruit assistance of objects, facilities, family, community resources.
   c. *Return* the patient if possible to previous supportive relationship.
3. Environmental manipulation
   a. *Remove* patient from noxious environment (to friends, family, emergency shelter).
   b. *Place* patient in protected environment: "asylum" concept. (This may be a hospital.)
4. Hospitalization: Indications

Patient:
   a. requires immediate intensive psychiatric observation and monitoring;
   b. requires specific psychiatric treatments best delivered in an inpatient setting (e.g., pharmacologic equilibration, introduction to new therapist);
   c. requires protection of containment in hospital because of dangerousness due to mental illness;
   d. requires asylum from deteriorating, chaotic, overburdened, or overwhelmed extrahospital support structures;
   e. requires intensive support during stressful interval (e.g., parents' vacation, loss of therapist).
5. Hospitalization: Contraindications

Patient:
   a. presents serious danger of nonconstructive regression;
   b. presents history of persistent failure to use appropriately or to benefit from hospitalization;
   c. desires to use hospital for nontherapeutic purposes (escape law, avoid final exams, as a place to sleep).

VII. SUGGESTED READINGS

A. INVOLUNTARY COMMITMENT

1. Appelbaum, P.S.: Civil commitment, in R. Michels, et al. (eds.), *Psychiatry.* Philadelphia, JB Lippincott, 1985.

2. Stromberg, C. D. & Stone, A. A.: A model state law on civil commitment of the mentally ill. *Harvard Journal on Legislation* 20:275–396, 1983.

3. Appelbaum, P. S.: Standards for civil commitment: a critical review of empirical research. *Int. J. Law. Psychiatry* 7:133–144, 1984.

4. Hiday, V. A.: Civil commitment: a review of empirical research. *Behav. Sci. Law* 6:15–43, 1988.

5. Treffert, D. A.: The obviously ill patient in need of treatment: a fourth standard for civil commitment. *Hosp. Community Psychiatry* 36:259–264, 1985.

6. Chodoff, P.: Involuntary hospitalization of the mentally ill as a moral issue. *Am. J. Psychiatry* 141:384–389, 1984.

7. Hoge, S. K., Sachs, G., Appelbaum, P. S., et al.: Limitations on psychiatrists' discretionary authority by the Stone and dangerousness criteria. *Arch. Gen. Psychiatry* 45:764–769, 1988.

8. Appelbaum, P. S.: Is the need for treatment constitutionally acceptable as a basis for civil commitment? *Law, Med. and Health Care* 12:144–149, 1984.

9. Cleveland, S., Mulvey, E. P., Appelbaum, P. S., et al.: Do dangerousness-oriented commitment laws restrict hospitalization of patients who need treatment? A test. *Hosp. Community Psychiatry* 40:266–271, 1989.

10. Miller, R. D., Maier, G. J. & Kaye, M.: Miranda comes to the hospital: the right to remain silent in civil commitment. *Am. J. Psychiatry* 142:1074–1077, 1985.

11. National Center for State Courts: Guidelines for involuntary civil commitment. *Ment. Phy. Dis. Law Rep.* 10:409–514, 1986.

12. American Psychiatric Association: *Involuntary Commitment to Outpatient Treatment.* Washington, DC, APA, 1987.

13. Mulvey, E. P., Geller, J. L. & Roth, L. H.: The promise and peril of involuntary outpatient commitment. *Am. Psychol.* 42:571–584, 1987.

14. Bursztajn, H., Gutheil, T. G., Mills, M. J., et al. Process analysis of judges' commitment decisions: a preliminary empirical study. *Am. J. Psychiatry* 143:170–174, 1986.

B. ASSESSMENT OF VIOLENCE

1. Monahan, J.: *The Clinical Prediction of Violent Behavior.* Rockville, MD, National Institute of Mental Health, 1981.

2. Mulvey, E. P. & Lidz, C. W.: Clinical considerations in the prediction of dangerousness in mental patients. *Clin. Psychol. Rev.* 4:379–401, 1984.

3. Webster, C. D. & Menzies, R. J.: The clinical prediction of dangerousness, in D. N. Weisstub (ed.): *Law and Mental Health: International Perspectives, Vol. 3.* New York, Pergamon Press, 1987.

4. Monahan, J.: The prediction of violent behavior: toward a second generation of theory and policy. *Am. J. Psychiatry* 141:10–15, 1984.

5. Wolfgang, M. E. & Weiner, N. A. (eds.): *Criminal Violence.* Beverly Hills, CA, Sage Publications, 1982.

6. Guze, S. B.: *Criminality and Psychiatric Disorders.* New York, Oxford University Press, 1976.

7. Monahan, J. & Steadman, H. J.: Crime and mental disorder: an epidemiological approach, in Tonry, M. & Morris, N. (eds.): *Crime and Justice: An Annual Review of Research, Vol. 4.* Chicago, University of Chicago Press, 1983.

8. Taylor, P. J.: Motives for offending among violent and psychotic men. *Br. J Psychiatry* 147:491–498, 1985.

9. McNiel, D. E. & Binder, R. L.: Predictive validity of judgments of dangerousness in emergency civil commitment. *Am. J. Psychiatry* 144:197–200, 1987.

10. Klassen, D. & O'Connor, W. A.: A prospective study of predictors of violence in adult male mental health admissions. *Law and Human Behavior* 12:143–158, 1988.

C. ASSESSMENT OF SUICIDALITY AND INABILITY TO CARE FOR SELF

1. Roy, A. (ed.): *Suicide.* Baltimore, MD, Williams and Wilkins, 1986.

2. Rosen, A.: Detection of suicidal patients: an example of some limitations in the prediction of infrequent events. *J. Consult. Psychol.* 18:397–403, 1954.

3. Goldney, R. D. & Spence, N. D.: Is suicide predictable? *Aust. N. Z. J. Psychiatry* 21:3–4, 1987.

4. Murphy, G. E.: On suicide prediction and prevention. *Arch. Gen. Psychiatry* 40:343–344, 1983.

5. Hendin, H.: Suicide: a review of new directions in research. *Hosp. Community Psychiatry* 37:148–154, 1986.

6. Hillard, J. R., Ramm, D., Zung, W. W. K., et al.: Suicide in a psychiatric emergency room population. *Am. J. Psychiatry* 140:459–462, 1983.

7. Pokorny, A. D.: Prediction of suicide in psychiatric patients: report of a prospective study. *Arch. Gen. Psychiatry* 40:249–257, 1983.

8. Pallis, D. J., Gibbons, J. S. & Pierce, D. W.: Estimating suicide risk among attempted suicides. *Brit. J. Psychiatry* 144:139–148, 1984.

9. Roy, A.: Family history of suicide. *Arch. Gen. Psychiatry* 40:971–974, 1983.

10. Dingman, C. W., & McGlashan, T. H.: Characteristics of patients with serious suicidal intentions who ultimately commit suicide. *Hosp. Community Psychiatry* 39:295–299, 1988.

11. Brent, D. A., Perper, J. A., Goldstein, C. E., et al.: Risk factors for adolescent suicide. *Arch. Gen. Psychiatry* 45:581–588, 1988.

12. Havens, L. L.: Recognition of suicidal risks through the psychological examination. *N. Engl. J. Med.* 276:210–215, 1967.

13. Weisman, A. D. & Worden, J. W.: Risk rescue rating in suicide assessment. *Arch. Gen. Psychiatry* 26:553-560, 1972.

14. Sifneos, P. E.: Manipulative suicide. *Psychiatr. Q.* 40:525–537, 1966.

15. Grisso, T.: *Evaluating Competencies*. New York, Plenum Press, 1986.

D. Managing Violence and Suicidality in Emergency Settings

1. Lion, J. R., Bach-Y-Rita, G. & Ervin, F. R.: Violent patients in the emergency room. *Am. J. Psychiatry* 125:1706–1711, 1969.

2. Skodol, A. W. & Karasu, T. B.: Emergency psychiatry and the assaultive patient. *Am. J. Psychiatry* 135:202–205, 1978.

3. Tupin, J. P.: The violent patient: a strategy for management and diagnosis. *Hosp. Community Psychiatry* 34:37–40, 1983.

4. Eichelman, B.: Toward a rational pharmacotherapy for aggressive and violent behavior. *Hosp. Community Psychiatry* 39:31–39, 1988.

5. Mattes, J. A.: Psychopharmacology of temper outbursts: a review. *J. Nerv. Ment. Dis.* 174:464–470, 1986.

6. Infantino, J. A. & Musingo, S. Y.: Assaults and injuries among staff with and without training in aggression control techniques. *Hosp. Community Psychiatry* 36:1312–1314, 1985.

7. Privitera, M. R., Springer, M. O. & Perlmutter, R. A.: To search or not to search: is there a clinical profile of a patient harboring a weapon? *Gen. Hosp. Psychiatry* 8:442–447, 1986.

8. Himmelhoch, J. M.: Lest treatment abet suicide. *J. Clin. Psychiatry* 48(12-suppl.):44–54, 1987.

9. Guggenheim, F. G.: Management of suicide risk in the psychiatric emergency room, in Guggenheim F. G. & Weiner M. F. (eds.): *Manual of Psychiatric Consultation and Emergency Care*. New York, Jason Aaronson, 1984.

3

Legal Issues in In-Patient Psychiatry

     5. Liability resulting from failure to comply with rules on patients' right to refuse treatment
        a. Battery
        b. Malpractice
        c. Civil rights violations
     6. Effects of patients' right to refuse treatment
     7. The future of the right to refuse treatment

D. Rights related to discharge from the hospital
     1. Voluntary patients
     2. Involuntary patients
     3. Conditional release
     4. Involuntary discharge
        a. For clinical indications
        b. On expiration of insurance coverage
        c. On expiration of court-ordered commitments
        d. After a dangerous or disruptive act
        e. After an infraction of the rules
        f. Following refusal of treatment

III. CLINICAL ISSUES

A. Implementing the right to treatment
     1. Aspects of hospital treatment
        a. Short-term intervention
        b. Long-term intervention
        c. Rehabilitation
        d. Custodial care
     2. Individual treatment plans
     3. Periodic review
     4. Use of multidisciplinary team
     5. Attention to environmental issues

B. Clinical aspects of patients' rights
     1. Rights versus economic realities
     2. Patients' rights in relation to clinical administration
        a. "Deprivation of freedom" versus the prescription of space
        b. Seclusion
        c. Least restrictive alternative
     3. Alternative models
        a. The "crime and punishment" model
        b. The behaviorist model
     4. Rights "versus" needs

C. Clinical aspects of treatment refusal
     1. Treatment refusal based on factors in the illness
        a. Denial
        b. Manic euphoria
        c. Projection
        d. Delusional guilt
        e. Other delusions and distortions
     2. Treatment refusal based on factors in the treatment
        a. Primary gain
        b. Secondary gain
        c. Specific factors in psychotherapy
        d. Specific factors in ECT
        e. Specific factors in medication

        i. Portal of entry
       ii. Dysphoric response
       iii. Side effects
       iv. Tardive dyskinesia (TD)
   3. TREATMENT REFUSAL BASED ON FACTORS IN THE DOCTOR-PATIENT RELATIONSHIP
     a. Transference
     b. Reality
     c. Intimacy
     d. Vacations
     e. Family pressures
     f. Autonomy
     g. Other elements
D. Clinical approaches to managing treatment refusal
   1. EXPLORATION OF ISSUES
   2. MAINTAINING THE ALLIANCE POSTURE
   3. AMELIORATION OF CAUSATIVE INFLUENCES
   4. ALTERNATIVES IN THE FACE OF PERSISTENT REFUSAL OF TREATMENT
     a. Discharge
     b. Commitment
     c. Role of ward staff in treating treatment refusal
     d. Use of formal mechanisms to adjudicate treatment refusal
E. Clinical approaches to involuntary treatment
   1. MAINTAINING ALLIANCE PRIMACY
   2. DOCUMENTATION
   3. RETURN TO VOLUNTARY TREATMENT
F. Clinical aspects of the request to leave the hospital
   1. EXPLORATION OF UNDERLYING ISSUES
     a. Anger or frustration at doctor, staff, or institution
     b. Fears, both real and paranoid, of other patients or staff
     c. Other dynamic issues
   2. THE ALLIANCE ISSUE
   3. THE DECISION TO COMMIT: CLINICAL IMPACT
     a. Clinical effects of decision to seek commitment
       i. Positive
       ii. Negative
     b. Clinical effects of decision not to seek commitment (to release patient)
       i. Positive
       ii. Negative
G. Clinical aspects of involuntary discharge
   1. CLINICALLY DETERMINED INVOLUNTARY DISCHARGE
   2. LAPSE OF INSURANCE AND ITS CLINICAL CONSEQUENCES
   3. EXPIRATION OF COURT-ORDERED COMMITMENTS
   4. INVOLUNTARY DISCHARGE FOR DANGEROUSNESS OR DISRUPTIVENESS
   5. INVOLUNTARY DISCHARGE FOR INFRACTION OF RULES
   6. INVOLUNTARY DISCHARGE FOR TREATMENT REFUSAL
IV. PITFALLS
  A. Countertransference factors in the right to treatment
  B. Countertransference factors in patients' rights
  C. Countertransference factors in treatment refusal
  D. Countertransference factors in involuntary treatment, hospitalization, and discharge
V. CASE EXAMPLE EPILOGUES

I. CASE EXAMPLES

A. Case Example 1

This 23-year-old man is tolerated by his family despite a slow slide into a withdrawn, catatonic state, until one day, after an argument, he assaults his father. The family then brings him to the hospital, insisting on his admission. At that time, he is found to be unwilling to undergo a mental status examination, saying to the examiner only, "Do whatever you want to me." He sits rigidly, appears to be hallucinating, and does not respond when asked if he is willing to sign himself into the hospital. He is admitted on an emergency 10-day commitment on grounds of dangerousness to others.

Once in the hospital, the patient begins to take antipsychotic medication, becomes a little less withdrawn, and is more open in expressing his fears that certain people are out to harm him. Now willing to talk with the ward staff and male resident in charge of his care, he steadfastly maintains that he is not ill and not in need of hospitalization. Nonetheless, he generally adapts well to the ward milieu. When his emergency commitment expires, he is committed by a court for a 6-month period, the judge agreeing that he represents an imminent danger to his family.

About 4 months into his stay, after a series of increasingly silent therapy sessions, the patient one day fails to appear for his appointment, and the resident goes to seek him out in his room. Attempting to engage the patient in conversation, the resident is surprised to find himself bodily picked up and carried to the door by the patient, who closes the door behind him and refuses to come out. From that point on, the patient also refuses to take his medication.

For nearly three weeks, the resident attempts to talk directly with the patient, but is continually rebuffed. Other staff members, with whom the patient will talk, report that he says that he hates his doctor, "for what he did to me, robbing me of my freedom." Recognizing that his patient is obtaining little benefit from a hospitalization now characterized by neither medication nor psychotherapy, the resident seeks out the supervising psychiatrist on the ward to discuss the situation.

B. Case Example 2

No one on the ward had expected that Mr. B. would be the average patient, yet no one was quite prepared for what is now occurring, and as the legal-psychiatric consultant hears the case presented to her, she frowns in thought.

Mr. B. is in his mid-twenties and bears the triple burden of recurring psychotic episodes, mental retardation, and a seizure disorder; surprisingly, however, none of these bears on his admission to the hospital. Instead, it is his tendency to set fires when distressed that has provoked a string of court-ordered evaluations, the last of which has now evolved into a civil commitment for dangerousness.

On the ward, however, fire setting has not been a problem; the patient has tolerated well being restricted from matches and has made no attempts to obtain them. The problem behaviors are, first, the patient's pattern of finding and swallowing an appalling number and variety of small metal objects, such as screws, tacks, and soda-can fliptops; and second, a tendency, when frustrated, to bang his head violently and repeatedly against the wall.

Even *these* behaviors are far from novel to the seasoned staff; what makes the situation intolerable (and provokes the consultation) is the fact that the patient is always smiling delightedly while engaged in these activities, treats them apparently as teasing games to be played with the staff, and appears to relish, with great enthusiasm, the dismay, consternation, and fury evoked in the ward personnel.

The chief resident relates how the treatment team initially responded to the first screw swallowing and head banging with aggressive medical, neurologic, and radiologic attention, but with each successive episode the enthusiasm for these procedures has waned. The medical liaison service has taken to sending back contemptuous notes after working up the patient yet again, suggesting that the psychiatric staff's failure to "keep this patient from harming himself" is probably grounds, as they see it, for malpractice proceedings.

The chief sums up the problem: "We could restrain the patient, but that could go on forever; there's no end point. Medication doesn't work; talking doesn't work; seclusion doesn't work; we can't just do *nothing!* What do we do?"

C. Case Example 3

The new psychology intern looks grimly around the closet-sized office to which he has been assigned for his supervised in-patient year of practical experience at the state hospital. After a strenuous but obligatory cleaning frenzy he is just beginning the laborious process of moving his books, papers, and equipment into place when the phone rings. Feeling a mixture of excitement and nervousness, he answers.

There is a short, heavy-breathing pause. Then a hoarse voice inquires, "Are you *my* therapist?"

The intern begins to explain that he has been assigned a few patients but has not yet had a chance to meet them; he is interrupted somewhat brusquely. "Look, I've been assigned to you. And what I wanna know is, what are my rights in this hospital? I wanna know what they are."

The psychology intern has no idea but recalls a handout from the orientation course just presented to all the interns. Groping for his briefcase, he fumbles out the patients' rights booklet distributed at orientation and begins to read aloud the state statute summarized therein. When he reaches the listing about the right to use the telephone, the caller stops him.

"That's what I thought. Listen, you know, I'm calling you on the hospital phone and they're standing right here. They aren't letting me use the public payphone up here in the locked unit, and I wanna call my girlfriend and my lawyer, and I wanna complain about this dump to somebody in authority down-town, and they won't let me. They won't even let me sign out!"

The psychology intern is nonplussed.

"Uh, okay, well, I'll tell you what, I'll come up to meet you, and we can try to figure this out. You're on the locked unit, you say?"

The patient grunts assent.

"Fine! Uh, I mean, I'll be right there."

Arriving somewhat winded on the fourth floor where the locked unit is, he urgently thumbs the buzzer for admission. For long moments he fidgets as noth-ing happens. Finally, the door is jerked open. A tall, burly man in jeans and a Grateful Dead T-shirt shushes him; he is disturbing the ward meeting. Abashed by the large surrounding audience, the intern asks to see the patient who called him. Rolling his eyes, the man points him to a hallway, from which someone is signal-ling to him. The intern goes to meet his first patient.

The psychology intern introduces himself to the patient, who is a short, slender man in his forties, whose features are marred by two scars extending into his cheeks outward from the corners of his mouth. Trying not to stare at this deformity, the intern obtains a repetition of the complaint with more details, couched in an unmistakable tone of blame for him, the intern. He is impressed by the fact that a violation of rights does, indeed, appear to be taking place. He promises the patient that he will investigate and try to right this wrong. A hurried check with a nurse in the hallway who is hastening to another task confirms the patient's complaint. Becoming annoyed at feeling thrust into the role of persecu-tor of a patient he has barely started with, he goes in search of the supervising clinician on the ward.

II. LEGAL ISSUES

A. The right to treatment

One of the most misunderstood of the legal doctrines that have affected psychiatric practice is the idea that psychiatric patients have "a right" to receive treatment. Although the concept has been used in various ways by the activist mental health bar, by the mental health professions, and by patients themselves, as it has been defined by the courts the "right to treatment" is a narrow and somewhat shaky formulation that has been limited in its impact on the mentally ill.

1. EARLY HISTORY OF THE DOCTRINE

The idea that treatment is due the psychiatrically ill patient as a right first arose as a theoretical construct in the early 1960s. Even in its initial appearance, the nascent right was limited to the involuntarily committed patient; the theory was that the involuntary patient was entitled, as a matter of fairness, given the deprivation of liberty that hospitalization entailed, to receive active treatment and not merely confinement and the barely adequate essential services that many large state facilities provided. The earliest court decision on the issue, *Rouse v. Cameron* in 1966, dealt with a patient who was committed after being found not guilty by reason of insanity, but was receiving no treatment. While the case was decided on statutory grounds, there were hints in the decision of a constitutional right to treatment.

Not until 1971, in the famed *Wyatt v. Stickney* class-action suit that challenged conditions in the Alabama state hospitals, was the right to treatment enunciated by a court on constitutional grounds. Failure actively to treat involuntary patients was deemed a deprivation of Fourteenth Amendment rights to due process and equal protection since treatment was due the patient as a *quid pro quo* for involuntary detention. It is important to note that this case was decided at the federal district court level and affirmed at the level of the court of appeals, but was never considered by the United States Supreme Court.

A case that did reach the nation's highest court was *O'Connor v. Donaldson.* This problematic 1975 decision considered a Florida case with a unique fact situation: a paranoid schizophrenic Christian Scientist was involuntarily hospitalized for 14 years despite the absence of dangerousness to himself or others, without treatment that he would accept (he refused medication, a fact usually overlooked in discussions of the case), and in the face of offers to care for him from responsible outsiders. He was judged to have been deprived of his right to liberty guaranteed by the Fourteenth Amendment, but the contortions of the Court to fit the scope of the decision to specific facts of the case reveal on what uncertain ground the right to treatment rested. The Court held that a non-dangerous, involuntarily committed patient could not be hospitalized, in the presence of viable alternatives in the community, without receiving treatment.

Notwithstanding *Donaldson,* numerous lower courts followed the lead of the *Wyatt* decision, finding a right to treatment for involuntary patients. The *Wyatt* court, in an approach later followed in other jurisdictions, issued a detailed decree implementing its decision, defining minimally acceptable treatment in precise terms, down to the number of square feet of floor space required for each patient and the number of cooks who must be employed in the kitchen.

Yet, as popular as this approach became, it was evident that the courts were having difficulty enforcing these decrees. When legislatures refused to appropriate sufficient funds to pay for the improvements, the courts were confronted with a constitutional crisis. In the end, it turned out that they had little power to coerce recalcitrant legislatures. Although the early right-to-treatment decisions clearly led to improvements in many state facilities, the limitations of the approach are evident from the subsequent history of *Wyatt.* The court continued to supervise its decree for more than a decade and a half. At no point, however, did Alabama facilities come fully into compliance with the initial judgment.

2. A SECOND PHASE: THE CONSENT DECREE

In an effort to avoid the adversary posture and heel-dragging by the state that characterized the *Wyatt* litigation, parties to litigation began to turn to consent decrees to resolve right-to-treatment suits. The decrees embody agreements between the two parties, typically the state's Department of Mental Health and a mental health advocacy group, that, without finding fault, specify the conditions to be changed and have the force of law. A master to supervise the administration of the decree can be appointed by the court. Prominent elements of the decree are usually the familiar numerical ratios for staff and facilities, plans for accelerating deinstitutionalization, and the promise of individualized treatment plans. The plaintiffs avoid lengthy litigation and gain the presumed cooperation of the state in implementing agreed-to changes, while the state avoids the risk of more sweeping judicially-ordered changes, and often gets to maintain administrative control of the system. In principle, then, the consent decree is to everyone's advantage.

But the consent decree, too, proved not to be a panacea. The executive branch of the state government signed the decree, but its implementation was still dependent on legislative appropriations, and they were not always forthcoming. Despite the hope of a cooperative effort raised by these decrees, many of the more prominent cases are still short of full compliance years after the decrees were issued.

3. *YOUNGBERG* AND THE RIGHT TO TREATMENT TODAY

The U.S. Supreme Court finally offered its view of the right to treatment in 1982 in a case involving a patient in a Pennsylvania facility for the retarded, *Youngberg v. Romeo.* Basing the right on patients' constitutional liberty interests, the Court ruled that involuntary patients were entitled only to that treatment required to assure freedom from unnecessary restraint and preventable assault. No more. To the extent that these rights conflicted with each other (e.g., to prevent a provocative patient from being assaulted one might have to restrain his freedom of movement) or had to be compromised for legitimate therapeutic reasons, patients were only entitled to a decision by a qualified mental health professional that abrogation of their rights was required.

The narrow ruling in *Youngberg* was read by many advocates as the death-knell of the right to treatment. In fact, the right has shown surprising resilience. Three factors have fed continued efforts to expand patients' right to treatment.

a. Broad readings of *Youngberg*

Lower courts have not found *Youngberg* as restrictive as many supposed they might. After paying obeisance to the Supreme Court's analysis, some lower courts have fashioned orders that look remarkably like the original decree in *Wyatt.* Some courts have also been creative in interpreting the requirement for professional judgments; one federal court, for example, declared that a facility that was unaccredited was presumed not to be making decisions according to accepted professional criteria.

b. State law rights

When revising their mental health laws in the 1970s, many states inserted broad language vowing to provide appropriate treatment to all mentally ill people. This language has formed the basis for a number of law suits accusing states of failing to keep their promises. Success has been variable. Some courts have agreed that the states imposed enforceable obligations on themselves, even with regard to voluntary patients and outpatients. Other courts have interpreted the statutory language as entirely hortatory and therefore non-enforceable.

State constitutions also provide a potential source of law supporting a right to treatment. Most states have provisions echoing the federal constitutional rights to liberty and due process, but state courts are not bound by U.S. Supreme Court interpretations of the federal constitution in deciding how far state provisions extend. These provisions have been employed in other patients' rights contexts (see discussion of the right to refuse treatment, Sec. II-C below), and they may yet prove to be important bulwarks of patients' right to treatment.

c. CRIPA

In 1980, Congress passed the Civil Rights of Institutionalized Persons Act (CRIPA). This enabled the Justice Department to investigate conditions in state institutions and bring suit against states found to be violating patients' or inmates' federal rights. Although few cases have reached the courts, a large number of investigations have been conducted, often ending with agreements by the states to improve institutional conditions. In theory, *Youngberg* defines—and limits—patients' rights under CRIPA, but the consent agreements that have resulted sweep fully as broadly as the *Wyatt* decree, including increases in staffing levels, controls on medication use, physical plant improvements, and more complete record keeping.

It may be, therefore, that *Youngberg* was read too narrowly by advocates who feared its impact on the right to treatment. The same kinds of conditions required to protect patients' liberty interests, and especially to insure that professional judgments are made when those interests must be compromised, may turn out not to be very different from the conditions envisioned as constitutionally required by the courts prior to *Youngberg*.

4. WHAT THE RIGHT TO TREATMENT IS NOT

Judicial activism on behalf of psychiatric patients has led many well-meaning individuals to misconstrue the impact of the catchphrase "right to treatment." The right is *not*:

a. A guarantee of treatment for all patients

Although state laws may provide otherwise, there has never been judicial extension of the constitutional right to treatment to voluntary patients or to outpatients. It applies only to involuntarily committed patients. For other classes of patients, states are free to decide whether they want to provide any services at all, and they can limit or expand them at their own discretion.

b. A guarantee of optimal treatment

Even those courts that have chosen to set highly specific criteria for institutions to meet have emphasized that they are concerned with achieving minimal, constitutionally required standards, rather than with requiring the best possible program.

c. A guarantee of effective treatment

The courts can require that professional staff be hired, but they cannot monitor this work so closely as to ensure that all patients receive the care that would be most efficacious in their situation. They can establish the preconditions for treatment but cannot guarantee that adequate treatment occurs. Similarly, courts are powerless in the face of conditions for which effective treatments do not yet exist (e.g., senile dementia). Other court actions establishing a "right to refuse treatment" may impact on the effectiveness of the right-to-treatment rulings (see section II-C below).

d. A guarantee of one's choice of treatments

Hospitals have not yet been required to provide a sufficient array of treatments that patients can decide which to select or refuse. Provision of a single accepted mode of treatment for each patient would seem to be adequate.

5. THE FUTURE OF THE RIGHT TO TREATMENT

For all the problems in implementing a right to treatment, there is no question that patients in many state facilities around the country are much better off today than they would have been without the court decisions and consent decrees based on that right. Even when imposed or agreed-upon standards have not been met in their entirety, substantial improvements usually have taken place. Those people who recognize that half-a-loaf indeed can be better than none can perceive the importance of litigation in this area. It has been, in addition, one of the few areas of mental health litigation in which clinicians and members of the mental health bar generally have been on the same side of the issue. The desire to improve hospital conditions unites almost everyone in the field.

Nonetheless, it is clear that certain costs are attached to this process. When right to treatment suits focus on only one part of a mental health system, they can force reallocation of limited funds in a fashion detrimental to those patients not among the class members covered by the suit. Judicial intervention into functions of the executive and legislative branches of government—including administration and funding of the mental health system—distorts the separation of powers that lies at the core of our system of government. And many constitutional scholars are profoundly concerned with unelected judges imposing on our elected representatives their views of how public monies should be spent.

The right to treatment, however, albeit in a stunted form, has achieved some security in legal doctrine. If elected legislatures fail to provide for the basic care and treatment needs of committed patients, unelected judges will continue to force some redistribution of funds to help this group. A recent decision of the U.S. Supreme Court (*Missouri v. Jenkins*) suggested that the courts' powers in this regard may be greater than previously assumed, perhaps extending to the actual imposition of taxes to raise funds needed to remedy constitutional deficiencies. Just how far the courts can go in this direction is, at this point, unclear. In sum, though by no means the panacea it was once thought to be, the right to treatment has been and will continue to be a useful weapon in improving the situation of the hospitalized mental patient.

B. Other rights of hospitalized patients

1. RIGHT TO THE LEAST RESTRICTIVE ALTERNATIVE (LRA)

The United States Court of Appeals for the District of Columbia, the source of many noteworthy decisions in mental health law under the stewardship of

Chief Judge David Bazelon, first applied the concept of the least restrictive alternative (sometimes called the least drastic alternative) to the psychiatric patient. In *Lake v. Cameron* in 1966, Judge Bazelon ruled that an individual could not be committed involuntarily to a psychiatric hospital if an alternative could be found that infringed to a lesser degree on her constitutional rights to liberty. The concept was picked up by other courts and appeared in such major cases as *Lessard v. Schmidt* (1972), an early case addressing mental patients' procedural rights in civil commitment. Since then the doctrine has become a commonplace in mental health litigation, and a feature of most "right to treatment" decisions, consent decrees, and most state statutes.

a. LRA in theory

"Least restrictive alternative" began, not as a rule designed specifically to answer the needs of psychiatric patients, but in a far-removed context. Its first use in an individual rights case, in *Shelton v. Tucker* (1960), was for the purpose of placing a limitation on the extent of the exercise of state powers, in this case striking down a law requiring Arkansas schoolteachers to reveal their membership in all outside organizations. From its birth, it was a doctrine that demanded that the state justify its activity on a linear scale: a lesser degree of state action to accomplish a given end was seen as always less restrictive than, and therefore to be preferred to, a greater degree of action: "Even though the governmental purpose be legitimate and substantial, that purpose cannot be pursued by means that broadly stifle fundamental personal liberties when the end can be more narrowly achieved" (*Shelton v. Tucker*). Further, and quite logically in the context, the action of the state was assumed to be the sole cause of the resulting restriction of liberty.

b. LRA in practice

The concept of LRA in mental health care has usually been applied in a rigid manner: a hierarchy of "alternatives" has been established using the model of more governmental action equaling more restrictions, independent of consideration of the individual patient's needs, and the patient has then been slotted into the "least restrictive" of those options. Hospitalization is considered ipso facto the most restrictive alternative and is therefore the least favored. Partial hospitalization will be given preference over it and outpatient treatment even more. In fact, if all services can be rendered in a "social service" setting (i.e., a vocational rehabilitation program) without any psychiatric input at all, that is sometimes considered better still. What has stopped this practice from making as much of an impact on mental health care in America as its advocates favor has been the absence in most states of realistic alternatives of any sort to the state hospital. Although the goal of many "right-to-treatment" class-action suits has been to compel the states to provide such alternatives, funding has been hard to generate and changes have come slowly.

c. The most therapeutic alternative

LRA doctrine has spawned a burgeoning literature of protest from the mental health professions. Objecting to the slighting of the varying needs of individual patients and to the therapeutic nihilism inherent in the selection of a setting that does the "least" to and for the patient, several commentators have suggested that mental health care be focused instead on the "most therapeutic alternative." This ideological shift would require rejection of the overly simplistic idea that a more intensive program is necessarily more restrictive. It would recognize instead that minimal treatment of a debilitating psychosis is likely to yield minimal liberty for the individual; effective, intensive treatment, though requiring a seemingly "more restrictive environment," will in the long run often leave the patient with a greater ability effectively to exercise his liberty. As much as some professionals would like to see such a substitution of doctrines, the choice rests in the hands of the courts. LRA is now well-established in civil rights law, and to argue for its inapplicability in the narrow area of mental health law will be a difficult task. Although the U.S. Supreme Court cast doubt on the constitutional underpinnings of LRA in mental health care in *Youngberg v. Romeo,* lower courts continue to embrace it, and as noted, it is now included in most state statutes. A more promising approach might be to infuse the doctrine with the notion that psychosis can be as restrictive as a locked ward and to permit a weighing of the degree of a patient's disability before deciding which environment is less restrictive for him or her.

2. RIGHTS IN THE HOSPITAL

a. A historical perspective

In order to understand why hospitalized psychiatric patients are often in the position of arguing for the right to do things that other members of society take for granted as their inalienable due, one needs to recall the theory that prompted the founding of the first major state psychiatric hospitals in the second quarter of the nineteenth century. Mental illness at that time was thought to be caused by the pressures and stresses of chaotic urban life, seen as an unstructured melange of sensation, that impacted with particular force on those with "hereditary defects of the mind." It was from this tumult and disorder that the first patients sought "asylum" in the new hospitals being built out in the peaceful countryside. The asylum, with its rigid routine and invariant schedule, was thought to exert its therapeutic effect by reestablishing a basic, health-promoting order within the individual. For this to be effective, the patient not only had to submit to the daily regimentation, but also to face isolation from the world he had left behind. At the beginning, therefore, the psychiatric patient in this country surrendered, usually involuntarily, the rights of association, speech, and privacy that his fellows in the community took for granted.

Long after the theory had withered and died, in fact well into the middle of this century, most patients remained bereft of their basic rights. Ideological fervor had given way to complacent torpor: in the understaffed and crowded caverns of the state systems of the late 1800s and first half of this century, it was easier to manage a regimented, tightly controlled mass of patients than to attempt to encourage individualistic exercise of basic rights and liberties.

b. The transitional period

This situation has been changing since the late 1960s when, in the light of the victories of the black civil rights movement, activist lawyers turned their attention to other "minority" groups, mental patients among them. By means of court decisions (mostly notably *Wyatt v. Stickney*), consent decrees, new state statutes, and departmental regulations, the legal status of psychiatric patients has been normalized. At the same time, some limitations on their rights remain, in part because of a different set of considerations: the nature of psychiatric illness and of its treatment, at least as we conceptualize it today, continues to require some restriction of patients' rights, both for their own protection and that of others. We may hope that at the end of this transitional period a new and fairer balance will have been struck, one that leans toward granting patients the free exercise of their rights, except in the presence of compelling reasons for withholding them.

c. Specific rights

Visitation.   Visits from relatives and friends, symbols of the environment left behind, outside the asylum walls, were anathema to the advocates of moral treatment who built the early asylums. These days, with the emphasis on maintaining the patient's ties with the community and on effecting rapid discharge and reintegration with life "outside," most facilities encourage visits. Therapists, in fact, often attempt to resolve family and personal issues that hinder such relationships.

There are occasions, however, when visits can be suspended "for cause": for a period shortly after admission while the patient is acclimating to the hospital, and the initial evaluation is being performed; during periods of extreme psychosis or agitation; when the previous visits of a given individual have been counterproductive (e.g., ending in a fist-fight) or have led to untoward consequences (e.g., a suicide attempt following a meeting with an estranged spouse). In addition, visitors who themselves disrupt the care of other patients on the ward, as by selling drugs, stealing valuables, or starting fights, legitimately can be restricted from visitation. Similarly, visiting hours can be limited to particular times of the day so as not to interfere with ward routine or activities.

State laws often specify that certain individuals have a right of free access without limitation. These may include lawyers, the clergy, and private or consulting physicians. Even here, though, the patient's clinical needs come first. If it is truly contraindicated for a visit to occur, as with a wildly excited manic patient, the clinician's obligation is to protect the patient from the stimulation that the visit would entail. While the patient's visitor always has the right to seek a court order mandating his admission, in most cases a careful discussion of the matter will lead to mutual agreement on what constitutes the patient's best interest.

More problematic issues are raised by other sorts of visitors. Does a hospital administration have the right to bar members of a "patients' liberation group" from organizing on an inpatient service? What if they are advocating that all patients refuse to cooperate with their care plans and refuse medications? Does a patient have a right to invite a reporter to visit her on the ward? Should an older man who "picks up" younger women after they are discharged be banned from visiting?

There are no easy answers. In general, and absent a statute to the contrary, the goal of regulation of visits should be to protect the patients' best interests, particularly their interest in regaining their health, but also their privacy. To the extent that this may sometimes interfere with First Amendment rights, that is regrettable, but the protection of those rights lies in the hands of the courts. The clinician should protect her patients first.

   Communication.   The right to free and open communication with the outside
world should be unaffected by hospitalization. Many hospitals, however, continue
to monitor and restrict their patients' communications, whether by letter or by
phone. They justify this practice by citing the need to protect the outside world
from potentially harmful contact with the "insane," whether of a threatening,
offensive, or prurient nature. Clearly there are instances in which communications
of this sort occur, as well as others in which the patient places himself at risk by ill-
considered, provocative, or foolish messages. Yet a blanket prohibition of all communication, or even uniform censorship, seems too broad a net to cast to trap the
few errant missives worthy of suppression. Hospitals that have taken the opposite
approach, namely permitting unfiltered communication except when protection
of the patient or of others seems indubitably to require curtailment of the privilege, have found little reason to regret the more liberal stance.
   Some state statutes grant explicit permission to the hospital administration
to censor communications. In other states the power rests on the need to act in
the patient's best interests or to protect third parties. Conversely, many states
mandate unlimited free communication with certain classes of individuals, often
including lawyers, government officials, and members of the clergy. Even in the
absence of such a provision, a maximal effort should be made to foster free and
private communication between a patient and his lawyer, if the patient's clinical
state at all permits it.
   Privacy.   Privacy means many things to many people. Implicit in the treatment of any illness in a hospital (even a medical hospital) is the sacrifice of much
of what is personal and private about one's daily life. It is coming to be increasingly accepted, however, that effective treatment is not incompatible with many
seemingly small measures that together help to protect the patient's sense of
uniqueness and inviolability. Patients' bills of rights, many of the right-to-treatment suits, and the more enlightened regulations require such steps as permitting patients to retain personal possessions and providing a secure locker for
them, furnishing private toilet and shower facilities, allowing a minimum number of square feet of floor space for each patient, and similar measures.
   Privacy also means protecting the confidentiality of patients (see Chapter
1), including not talking about patient matters within earshot of other patients or
nonprofessional staff, and restricting access to patients' records to authorized
personnel with a need for it.
   The most famous "privacy" case concerning a state facility arose in the
context of Frederick Wiseman's filming of *Titicut Follies* at the old Bridgewater
State Hospital for the Criminally Insane in Massachusetts. Wiseman's film, a
severe indictment of conditions at the hospital, was banned from public display
in Massachusetts on the grounds that it invaded the privacy of those patients who
were portrayed in it. Needless to say, the ban also protected the public officials
who were responsible for conditions at Bridgewater from facing the wrath of an
informed public. The case illustrates the often delicate trade-offs between various rights, here the right to privacy posed against freedom of speech and the
right of the public to know, that one faces in this complicated area.
   Rights to protection from harm.   Among the few treatment-related rights that
the U.S. Supreme Court has been willing to recognize has been the right of
committed patients to be free from physical assault. Patients' bills of rights in
many states extend this right to all patients. Implementing the right to freedom

from harm requires attention to those patients who may be violent toward others and to appropriate intervention, including medication, space restriction, and seclusion or restraint when necessary. In so far as the common law recognizes a similar right as a component of the standard of care for hospitalized patients, failure to protect patients appropriately can lead to actions for malpractice.

It is not only other patients who may inflict injury; staff members can be abusive as well. Patients are entitled to be protected from staff abuse by careful screening of employees and appropriate supervision. Complaint mechanisms with adequate means for investigation are also necessary. Particular attention needs to be given to staff members who work shifts with little supervision, such as on nights and weekends. Often training and support of these staff members, who can feel neglected by the institution, can prevent abuse from occurring.

Rights to freedom of movement. Along with the right to be free of harm, the U.S. Supreme Court found a constitutional liberty interest in freedom of movement. As they interpreted this right, movement within the hospital cannot be arbitrarily restricted—as by the use of seclusion and restraint for the convenience of the hospital staff—but limitations must relate to legitimate therapeutic needs.

State restrictions on the use of seclusion and restraint, however, are even more rigorous. Many states now recognize the prevention of harm to the patient or others as the sole legitimate basis for seclusion or restraint. Possible therapeutic uses (e.g., limiting stimulation of disorganized patients) are no longer considered acceptable in many jurisdictions. This is unfortunate, but in some ways is in keeping with the tendency to view hospitalization as a means of preventing physical harm, rather than as a means of treating mental illness.

There are also procedural requirements attending the use of seclusion and restraint that vary from state to state. These include constant observation or frequent checks of the patient, thorough documentation, periodic examinations by a physician while the patient remains secluded or restrained, and periodic time outs to allow the patient to use toilet facilities and stretch his limbs. Failure to observe these requirements can result in civil penalties or licensure revocation for facilities, and the possibility of administrative sanctions or law suits against clinicians.

Economic rights. As it has become more generally accepted that the disabling effects of mental illness are often quite specific in their impact, frequently leaving large areas of a patient's functional capacity unimpaired, there has been an increasing tendency to permit psychiatric patients to manage their own financial affairs (and often matters of personal status such as marriage, divorce, and custody). Almost all facilities allow patients to hold and spend small amounts of money, and many jurisdictions require, absent a finding of incompetence, that patients be given the opportunity to handle important financial matters even while hospitalized. No states follow the old practice of equating commitment with a finding of incompetency to manage one's affairs.

On the other hand, there are instances in which the restriction of the right to spend money is in the patient's best interest and where a failure to so restrict places the clinician at risk of being found negligent. A patient who is not capable of rationally dealing with his assets, even if he is not officially declared incompetent by the court—for example, a manic patient who, if permitted, would spend his family's savings on frivolities—might have a legitimate cause of action at a later date against any caretaker who permitted such profligacy to occur. Ideally, a determination should be made soon after admission as to the patient's ability to manage his financial affairs. Guardians, conservators, or representative payees, as appropriate, should be sought to act on the patient's behalf. Nevertheless, in those circumstances (and they will be frequent) in which such individuals are unavailable, or in which the incapacity is likely to be of sufficiently short duration that such appointment of proxies would not be useful, the inpatient clinician must continue to step in to protect the patient's needs. While abuse of this discretion is always possible, the patient's ultimate right of appeal to the courts, combined with a healthy bias in favor of the patient managing his affairs whenever possible, should minimize this problem.

Right to be paid for work.   A good example of the difficulties that arise in mixing a "rights" model with a "therapeutic" model is the muddled state of the law concerning patients who perform work in the hospital. Work was a cornerstone of nineteenth-century moral treatment. State hospitals were deliberately located in the countryside, with ample farmland surrounding them, to give patients an opportunity to perform "therapeutic" labor. Over time, however, the therapeutic nature of the labor became obscured by the need of the underfunded hospital to utilize patient labor in order to stay within its budget. Patients were often forced to work for reasons that had little to do with treatment.

In reaction to this abuse, some courts have ruled that this uncompensated labor violates the Thirteenth Amendment's ban against involuntary servitude. Other courts have applied the Fair Labor Standards Act to require that work be compensated at minimum wage levels, and that overtime provisions be applied. The only exceptions allowed are for patients who are rated as proportionately less productive than non-handicapped workers. The result of these two lines of decisions has been to require that work assignments be "voluntary," that patients usually be paid for their work at market rates, or, in some cases, that unpaid work be limited to "therapeutic" labor, tasks not required for the maintenance of the hospital. Difficult as it is to distinguish between therapy and slavery when it comes to washing floors or folding linen, it is even more difficult to persuade tight-fisted state legislators to appropriate funds to pay patients who usually are receiving free treatment in a state facility.

Thus the end result of seeking a legal remedy for an admitted and shameful abuse is the threat of depriving all patients of the benefits of a chance to work. The benefits of work include a badly needed boost to self-esteem, the ego-integrative effects of applying oneself to a task, improvement of attention span, a relief from the monotony of life in many hospitals, and the real improvements in the milieu that can be made by patient labor.

On therapeutic grounds alone, one would favor paying patients for the work they do. But until the legislatures agree, there appears to be no good solution to the problem. Work programs have ground to a halt.

The civil rights officer (CRO).   The discussion above should have demonstrated how problematic in practice may be the appealing notion of "patients' rights"; doing away with all rights and returning to the snake-pit days when our hospitals were "the shame of the states" is hardly the solution. Rather a method needs to be found for settling disputes over patients' rights short of recourse to the courts. An effective means for both maximizing patients' rights and minimizing disruption of the hospital's therapeutic functions is the appointment of a civil rights officer (CRO).

Mandated by statute or regulation in some areas, the office of CRO provides an ombudsperson for patients when concerns about their rights arise. The position should be filled by someone who is familiar with patients' needs and with ways of getting things done in the hospital bureaucracy, but someone who is outside the direct line of responsibility for patient care. The CRO should be available to patients to answer their questions about the extent of their rights and to help find a solution for problems that arise. The CRO is not responsible for resolving disputes, but for bringing problems to the attention of the appropriate officials and for aiding patients in presenting their complaints. Though the CRO will often be able to settle issues raised by patients by exploration or mediation, there will be times when the most appropriate step will be to refer patients to outside legal assistance. To avoid conflicts of interest, the CRO should not serve in a similar advisory role to staff members; they should be able to obtain assistance with legal issues from their own consultant.

Protection and advocacy services. Despite growing attention by psychiatric facilities to patients' rights, and the proliferation of internal mechanisms to protect patients, such as civil rights officers, there is a belief among mental health advocates that widespread abuses remain. This belief led states to establish—and more recently, Congress to require—protection and advocacy services (known as P&As) for mentally ill patients. P&A services, usually staffed by attorneys and paralegals, operate independently of the mental health system. Although models differ from state to state, P&As usually station representatives at major psychiatric facilities, where they inform patients of their rights and solicit complaints. Efforts may be made to resolve complaints through negotiation with the facility, often through the civil rights officer. If these attempts fail, P&As have the capacity to file suit against individuals, private facilities, and the state. Congress has appropriated some funding for P&As in each state, with additional money coming from state budgets. P&As can be awarded attorneys' fees by the courts at the conclusion of many types of successful litigation.

The P&A model entered the mental health system from the mental retardation system, where it has functioned for much longer. Its efficacy is a matter of dispute. Advocates point to the need for some external check on the authority of administrators and clinicians in facilities where they would otherwise have unchallenged power to control every aspect of patients' lives. Opponents argue that in a situation of limited funding, a chronic characteristic of the public sector, P&As distort the allocation process by forcing resources to be devoted disproportionately to the problems they target for attention. Some clinicians believe that P&As were created as a substitute for adequate funding of mental health programs. There is also little question that hospital staff, already operating under considerable stress, view the presence of P&A attorneys, and the implicit threat of a lawsuit that they carry in their negotiating arsenal, as an additional unpleasant aspect of their job. Nonetheless, recent trends suggest that P&As will remain a permanent fixture on the mental health landscape. (See Chap. 7, Secs. II-A-4 and II-B-1-d-ii for further discussion of the relationship between clinicians and P&As.)

C. Right to refuse treatment

As part of the more general movement to afford mental patients the rights enjoyed by other members of society, a good deal of attention has been given to their right to refuse psychiatric treatment. This right has now been recognized in various forms in a large number of court decisions, and some right of refusal is granted by many state statutes or regulations.

1. HISTORY OF THE RIGHT TO REFUSE TREATMENT

In principle, voluntary inpatients have always had the right to refuse treatment they did not desire, if in no other way then by leaving the facility. The situation for involuntary patients, however, was rather different. Since commitment was based on their need for treatment (see Chap. 2, Sec. II-D-1), it was presumed that the procedures required to detain them were also sufficient to allow them to be treated against their will. In this context, the right to refuse treatment was not even imagined.

When commitment statutes changed to emphasize dangerousness criteria, however, the question began to be raised as to where the state derived its power to treat over patients' objections. If preventing dangerous behavior was the goal, and that could be accomplished by detaining the patient under supervision, it was argued that the state had no compelling interest in overriding the refusals of unwilling patients. Further, it was maintained, patients had substantial interests in having their refusals honored. These interests derived from common law rights to control what was done to their bodies, and constitutional rights to privacy, liberty, equal protection, and due process.

Early cases, in the 1960s and 1970s, focused on patients' right to refuse treatments that were thought to be exceptionally intrusive: aversive therapy with drugs that induce nausea or paralyze respirations, psychosurgery, electroconvulsive therapy. Beginning in the late 1970s, more than a score of courts extended this analysis, granting some version of a right to refuse treatment with antipsychotic medications. These decisions are often premised on a distorted view of the risk/benefit balance of these drugs, but the legal rationale derives from the idea that mental patients do not lose the right to decide what should befall them merely because of involuntary commitment.

2. CURRENT APPROACHES OF THE COURTS

Although the right to refuse treatment with antipsychotic medication is often spoken of as a unitary concept, the courts have defined the right very differently across jurisdictions. Two broad approaches have been followed, with several variations of each.

a. Treatment-driven models

Courts adopting this approach have tended to recognize patients' interests in limiting inappropriate medication but not in refusing indicated treatment. Thus, when patients object to treatment, these courts require that the objection be reviewed by either the treating physician (a minimalist approach) or an independent consultant. If the recommended treatment is found to be appropriate, it is permitted to proceed. One might characterize this model as endorsing a right to object to treatment but not a right to refuse it.

Federal courts have tended to favor this approach. At this writing, the U.S. Supreme Court has not decided the contours of a federal constitutional right to refuse treatment in civil facilities, but it has given some hints of its views. The

Court remanded one of the cases that reached it on this issue (*Rennie v. Klein*), indicating to the lower court that it should reconsider its decision in light of *Youngberg v. Romeo* (see Sec. B-3 above). *Youngberg* had noted that patients' rights could be limited in the interests of treatment as long as a professional judgment was made by qualified personnel in this regard. This action of the Supreme Court seemed to suggest that it favored a similar approach here. Many federal courts (and a few state courts) have operated under that assumption, endorsing treatment-driven models.

More recently, the U.S. Supreme Court has taken a similar approach in a case involving the right of prisoners to refuse treatment (*Washington v. Harper*). It held that Washington state's procedures for reviewing prisoners' objections to treatment, which included review by a three-person clinical/administrative panel, with rights to present evidence, to have lay representation, to appeal, and to regular review was sufficient to vindicate prisoners' rights. Substantively, if a prisoner met the state's commitment criteria, and treatment was in his interests, the medication could be administered. It is unclear to what extent the Court was carving out a special exception for prisons—to whose needs it has always been deferential—or whether it would endorse an approach of this sort in a civil setting, as suggested by some of the analysis in the opinion.

Advocates of a right to refuse treatment, however, argue that this model misses the point. Although it may improve the quality of care, it does nothing to insure that patients have the right to determine whether or not they will receive medication in the first place. Thus, they argue for an entirely different, rights-driven approach.

b. Rights-driven models

This model views patients' rights to determine whether or not they are treated as primary. Those rights may be based on the federal constitution, despite the U.S. Supreme Court's *Youngberg* decision, but increasingly they are not. State courts, which have taken the lead in adopting rights-driven models, often base their decisions on common law rights to control what happens to one's body, state statutory law, or state constitutions. This renders their decisions non-reviewable by federal courts, allowing them to extend patients' right to refuse treatment well beyond what the U.S. Supreme Court is willing to recognize as required by the federal constitution.

The key to the rights-driven approaches is to minimize the differences between the rights of involuntarily committed patients and other persons. Since non-committed persons cannot be treated against their will unless they have been found to be incompetent to make decisions for themselves, rights-driven models incorporate a similar determination for committed patients. Some variation is evident, however, in the identity of the decisionmaker and the degree of procedural protections afforded.

The simplest of the rights-driven models calls for an independent evaluator or panel to assess the refusing patient's competence, along with the need for treatment. If found to be incompetent, and if the suggested treatment is deemed to be appropriate, the patient can be treated over her objections. Although this model has the virtue of avoiding lengthy court proceedings, that is precisely the aspect that concerns many patients' rights advocates. They contend that this continues to grant a lower level of protection to committed mentally ill persons than that afforded to others, who would have their incompetence determined by a judge. On the other hand, clinicians are concerned that this model allows some committed patients to refuse treatment, putting the clinicians in the position of being responsible for the care of patients whom they cannot treat effectively.

A proposal that would respond to both these problems would limit involuntary commitment to patients who are found by a judge to be incompetent to make decisions about treatment. (See Chap. 2, Sec. II-F-1-a.) This would grant patients the right to a judicial determination of incompetence, while eliminating the possibility that committed patients could refuse appropriate medication. Utah is the only state to have adopted this model for all committed patients; after commitment, physicians are allowed to prescribe for patients those medications they believe are needed. Decisionmaking power might, of course, be conferred on other parties, for example family members, a guardian, or even a judge.

The most popular of the rights-driven models, though, now being adopted by one state after another, does not restrict the scope of civil commitment in this way. If a committed patient refuses treatment, he is subject to a court hearing on his competence. If found competent, his refusal stands. If found incompetent, the court will make a decision as to whether treatment should be permitted. Some courts will ground this determination in their view of whether treatment is in the patient's best interests. Other courts will rely on their perception of what the patient would have wanted if he were competent to make a decision—the so-called "substituted judgment" approach (see Chap. 5, Sec. II-D).

3. Statutory and Regulatory Approaches

As in so many other areas of patients' rights, it has been the courts that have taken the lead in fashioning the right to refuse treatment with medication. But almost all of the states have responded by now with statutes or regulations that echo one of the models described above. Generally, states attempt to adhere to treatment-driven models unless compelled by the courts to adopt a rights-driven approach. They have been fairly creative in establishing procedures for review of refusals, including interdisciplinary panels, and multi-layered review, beginning in the facility and then moving to regional or state administrative levels. Challenges to some of these procedures, however, have led to a number of court decisions imposing a judicially-run, rights-driven model.

4. Emergencies

The court decisions have acknowledged the traditional prerogative of clinicians to take whatever steps are necessary to deal with emergencies, including the use of seclusion, restraint, and involuntary medication. The term "emergency," however, has tended to be rather narrowly construed. Some courts, for example, reject a clinical definition of emergency that encompasses such criteria as severe suffering on the part of the patient and the likelihood of rapid deterioration in favor of a narrower, more legalistic definition limited to the occurrence or threat of significant bodily injury to the patient or others or the likelihood of irreversible deterioration. Within that scope, medication is permitted, but only to the extent necessary to control the emergent situation. That is, if a single injection of a neuroleptic is sufficient to sedate or to diminish the frightening hallucinations of an assaultive patient, further treatment is not permitted, even though the patient remains psychotic, and the long-term risk of recurrence is present. This is consistent with a non-clinical view of the use of medication as a means of controlling behavior rather than as a treatment for illness; this view is analogous to defining dangerousness rather than need for treatment as the sole criterion for involuntary commitment.

Even with these "tight" criteria, the point at which an emergency begins and involuntary treatment may be initiated is often an uncertain one and requires a large amount of clinical discretion. For example, a patient who is refusing food and fluids will, at some point, become an emergency case; careful electrolyte or blood pressure monitoring may be necessary to satisfy a court that this point has been reached. The medical conservativism that may inevitably result from such legalistic criteria may place the patient at significant risk. On the other hand, a repetitively assaultive patient with a regular pattern of building up to an assault (such as cursing loudly at hallucinatory images) need not be allowed to strike someone, even under the strictest definitions of emergency, before medication may be administered. Many facilities will undoubtedly continue to use more clinically oriented definitions of emergency. In the absence of statutes or court rulings to the contrary this is acceptable. Clinicians acting in good faith and in their patients' best interests are unlikely to be held personally liable in such a situation.

5. LIABILITY RESULTING FROM FAILURE TO COMPLY WITH RULES ON PATIENTS' RIGHT TO REFUSE TREATMENT

There are three general categories in which liability could accrue for non-consensual treatment in violation of legal rules in a given jurisdiction.

a. Battery

A criminal charge of battery (performing an unconsented touching) along with the related charge of assault (inducing the apprehension that a battery will be committed) are possible consequences of involuntary medication practices. Along with the criminal charge, a civil suit for damages resulting from the alleged battery can also be filed. Courts, however, are usually reluctant to introduce criminal issues into the hospital setting, where unconsented touchings are a routine part of daily work with the severely ill. The availability of other remedies, considered below, contributes to this reluctance, as does the general trend of considering issues of consent as an element of malpractice, rather than as battery. Nonetheless, such a criminal or civil action remains a possibility, particularly where circumstances suggest that medications were administered for purposes other than treatment.

b. Malpractice

The usual benchmark for judging malpractice liability is a failure to conform to the standard of practice of the profession (see Chap. 4, Sec. II-A-1-b). Thus, as non-consensual treatment becomes less common, the practitioner who administers medication against his patient's desires places himself at increasing risk. This assumes, of course, that such action is not sanctioned by state statute or regulation. Already the doctrine of informed consent (see Chap. 4, Sec. II-B) has been sufficiently elaborated in nonpsychiatric medical cases to provide ample precedent for suits against mental health clinicians claiming a failure to obtain informed consent. An additional caveat is warranted: the usual standard of liability, the extent of deviation from accepted practice, can be rejected by the court if it feels that the standard of the profession itself is improper. It was through just such means that malpractice suits over informed consent became prevalent in a medical community that had generally paid little heed to such formalities. Precedents in other jurisdictions are important barometers for judging how acceptable even a widely followed standard of care is likely to be to a court. Recent decisions certainly point in the direction of decreasing acceptability of involuntary medication. The old practice of obtaining the consent of next-of-kin in place of the patient's is similarly falling into disfavor. Rather, except in emergencies, the substituted consent of a statutorily or judicially authorized decisionmaker is preferred.

c. Civil rights violations

Section 1983 of Title 42 of the United States Code provides that anyone who, acting under color of state law, deprives an individual of his federal civil rights is liable for suit for damages resulting from his acts (see Chap. 4, Sec. II-C-5). Such suits are particularly likely to be filed against employees of a state system, but even private facilities authorized by the state to detain patients involuntarily are potential targets. The crucial element here is the definition of involuntary medication as a deprivation of civil rights. Unfortunately, the same court that decides that a right has been violated will be the one to determine that damages are due. Herein lies the practical import of the Federal constitutional arguments for a right to refuse treatment outlined above. To the extent that these become widely accepted, the practitioner is at risk for a federal suit. Most malpractice insurance policies, incidentally, cover neither the expenses of contesting such a suit nor the monetary damages that may result.

6. EFFECTS OF PATIENTS' RIGHT TO REFUSE TREATMENT

A large number of studies have been published evaluating the effects of rules allowing patients to refuse treatment with medication. When the initial judicial opinions on the matter began to appear in the late 1970s, many clinicians expressed fears that inpatient facilities, particularly in the public sector, would be swept by epidemics of refusal, rendering efforts to treat the mentally ill completely unavailing. Fortunately, that has not been the result. Studies demonstrate that, when refusal is permitted, about 10% of patients will refuse medication for at least one day at some point during their hospitalization. These numbers vary according to type of facility (forensic facilities have higher refusal rates) and other factors. Although this represents a sizeable number of patients, it is not the epidemic that was feared.

The few studies that have followed patients from the point of refusal (rather than identifying them when efforts are made to override their objections) indicate that the majority of refusers will reaccept medication voluntarily within one week of refusal. This speaks to the importance of the negotiation process between clinician and patient, rather than the legal system, as the primary means of resolving refusals. (See Sec. III-D below.) Only a minority of refusals result in recourse to formal review, and most studies suggest that almost all of those patients ultimately get treated. This is true regardless of the review mechanism, although ironically judges appear to approve a higher percentage of treatment requests (90–100%) than independent clinical reviewers on in-house committees. One study found that about one-fifth of refusals resulted in a permanent discontinuation of antipsychotic medication, but in none of these cases did clinicians believe that medication was essential to the patient's care.

The outcome of treatment refusals thus appears to be rather benign, but the costs of the process are extensive. Judicial review, in particular, results in lengthy delays (up to several months) prior to hearings, and costly investment of clinical and legal time. In the meantime, refusing patients are significantly more likely to commit assaults and require seclusion than non-refusers, and are rated as highly disruptive to the therapeutic milieu. Independent, non-judicial review is much faster and less costly, but as described above, is losing popularity in the courts.

One area in which little research has been done concerns the efficacy of involuntary treatment. Comparisons of voluntary and involuntary patients show similar rates of improvement at the end of hospitalization, but most involuntary patients take medications willingly once hospitalized. Reports of refusers treated against their will with medication suggest that many of them improve, and this is confirmed by clinical experience. What remains unknown is the long-term effect of involuntary treatment: do patients treated without their consent improve while in the hospital only to stop medications and relapse once released? Are they then less willing to seek voluntary hospitalization because of their previous experiences? These are important areas for careful empirical investigation.

7. THE FUTURE OF THE RIGHT TO REFUSE TREATMENT

Granting involuntarily committed patients a right to refuse treatment with medication, the major modality for restoring many patients' mental health, poses something of a dilemma for the mental health system. If the justification for involuntary commitment is derived solely from the state's police powers and is limited to the prevention of harm to others and to the patient herself, then perhaps allowing committed patients to refuse treatment makes some sense. As suggested earlier, however, (see Chap. 2, Secs. II-D-2-c), it is difficult to justify involuntary commitment solely on a police powers' basis. The only discernible rationale for allowing detention of the mentally ill when similar interventions can not be undertaken with the non-mentally ill is the *parens patriae* rationale that they will benefit from treatment. To permit committed patients to refuse treatment, with the implicit consequence of indefinite detention, is inconsistent with the underlying purpose of the civil commitment system. Further, since indefinite detention is probably a more severe deprivation of liberty than is time-limited treatment with a medication that restores the patient's ability to deal with the world, if the state has the power to impose the former, it almost certainly has the right to impose the latter too.

This argument, though occasionally recognized by the courts, has been largely neglected in the flight from acknowledgement of *parens patriae* rationales for commitment. But the common sense idea that, in the words of one court, "Nonconsensual treatment is what involuntary commitment is all about" makes its way to the surface through more indirect channels. As noted above, decision-makers who are asked to rule on whether refusing patients should be treated allow treatment in the vast preponderance of cases. This would appear to reflect the belief that it makes no sense to commit patients because they are mentally ill and then allow them to refuse the only treatment that provides a hope of returning to the community.

Where does the right to refuse treatment go from here? With the tendency of state courts to adopt rights-driven models of resolving objections to treatment, a fairly strict version of the right is likely to be with us in many jurisdictions for some time. But it is probable that decisionmakers in those states will limit the impact of the right by allowing treatment of refusers in the majority of cases. Only when, as a society, we once again accept *parens patriae* justifications for governmental intervention can we expect to see treatment-driven approaches become dominant. In the meantime, a recognition by policy-makers of the inefficiency of judicial review and of the desirability of substituting a non-judicial process would be most welcome.

D. Rights related to discharge from the hospital

In many ways the most important right a patient has, the one that makes all the others meaningful, is the right to leave a hospital if the situation becomes unacceptable to her. The exercise of this right differs for voluntary and involuntary patients.

1. VOLUNTARY PATIENTS

As noted above (see Chapter 2, section II-C-2), there are two classes of voluntary patients. The "pure" voluntary patient can leave the hospital at will, limited only to reasonable hours, such as daytime hours, or to weekdays. "Conditional" voluntary patients (the terms differ in different states) may be required to give notice, often amounting to several days' notice, before they are permitted to leave. This period is designed to provide an opportunity for the hospital staff to evaluate the patient's potential committability or suitability for discharge. These patient-initiated discharges are often referred to as discharges "against medical advice" or "AMA." Strictly speaking, however, this is not always the case, as there will be instances in which, for a variety of clinical reasons, the patient's caregivers will acquiesce in the decision to leave. When the discharge is occurring over the strenuous opposition of the clinical staff, it is sometimes useful to acknowledge this by having the noncommittable patient sign a second form, similar to that used in medical hospitals, indicating that the patient is aware of the grounds for the hospital's opposition to her departure. In addition to the potential positive clinical effects of such a procedure, the additional documentation may be useful in the event that harm befalls the patient or a third party as a result of the premature cessation of inpatient treatment.

2. INVOLUNTARY PATIENTS

Patients who have been civilly committed by the courts, hospitalized by virtue of an emergency, or committed under any one of a number of criminal statutes, or conditional voluntary patients who are unwilling to wait the mandated time prior to discharge, all share a common remedy, a writ of habeas corpus. This traditional means of limiting the power of the state to detain individuals, protected in our constitution, dates back to medieval England and means literally "may you have the body." Issued on request to a court, it provides for the immediate appearance of the patient in court (same day or next day hearings are not uncommon) to review the ground for detention. If the state is unable to make a showing that the patient is being legally detained, that is, that he had been found to meet the criteria for commitment, immediate release may be ordered.

Although the writ is supposedly concerned more with procedure than with substance (in other words, that a fair procedure for the determination of commitability has been followed rather than with the outcome of that procedure), in these contexts it almost inevitably turns into a hearing at which the merits of the commitment decision are reargued. The basis for this is the frequent assertion by the patient that his condition or circumstances have changed so substantially since the original determination that a rehearing on the facts is required. The power of the writ lies in the immediacy of the response to it. Properly, it should be reserved for remedying egregious errors or for situations in which continued hospitalization is seriously damaging to the patient, lest hospital staff be overwhelmed with the necessity of responding to a large number of writs to the detriment of patient care. Concerned lawyers can often accomplish as much through negotiation with the hospital staff, assuming that, in fact, an error has been made, as they can by turning to one of the major weapons in the legal arsenal.

3. CONDITIONAL RELEASE

Not all patients who leave psychiatric hospitals are discharged outright. Many are given some form of conditional discharge, sometimes referred to as "visit" or "trial visit" status. This device allows the patient to retain technical inpatient status while residing for a time outside of the hospital. Advantages of the procedure include the greater ease of readmitting the patient should she require it; the sense of support imparted to the patient, who knows at this difficult time that she has not been abandoned by the institution; and the ability to continue to provide services that are restricted to those who are formally inpatients, such as the provision of free medication to a financially shaky patient or continued access to facilities for occupational therapy. There is, of course, a potential for abuse in that the hospital can recall the patient against her will for rehospitalization, although the courts have generally required that some sort of hearing take place at which the patient has an opportunity to challenge the change in status. Examples of abuse are difficult to find, as the chief difficulty with the system in many areas appears to be the lack of sufficient staff to monitor the conditionally released patients. Even patients whose clinical conditions warrant rehospitalization may therefore not be identified, and the promise of early intervention and prompt treatment often goes unfulfilled. (See the related discussion of outpatient commitment in Chap. 2, Sec. II-F-4.)

4. INVOLUNTARY DISCHARGE

There are many instances in which a patient desires to remain in a psychiatric hospital even though his clinician is recommending discharge. If the impasse persists, the clinician may resort to an involuntary discharge. (See Sec. III-G below, and Chap. 2, Sec. III-E-5.) The legal implications of such a measure vary with the specific circumstances that induce it.

a. For clinical indications

This is the most clear-cut case of involuntary discharge from the clinician's point of view. The patient has benefited maximally from hospitalization, or faces the danger of dependency and regression, and discharge is therefore clinically indicated. Since the idea that a patient might want to remain in a psychiatric hospital longer than necessary is counterintuitive to most laypeople, the clinician can find herself in the position of being accused of negligent and callous treatment should anything befall the newly discharged patient. Careful documentation of the clinical basis for discharge is therefore essential, and predischarge consultation with family members can be useful as well.

b. On expiration of insurance coverage

Private facilities cannot, in general, afford to continue to treat patients whose insurance has expired. This constitutes a reason for discharge, as long as the patient is not abandoned. Transfer of care to a state facility or to an outpatient clinician who is willing to accept the patient is essential before responsibility for the patient's care is relinquished.

c. On expiration of court-ordered commitments

This situation is similar to that considered in Section a above, except that the decision must be justified somewhat more rigorously. Before discharge the clinician should document both the clinical grounds for overriding the patient's desire to remain and the resolution of those factors, whether dangerousness or inability to care for self, that motivated the original commitment.

d. After a dangerous or disruptive act

In moving from a simple consideration of the patient's best interest, as in Sections a and c above, to a response to an act that endangered other patients or staff members, additional safeguards should be imposed to protect the patient. The patient should have an opportunity to respond to the charges that she committed the act in question, and an impartial fact finder, out of the clinical chain of command, might be useful. However, since it is beneficial neither to the potentially dangerous patient nor to the other patients or staff to retain her on a ward that is not equipped to handle violence, if the charges are substantiated, further action is justified.

This can take a number of forms. Patients who are not likely to be assaultive on the outside and who can care for themselves can be discharged outright. Patients who cannot care for themselves or who are likely to be dangerous to others outside of the hospital can be transferred to state facilities for dangerous mental patients. In those cases in which psychosis is absent or is unrelated to the violence, the patient can be held criminally responsible for her acts. Charges can be filed for the initial act of violence, and discharge to the street with notification to the police is possible. A psychiatric hospital is not required to detain any person who is liable to be dangerous to others unless that dangerousness results from mental illness. Adequate notice to the police provides sufficient protection for the community. Careful documentation of all steps is, or course, vital.

e. After an infraction of the rules

A nonthreatening infraction of the rules may serve as a basis for discharge if it is in the patient's best interest for such violations to be responded to seriously or if the patient is able to care for himself outside of the hospital and the needs of the other patients that have been infringed outweigh his need for continued hospitalization. An informal, impartial review of the circumstances is appropriate here, too.

f. Following refusal of treatment

This is a sensitive situation, since it may appear that this step is being taken in retaliatory response to the narcissistic insult that refusal of treatment entails for the clinician. It is justified when the patient is not committable, means of overriding refusal are unavailable or contraindicated, and it is in the patient's long-term best interest. This latter requires a delicate clinical appraisal of the benefit to the patient of a clear-cut statement of the clinician's stance with regard to the need for medication or other treatment balanced against the harm likely to result from discharge. One of the most difficult clinical decisions, its basis should be carefully documented. Of course, if the patient can survive safely outside the hospital and is unlikely to benefit from a prolonged stay without the recommended treatment, discharge becomes clinically indicated.

III. CLINICAL ISSUES

A. Implementing the right to treatment

The treatment of a psychiatric patient sick enough to require hospitalization has become a subspecialty of the field: inpatient psychiatry. While the topic has been explored elsewhere (see Suggested Readings—Principles and Problems of Inpatient Psychiatry) and clearly merits a book in itself, certain general points might here be made under the rubric of clinical aspects of the right to treatment. Four broad aspects of hospital treatment may be defined (with some overlap): acute, short-term intervention; long-term intervention; rehabilitation; and custodial care.

1. ASPECTS OF HOSPITAL TREATMENT

a. Short-term intervention

The patient may be admitted in crisis, overwhelmed by internal and external stress, and require a brief hospitalization aimed at support, crisis intervention, and plans for future, definitive outpatient intervention. The major result achieved by such intervention may be, in fact, "hooking up" the patient with a therapist; at other times hospitalization may serve as a collective consultation to an ongoing therapy. Examples of clinical conditions suited to such intervention are acute but transient suicidality, severe pan-anxiety, and toxic states without sequelae. The goal of hospitalization is to return the patient to outpatient status and functioning as rapidly as possible.

b. Long-term intervention

Here the patient may be admitted for definitive treatment of major mental illness that is not expected to respond to short-term interventions. Examples of clinical conditions appropriate for such interventions include the major psychoses (the schizophrenias and the affective disorders), other severe depressions, mental illness complicated by medical disease, persisting suicidality, personality disorders, and major antisocial acting out as symptomatic behavior. The goals of hospitalization are active treatment of the disease in question and a return (usually on a gradual, stepwise basis) to previous or optimum possible levels of functioning outside the hospital; ongoing aftercare and outpatient treatment are often indicated.

c. Rehabilitation

A patient may be admitted after evaluation reveals an illness of such severity or chronicity, or of such a nature, as not to be likely to respond to any great degree to the kinds of definitive interventions listed above. The interventions for such patients may partake less of the character of active treatment than of rehabilitation; the goals of hospitalization are vocational assessment and training, instruction in marketable skills, placement in workshops, instruction in personal hygiene and activities of daily living (ADL), and the like.

d. Custodial care

Despite the best efforts of the psychiatric profession, there remains a small but ineradicable population of patients whose problems—whether secondary to regression, chronicity, organicity, or a combination of these states—simply do not respond to treatment. This population requires lifetime hospitalization or institutionalization. Misguided attempts at deinstitutionalization make these patients their primary victims; the problems of these patients cannot be voted away by the political process. The goals of hospitalization are maintenance of human dignity; food, clothing and shelter; activities, exercise, and entertainment as indicated; and fostering of human relations in a structured, caretaking environment.

With the above models in mind, we may consider implementation of the right to treatment.

2. INDIVIDUAL TREATMENT PLANS

Hospitalization per se accomplishes the goal of asylum for individuals and, if dangerousness is an issue, protection of the community. Clearly if treatment is to occur beyond these rather limited goals—i.e., beyond basic custodial care—it must be carried out in accordance with a plan that systematically addresses the needs of the patient in accord with a biopsychosocial model. This plan must, of course, be clearly documented in a record.

> **Example 1:** A twenty-year-old "street schizophrenic" who lived in doorways, eating from garbage cans, was admitted actively hallucinating. Her biologic needs included nutrition and treatment for her tuberculosis; her psychological needs included treatment of an acute exacerbation of a chronic schizophrenic process; her social needs included group home placement and a structured day program aimed at rehabilitation, hygiene, and interpersonal skills. The patient's abilities as a seamstress served as the nucleus of her vocational rehabilitation.

The example above implies the necessity for individualizing the plan to the specific strengths, deficits, and needs of the patient.

3. PERIODIC REVIEW

Since hospital treatment of major mental illness is often a long-term process inducing a generally slow rate of change, there exists a danger that treatment processes will be instituted on the basis of admission symptomatology, and that this treatment will proceed unaltered and hence unresponsive to subtle (or even gross) improvement (or deterioration) in the patient's clinical state.

This danger may be largely avoided by regular review of the treatment plan, addressing in particular whether or not the specific goals of the interventions have been achieved. This means, quite simply, deciding what is not working, and changing or stopping it, and deciding what *is* working and continuing that.

In order to prevent stagnation of the treatment program into sterile or rigid routine, regular consultation "from the outside" is helpful in providing new perspectives on patient care. Both such external review and regular internal review must be documented in detail, not only to maintain high standards of treatment, but to provide data essential for quality control, research, utilization review, and reimbursement by third parties.

4. USE OF THE MULTIDISCIPLINARY TEAM

Most inpatient treatment is now carried out by a staff drawn from the disciplines of psychiatry, psychology, social work, nursing (including attendants or aides), and occupational therapy (including ADL, vocational, recreational, expressive, and activities therapies). It should be emphasized that this use of a team is not merely a method of compensating for the relatively small number of psychiatrists; rather, it is a means of utilizing specific abilities that are inherent in each discipline. The value of the unique contributions of the individual disciplines depends in large part on their successful orchestration by skilled team leadership into coordinated action in carrying out the treatment plan.

5. ATTENTION TO ENVIRONMENTAL ISSUES

The intensity and specialization of inpatient psychiatry may breed a parochialism of attitude that scants attention to the impact of the external environment, i.e., the community. The community may provide pathogenic forces in the form of crime, intolerance of deviance, extrusion of the patient, and massive disruption of structure such as displacement and forced relocation of citizens. In addition the community may offer constructive forces such as halfway houses and group houses, activities and support systems for discharged patients.

The hospital ward itself is also an environment deserving of attention in relation to the right to treatment. It is not only human dignity and decency that suffer from dirt, disorder, lack of privacy, crowding, unavailability of essentials, and other dehumanizing factors; it is also the patient's clinical state that suffers, since such surroundings promote regression, apathy, and "institutionalism" in its various forms. While clinical personnel often have little control over the ward environment, the critical importance of a humane and safe milieu in promotion of the right to treatment must be emphasized.

B. Clinical aspects of patients' rights

The patients' rights movement represents an important effort to raise popular consciousness about a markedly disenfranchised population. At present, in many institutions, patients are given brochures or leaflets on admission that define their rights in simple language—a laudable approach, although at the point of admission many patients are in no condition to read leaflets. Patients' rights issues may have clinical impact on patients and treaters as well.

1. RIGHTS VERSUS ECONOMIC REALITIES

A number of patients' rights are related to certain aspects of the milieu, such as the rights to adequate privacy, toileting facilities, clothing and supplies, etc. Unfortunately, in many institutional settings (especially in the public sector) the presence of these facets of the milieu depends almost totally on public funding of various kinds, often controlled by economy-minded legislatures and processed through creaky civil service bureaucracies. When such basic necessities are unavailable to patients, many patients and naïve legal activists tend to blame the clinical staff, often the ones with the *least* control over, say, the availability of toilet paper (a scarce commodity in many a state hospital). From this fallacious point of view, treatment staff are seen as withholding essential needs from patients or depriving them of their rights—a picture that casts the staff in a clearly adversary posture.

2. PATIENTS' RIGHTS IN RELATION TO CLINICAL ADMINISTRATION

Clinical administration refers to a body of practices that determines the immediate moment-to-moment management of the inpatient; included are the use of medications, space restrictions and expansions (staying in room, leaving on pass, etc.), use of emergency treatments (seclusion, physical restraints, etc.), and other similar interventions not appropriately subsumed under the psychotherapies (see Suggested Readings—Gutheil, "On the Therapy in Clinical Administration").

Correct use of these interventions requires a specialized understanding of the problems unique to persons in states of severe psychic disturbance. Without such understanding, interventions may not be understood, or their intent may be misinterpreted.

a. "Deprivation of freedom" versus the prescription of space

An important and ubiquitous aspect of inpatient work is the clinical administration of space. This term refers to the way space and freedom of movement are prescribed for the patient on the ward; the range of possibilities includes, at one end of the spectrum, discharge to the outside, and at the other, seclusion or restraint. In between, the patient may be required to stay in a room, stay on a ward or on part of a ward, or stay within the hospital proper. Passes and visits home are also part of this system.

The rationale for this prescriptive approach rests on an understanding of the severely disturbed patient's experience of space. Patients in a number of clinical states experience a markedly increased sensitivity to sensory input in all modes; what would ordinarily be experienced as normal perception becomes sensory bombardment. The wider the space and the more activity going on in it, the greater this kind of input overload for the patient.

In addition a greater range of movement provides more opportunities for encounters with others, unexpected experiences, and new demands for coping and mastery of one's own impulses. Conversely, a known space, thoroughly explored and thus exhausted of surprises, becomes comfortably familiar and thus supportive; the paranoid patient need not fear the hidden attacker around the unknown corner.

Finally, space may be used to support internal controls by decreasing stimulation or temporarily providing isolation for the patient who is struggling to control anxiety-based assaultiveness. The concept at issue is that of "limit-setting," whereby a patient who feels internal controls giving way—an extremely frightening experience—can be reassured that external controls (like limited space or sufficient numbers of staff) are available. Deprived of such controls, many patients in these states become increasingly agitated or assaultive. (See Example 4, below.)

With this in mind, one can grasp how in certain clinical states, the patient's experience of "greater freedom" (more room in which to move around) may be paradoxically stressful and anxiety producing, while "less freedom" may be reassuring and calming.

b. Seclusion

One area of frequent misunderstanding at the legal/clinical interface is the use of seclusion (see Suggested Readings), a technique that represents clinical use of *minimal* space. The locked door connotes to legal sources an analogy with solitary confinement, as in a correctional system. In fact, despite the potential for abuse, seclusion offers several advantages for treatment of the seriously ill.

Seclusion offers: *containment* of the out-of-control patient, dangerous to self and others, for that patient's protection and that of other patients; *isolation* from interpersonal relationships that, due to the illness, may be threatening, overstimulating, or enraging; and *decrease in sensory input* for those patients in states of sensory bombardment whose sensitivity to, and distortion of, sensory input is preternaturally high.

Seclusion is misused if it is employed as punishment, as a substitute for staff attention or time, or as an expression of countertransference feelings not related to the patient's actual clinical state. An important step toward the appropriate use of seclusion was the publication of a task force report by the American Psychiatric Association addressing professional standards for seclusion and restraint (see Suggested Readings—Tardiff). This publication represents a milestone for the profession in shedding its ambivalence over this politically controversial treatment modality and in articulating appropriate standards for its use.

The topic of restraint was also addressed by the task force report. Different facilities vary widely in their choice of preferred restraints, with differences based largely on tradition and experience. Restraints in general range from wrist and ankle leather bracelets to wet sheet packs, camisole jackets, posey belts, and variations on these themes. As a rule of thumb, facilities should select a form of restraint with which they are the most familiar and in application of which staff are most practiced; other considerations are arguably secondary.

c. Least restrictive alternative

This doctrine relating to involuntary commitment has gained in popularity with time (see Section II-B-1 above). It represents, as noted, an application of a legalistic frame of reference to treatment by arbitrarily focusing on degree of restriction as the most important vector and locating the options along it.

Although one treatment modality may have in some way less inherent restrictiveness than another, it may not necessarily be optimal in other (perhaps more important) ways, such as the amount of observation and monitoring possible; access to specialized examination and testing; and so on. Ironically, certain clinical and institutional issues conspire to make restrictiveness less straightforward than may appear, as in Example 2.

> *Example 2:* The combination of mild retardation, temporal lobe epilepsy, and schizophrenia burdened a young man who was prone to unpredictable, terrifying, violent attacks against women. When an inpatient in an inner-city community mental health center, he spent almost all of his time restricted to his room or in seclusion, for the safety of patients and staff.
>
> After the last in a series of attacks, he was sent to a maximum security psychiatric hospital. There he was free to go outdoors, walk freely about the courtyard, and otherwise enjoy what amounted to *greater* freedom and *less* restriction because of the high level of security provided by the "more restrictive alternative" hospital. These freedoms were unattainable in the ostensibly less restrictive community setting. In addition, the all-male security environment markedly diminished the patient's anxiety about losing control of his impulses toward women—an anxiety that returned full force when he was returned after a time to the sexually mixed community setting.

3. ALTERNATIVE MODELS

This approach to the seriously ill patient (i.e., clinical administration) has been clinically validated in contemporary hospital practice. Those unfamiliar with the effects of major mental illness, however, are prone to two common misunderstandings of these principles and misinterpretations of the rationale for their application. These modes of misinterpretation may be styled the "crime and punishment" model and the "behaviorist" model.

a. The "crime and punishment" model

The adoption of the crime and punishment model represents an occupational hazard to which lawyers are particularly prone, in light of their immersion in the adversary structure of the criminal justice system. This model may be misapplied to clinical administration.

The following example illustrates how the same clinical event is perceived in different ways through application of the legal and clinical models.

> *Example 3:* Flooded by psychotic panic, a young patient fled the ward and was returned from escape by the police. Back on the ward, he was secluded for his dyscontrol and calmed rapidly over a day or so.
>
> Months later, during a habeas corpus hearing demanding his release, his attorney portrayed this episode as if the staff, "angered" by the patient's escape, had "punished" the patient by putting him in "solitary."

b. The behaviorist model

The behaviorist model, employed in some institutional settings and by some legal authorities, gives the appearance of similarity to the practices of clinical administration; however, the differences are extremely significant.

According to this model one "reinforces" adaptive or desirable behaviors by giving "rewards" (or removing noxae) and one "extinguishes" undesirable or maladaptive behaviors by applying "punishments" (or removing rewards). The patient learns to conform behavior to the relevant standard.

There are three problems posed by this model in relation to inpatient care. First, the model is moralistic in tone, rather than clinical. Second, it deals with the patient as an exterior, as an emitter of behaviors, rather than as a person with an internal experience as well. Finally, the model is often distorted when applied to prescription of space: behavioristically, decreased space is seen as punishment for bad behavior and increased space, as reward for good. While such experience of space might conceivably apply to the average person, patients in psychotic states may, as noted above, react in the very opposite manner, whereby increased space, for example, may be terrifying rather than rewarding.

The behaviorist paradigm is thus susceptible to the charge that it infringes on patients' rights in ways that do not always offer *immediate* benefit to the patient; that is, this paradigm is designed to effect long-term behavioral change. The legitimacy of such an approach, particularly with the nonconsenting patient, is problematic. Clinical administration, on the other hand, always looks to the procedure that will most immediately benefit the patient, either as treatment, protection, or both; immediate benefit is never sacrificed for long-term behavioral change, although, of course, the latter may well result from a properly administered clinical approach.

4. RIGHTS "VERSUS" NEEDS

Legal authorities understandably place *rights* in the foreground of their perceptions of the patient, the institution and patient care (see Chap. 7, Sec. II-A-2-C). This, however, has the effect of placing the legal authorities on a slightly different track from members of the treatment team, who are mandated to minister to the patient's *needs*. This difference in vector, as it were, may lead to clashes of priorities between the legal and the medical systems.

> *Example 4:* An acutely manic, agitated woman had been room-restricted despite her protests that she wanted "to walk around and get some exercise." A young law student assigned to her case aggressively demanded that she be allowed the "right to this freedom." An inexperienced staff member, intimidated by the lawyer, let the patient out. Panicked, the patient stripped and set fire to her clothing. Now facing a life-threatening emergency, the staff was forced to seclude her.

In this example neither legal nor clinical personnel grasped the fact that in certain clinical states the *right* to a freedom can be extremely dangerous or injurious to a patient whose *need* is for external controls.

Ideally, a patient's needs are met within a context respectful of a patient's rights. But Dr. Alan Stone's cogent comment should be recalled (see Suggested Readings, "The Myth of Advocacy"): "[Legal advocates] have not been willing to consider seriously the needs of the mentally ill and to formulate those needs as rights; [instead] they have treated rights *as if they constituted* the needs of the mentally ill." (Emphasis added.)

This area of potential misunderstanding requires ongoing attention by legal and clinical agencies to ensure synergy between efforts to honor the rights *while* meeting the needs of the mentally ill.

C. Clinical aspects of treatment refusal

From a clinical perspective the origins of treatment refusal are manifold; in addition, the psychology of refusal of medication is not necessarily similar to the psychology of refusal of psychotherapy or of electroconvulsive therapy. Despite this heterogeneity, certain empirically useful generalizations can be proposed about the psychodynamics of treatment refusal. For convenience we might divide the topic into illness factors, treatment factors, and alliance factors.

1. TREATMENT REFUSAL BASED ON FACTORS IN THE ILLNESS

a. Denial

The patient whose illness leads him to *deny* illness, claiming to be in the hospital "for a rest," "to help the other patients," or as a "researcher" or "volunteer," may refuse treatment on this basis; the patient takes the position, "Treatment for *what*? I'm all right."

b. Manic euphoria

In a manner related to denial, a patient in this state presents the position "Everything is wonderful, there are no problems, I feel fine," leading to treatment refusal on that basis.

c. Projection

Clinical states partaking of paranoid mechanisms may demonstrate projection onto others of responsibility for the patient's thoughts, feelings, or experiences; the patient takes the position, "Why should *I* take treatment? *They* are the ones persecuting me."

d. Delusional guilt

In schizophrenia and the psychotic depressions where delusional guilt often plays a prominent role, a patient may feel unentitled to, and undeserving of, help. The innate pessimism, inseparable from the depressed state, moreover, may vitiate any hope of relief, leading to nihilistic despair. The patient's positions may be, "I don't deserve help; I am meant to suffer; I must atone; it's no use and nothing can help."

e. Other delusions and distortions

In various psychotic states patients may refuse treatment on the basis of the specific content of the delusion; for example, "I am the messiah," "People are trying to poison me," etc. Medication seen as a symbol (or seen in terms of a distorted interpretation of its direct effects or side effects) may be incorporated into the delusional system. Similarly, psychotherapy may be experienced delusionally as spells being cast or as being put in someone's power. ECT may be delusionally seen as punishment, execution, or electrocution.

2. TREATMENT REFUSAL BASED ON FACTORS IN THE TREATMENT

Certain aspects of psychiatric treatment itself (not necessarily deleterious ones) may evoke treatment refusal.

a. Primary gain

Since major mental illness often serves restitutive functions, a patient may resist alteration of this "equilibrium"; a typical example is the manic patient who, when treated for her elation, will probably become depressed (or at least less "high") and may resist this transformation, no matter how therapeutically necessary or indicated it may be. Similar points may be made for psychoses as restitutive attempts to deal with psychic pain.

b. Secondary gain

The "sick role" has certain sanctions and gratifications that may be prized by the patient (or family), such as being entitled to attention or special consideration; or receiving "license" to act out, abuse the family, or be taken into a hospital and cared for. Treatment may be refused in order to preserve this role and its special considerations, one of which may be the simple fact of meriting the staff's and the hospital's attention.

c. Specific factors in psychotherapy

By its nature and purpose, psychotherapy addresses in part uncomfortable, unpleasant, or painful aspects of one's experience, and may be resisted on these grounds.

> *Example 5:* A manic patient refused to meet with her doctor for a second appointment, explaining this by shouting, "I don't feel like meeting with you; all you want to do is bum me out [make me depressed]!" This accusation, of course, was partly true, since patients in florid mania cannot truly participate in therapy until returned toward baseline or even to mild depression.

In addition, psychotherapy is inherently slow and time-consuming and may readily evoke impatience and consequent refusal. Finally, it may be refused out of hand on the grounds that "talking won't help."

d. Specific factors in ECT

Despite an efficacy rate in the treatment of major depressions approaching 90% in some studies—an index of success far exceeding that of other remedies—as well as an impressive safety record, ECT remains a frightening prospect, inspiring fantasies comparable to, or greater than, those evoked by major surgery (which it resembles in some ways; e.g., both involve anesthesia). In addition to refusing treatment on the basis of guilt (as noted above), a depressed patient may understandably fear (and hence refuse) the procedure. (We might note, however, that an occasional depressed patient *requests* ECT in part because it is viewed delusionally as "punishment" for depressive guilt.) These fears are augmented if the depression features paranoid elements.

The above-mentioned concerns, coupled with a history in this country of overzealous use (and abuse), have tended to provoke legal authorities to treat ECT in a manner quite different from medication, despite the greater safety and efficacy of ECT in many situations.

e. Specific factors in medication

Portal of entry.   As something ingested or received by injection, medication may evoke refusal in relation to conscious or unconscious conflicts, related to the particular portal of entry into the body.

> *Example 6:* A patient refused nighttime medication but took the same drug and dosage freely during the day. Careful exploration revealed that a fatherly night staff member stirred up profound and conflicted oral yearnings in the patient, making it impossible for him to take anything into the mouth.

> *Example 7:* A violent male patient required intramuscular medication. Weeks later, when improved, he described having interpreted the experience as a homosexual assault which, though administered by a female nurse, came "from the doctor."

Dysphoric response.   There is a category of schizophrenic patients described in the literature who have a dysphoric response to medication, a situation characterized by poor compliance and a poor prognosis. Although it is unclear how many patients respond in this way, refusal may be based on this idiosyncratic reaction.

Side effects.   Like almost all powerful pharmacologic agents, psychotropic medications produce a variety of side effects. These effects, though in general not disproportionate to the efficacy of the medication, can nevertheless be quite disturbing and can prompt drug refusal. The degree of disturbance is greater if the patient has not been prepared to expect them.

The side effects that most commonly produce subjective discomfort fall into several groups, briefly (and not exhaustively) reviewed here (see also Suggested Readings). The nature of the psychological response to the distress occasioned by a given side effect may be idiosyncratic and dependent on the patient's concerns.

- The anticholinergic effects include dry mouth, blurred vision, constipation, and urinary retention, each of which can be variably disturbing. Some patients find visual blurring particularly disturbing; others are more distressed by alteration in bowel regularity.
- The autonomic side effects include postural hypotension, leading to dizziness on abrupt rising to a standing posture.
- The extrapyramidal side effects are often the most subjectively disturbing. These include dystonias and dyskinesias (spasms and abnormalities of movement); akathisia (motor restlessness, occasionally experienced as discomfort

without a movement component); akinesia or stiffness; or tremor and incoordination. When these movement disturbances affect eye muscles and tongue or pharynx musculature, they can be especially upsetting, as the eyes may roll upward, and speech and swallowing may be interfered with.

Fortunately these side effects can almost always be corrected by a change in medication, a change in dosage, or the administration of a second medication to counter these effects. However, the fear of these effects or their actual appearance may promote medication refusal.

Tardive dyskinesia (TD).   This side effect is the most problematic for the psychiatric profession and is the one most seized upon by legal and other opponents of pharmacotherapy. The term refers to lasting (tardive) effects of medication that may involve movement disorders (dyskinesias) of face and tongue musculature, as well as muscles of the extremities and more rarely other parts of the body. Fear of, or the appearance of, this effect may lead to medication refusal, although patients are often not conscious of the existence of the abnormal movements.

This deleterious effect of antipsychotic medication use poses several problems. First, in terms of diagnosis, a careful reading of Kraepelin's observations of schizophrenics, in the century before phenothiazines were first synthesized, reveals descriptions of movement disorders appearing in late life and strikingly resembling TD. Second, concerning prevention, this effect appears at times to occur even following relatively brief exposure to medication at low doses. Third, treatment response for TD has been variable but generally poor; at present, research in treating TD, though extremely active, remains at an embryonic stage.

Given the current irreplaceable importance of medications in the treatment of major mental illness and in facilitating the return of patients to the community, tardive dyskinesia must be viewed as a risk to be carefully weighed against the benefits, as with all treatments.

3. TREATMENT REFUSAL BASED ON FACTORS IN THE DOCTOR-PATIENT RELATIONSHIP

Compliance with treatment (see Suggested Readings) has repeatedly been shown to correlate directly with the quality of the doctor-patient relationship; a durable therapeutic alliance based on mutual trust and respect appears to be one of the best treatment-motivating factors. Conversely, distrust, hostility, or other alliance-threatening feelings may express themselves in the refusal of proffered treatment (a mode of expression, of course, not limited to psychiatry but true of medical practice in general). The major areas of difficulty follow.

a. Transference

During intensive therapeutic work, powerful feelings deriving from early, including infantile, experiences may be stirred up and may fasten upon (be "transferred" to) the therapist; these so-called transference feelings may represent the inappropriate application to the therapist of either *realistic* assessments of the primary object ("the therapist seems to me to be as mean and cold-hearted as my father") or frankly *delusional* perceptions ("I am the Messiah and the therapist is my apostle, Peter") that distort, through imagination, the early relationships.

On the basis of these transference feelings, a patient may refuse to accept treatment offered by the object of such emotions.

b. Reality

In addition to the transference elements noted above, reality factors of all descriptions may interfere with the collaborative mutuality of the doctor-patient relationship; these interferences may breed treatment refusal in readily comprehensible ways.

Trust failures represent major interferences: the therapist who deceives, financially or sexually exploits, or knowingly misinforms the patient; who breaches confidentiality without permission; or who acts in other ways contrary to the patient's best interests may forfeit the patient's trust and cooperation with the treatment plan.

Chronic irritation may precipitate treatment refusal. A therapist who is always late, too forgetful, cancels appointments repeatedly, is often unavailable without coverage, and commits similar recurrent peccadilloes may engender sufficient anger that the patient refuses treatment.

c. Intimacy

The intensity, shared confidences, and depth of emotional involvement in the therapeutic relationship naturally breed intimacy but may breed conflicts as well, as in Example 3, above; treatment refusal may represent a patient's mode of withdrawal from conflicts around closeness.

d. Vacations

The therapist's vacation, a common occurrence in therapy, deserves special mention as a factor in treatment refusal from the viewpoints of both transference and reality. Issues of separation and abandonment mobilized by the vacation may unleash powerful feelings of rage, terror, and sorrow, barely credible to the non-clinician. Vacations are a familiar cause for patients, normally treatment compliant, suddenly to discontinue their medications, occasionally to the point of decompensation and of need for hospitalization. The psychological issue, conscious or unconscious, often takes a retaliatory form: "If you won't stay around, I won't take 'your' medication."

e. Family pressures

Families of inpatients may interfere in the doctor-patient relationship from a number of motives: jealousy of the doctor-patient intimacy, competition with the treatment team over who is more helpful, struggles over the patient's loyalty to hospital versus family, and so on. Family rivalry over who "feeds" the patient better may play itself out in relation to medication, the doctor's "special food." Treatment refusal may express a patient's response to these family pressures.

f. Autonomy

This element enters into the doctor-patient relationship in both direct and transferential ways. A patient may feel an intense need to maintain the boundaries of his own self against the actual or experienced incursions of intrusive family members and, by extension, of the intrusively experienced clinician. The patient may thus attempt to defend his embattled autonomy by saying "no" to treatment (and commonly to other expectations, such as taking showers, eating hospital food, changing clothing, and participating in groups).

An irony of this element lies in the fact that the drive toward autonomy is an essential positive factor in the recovery process—a factor that here may operate in the reverse direction, toward maintaining the pathologic status quo. The clinician is challenged to preserve the patient's autonomous strivings while, paradoxically, attempting to contravene them in the service of treatment.

g. Other elements

An early study of drug refusal revealed that refusal was often used by chronically ill, severely thought-disordered patients as a nonspecific method of communicating individualized distress from a wide variety of causes, such as frustration and as a means of expressing a wish to talk with staff, a request for attention, and the like.

D. Clinical approaches to managing treatment refusal

1. Exploration of issues

The psychodynamics of an individual patient's refusal of treatment are fully as legitimate a topic of therapeutic investigation as those matters that brought the patient to the hospital. The patient's posture of denial, persistence in repetitive patterns of self-defeating behavior, delusional guilt, or other problems should be explored in the customary manner in relation to treatment refusal. At times the legalistic atmosphere now surrounding the "right to refuse treatment" issue can obscure the fact that refusal is, at base, far more nearly a psychological problem than a legal one; the clinician must attend to the issue in treatment. In particular, clinicians must actively resist the temptation to shift immediately into an adversarial posture and to invoke too readily the legal mechanisms for "processing" treatment refusal cases before careful clinical exploration has taken place.

2. Maintaining the alliance posture

The patient's refusal of the therapist's recommended treatment places the two parties in an oppositional stance that represents, most significantly, a threat to the treatment alliance. Faced with this problem, the clinician must address and recruit the highest level of the patient's functioning that remains available; the clinician allies himself with this level. Practically, such an approach requires seeing refusal as a problem facing the *dyad,* not the therapist or the patient alone.

3. Amelioration of causative influences

In addition to the psychotherapeutic investigation/intervention described above, specific influences leading to refusal may be identified and ameliorated directly. Subjectively troublesome side effects may be managed in the usual ways; ventilation of unexpressed hostility may be encouraged; misinformation about the medication may be corrected through education; conflicts and impasses on the ward may be resolved; family members may be involved constructively; and interpersonal attention may be paid in various ways. All these responses may correct the problematic situation that sparked refusal.

4. ALTERNATIVES IN THE FACE OF PERSISTENT REFUSAL OF TREATMENT

The clinician faced with a patient whose refusal does not respond to the approaches described above has a number of options available, though none is totally satisfactory.

a. Discharge

As in other medical situations an inpatient who refuses recommended treatment may be discharged. This otherwise equitable solution regrettably is often precluded by the fact that the patient may not be in a clinical condition that allows discharge (as is often the case in the very population most likely to refuse). When clinically and ethically feasible, however, discharge presents an acceptable response to persistent refusal.

b. Commitment

In some jurisdictions, committed patients may be involuntarily treated while voluntary patients are not. In these cases, clinicians may petition for commitment of a voluntary, refusing patient under the statutes that apply. Permission to treat may be thus directly or indirectly granted (but see Sec. II-C-2).

c. Role of ward staff in treating treatment refusal

An early study on overt drug refusal revealed a finding nearly ignored in the literature on drug treatment: the critical importance of the *nurse*-patient alliance in resolution of refusal. Therapeutic work, reassurance, coaxing, and persuasion on the part of the medication nurse proved to be pivotal influences in reducing medication refusal to a mere 24-hour problem in most instances. In similar ways, nursing and other ward staff may play vital roles in reversing refusal by means of positive, caring relationships with the patient.

d. Use of formal mechanisms to adjudicate treatment refusal

As indicated in Section II-C, the states have put in place—through case law, statute, or regulation—a wide variety of mechanisms to adjudicate the issue when the patient refuses treatment. These mechanisms usually involve determination of the patient's competence and the invocation of a number of vicarious decisionmakers, ranging from the treating psychiatrist to a judge, to decide about treatment. Clinicians are expected to familiarize themselves with current rulings in their own jurisdictions.

Clinicians should, however, remember the importance of an alliance-based relationship with the patient, even when acting so as to contravene her expressed wishes. In addition, in legal or quasi-legal settings such as hearings and formal consultative processes, clinicians should do their homework. They should prepare themselves appropriately by familiarizing themselves with the patient's history, especially in terms of previous responses to treatment, and present the material confidently and forthrightly. Pre-hearing conferences with hospital attorneys or similar individuals are an essential part of the clinician's preparation.

In some jurisdictions, legal guardianship for the incompetent patient is the mechanism invoked to respond to the problem of treatment refusal. This issue is addressed in detail in Chapter Five. If the vicarious decision-making mechanism results in the finding that the patient may indeed refuse treatment, clinicians should not view this outcome as a defeat. Clinical efforts at persuasion and recommendation should continue, and every effort should be made to invoke the other modalities of treatment of the modern milieu. The patient's further deterioration should trigger a prompt return to the decision-making body for a rehearing and reassessment. Clinicians may also consider reapplication (i.e., repetitioning) when a different judge is sitting or even, under particularly egregious circumstances, appeal of lower court decisions. While, as noted above, treatment refusal may trigger questions about discharge, such discharge should never be merely retaliatory in response to a negative legal finding.

E. Clinical approaches to involuntary treatment

Formal review of patients' refusal of treatment may result in authorization to begin involuntary treatment, which raises a number of clinical issues.

1. MAINTAINING ALLIANCE PRIMACY

Even in a clearly oppositional situation in which the patient's stated (albeit delusionally founded) refusal is being overruled, the therapist should still attempt to speak to the healthy side of the patient's ego, emphasizing the rationale for this course of action and including exploration of the patient's feelings and reactions as a legitimate part of the procedure. The patient's attention is directed to previous positive effects of medication, if any, and to the role of treatment in rapid release from the hospital. Efforts directed toward involuntary treatment should be described candidly in terms of their purpose in serving the patient's *interests*, though contrary to the patient's *wishes*. The clinician should take an unequivocal stand against psychotic distortions of the treatment situation and maintain a realistic view of the patient's medical needs.

2. DOCUMENTATION

It should again be emphasized that at all stages of the proceedings there must be careful documentation of all facts pertinent to the decision to institute involuntary treatment. These include:

- Diagnosis and validating information
- Indications for use of treatment and rationale for appropriateness of that particular treatment
- History, if any, of previous treatment(s) and success/failure of same
- Grounds for belief that refusal is clearly a product of the illness; i.e., refusal is incompetent
- Legal proceedings and outcomes
- Progress of treatment once initiated

3. RETURN TO VOLUNTARY TREATMENT

As soon as possible and clinically feasible a patient should be invited to participate voluntarily in treatment; this change should be discussed in anticipation of its arrival, and the subject should be kept open during the changeover.

The opportunity should not be lost to explore in detail the dynamic and environmental bases for refusal to render them explicit, not only for therapeutic understanding but for future reference in case of relapse and rehospitalization. Since a number of mechanisms for deciding about treatment refusal employ a model based on what the competent patient wants, careful notes should be made about the patient's reasoning in deciding to resume treatment. These data may be of central import at later legal proceedings. (See also Chapter Five.)

F. Clinical aspects of the request to leave the hospital

The freedom to leave the hospital is an important right for the patient that must be honored to preserve the voluntarity of hospitalization whenever possible. It should be a matter of course, however, to treat the request to leave the hospital as legitimate material for clinical exploration which, like any other topic, offers an opportunity to understand the dynamic context in which it arises. We refer here to formal requests to leave as provided by law, rather than simply the patient's verbal initiation of the subject of discharge.

1. EXPLORATION OF UNDERLYING ISSUES

On an inpatient ward, submission of a request to leave (often by means of a form that gives a few days notice of the wish to leave) commonly heralds the emergence of the affects of anger or fear in the patient. Some of the precipitants to these affects include:

a. Anger or frustration at doctor, staff, or institution

Example 8: Feeling considerable distress, a patient came to the medication station urgently requesting an optional dose ("p.r.n.") of medication. The medication nurse, busy with another patient, said she would have to wait. Angered, the patient loudly demanded a discharge request form. After signing it, the patient spoke at length to the med nurse and resolved her anger. She then signed a retraction of her request.

b. Fears, both real and paranoid, of other patients or staff

Example 9: When a patient witnessed an attack on staff by a violent patient, barely controlled by available personnel, she was extremely frightened by this display; she impulsively signed a discharge request and, at its expiration, left the hospital.

Example 10: A patient developed the delusion that the other patients on the ward were discussing him telepathically in a pejorative way. Fearing that they were conspiring to harm him, he signed a request to leave. Medication and active reality testing by staff corrected the delusion and the patient retracted his request.

c. Other dynamic issues

These include conflicts around closeness and intimacy; fears of being trapped; and dread of disloyalty to, or separation from, the family.

2. THE ALLIANCE ISSUE

From the viewpoint of therapeutic exploration the formal request to be discharged represents a potential strain on the alliance; the patient's leaving in this way derives from a unilateral exercise of legal rights, in contrast to the collaborative negotiation of the jointly planned and explored discharge. In other words, while the patient's formal request to be discharged is sanctioned by law (and discharge may be clinically indicated), the opportunity has been lost to accomplish this step within the alliance.

Therapeutic exploration should be directed to this lost opportunity: what feelings, thoughts, assumptions kept doctor and patient from working in concert toward the goal of a planned discharge, just as other goals in treatment are jointly explored and achieved?

3. THE DECISION TO COMMIT: CLINICAL IMPACT

This issue was explored in Chapter 2, but we might in summary review the issue here from a clinical standpoint.

a. Clinical effects of decision to seek commitment

positive: alliance improved through demonstration of concern; provision of "holding," "containing" patient's impulses, etc.

negative: decrease in autonomy and responsibility, feeling trapped (panic, regression); interpreting commitment as seduction, aggression, etc.

b. Clinical effects of decision not to seek commitment (to release patient)

positive: enhancement of autonomy, turning over responsibility to patient, avoiding regression, etc.

negative: rejection, separation fears, failure of concern ("They don't care about me"), etc.

G. Clinical aspects of involuntary discharge

Involuntary (also termed mandatory or administrative) discharge may occur in different ways that require individually distinct modes of reasoning, documentation, and clinical management (see also Chap. 2, Sec. III-E-5, and Sec. II-D-4 above.)

1. CLINICALLY DETERMINED INVOLUNTARY DISCHARGE

The most common type of involuntary discharge occurs when an inpatient is restored to the level of health or functioning clinically consonant with being an outpatient, in consequence of which the doctor recommends discharge. However, the patient may feel (as often happens) dependent on or attached to the hospital; fearful of, or reluctant to face, the difficulties of the world "outside"; resistant to the loss of regressive gratifications and to the demands of autonomy; or unwilling to return to family. Profound feelings of separation, loss, and abandonment may be evoked by even an optimal discharge. Thus, from the patient's point of view, the planned discharge is involuntary.

It should be noted that these feelings of reluctance to leave the hospital are not necessarily indices of the inappropriateness of the initial hospitalization, the inpatient management of the case, or the length of stay, or of the inefficacy of the treatment modalities utilized. The flywheel of human inertia turns ponderously, and many persons, not all ill, resist alteration in the status quo. Surprising as it may seem to the layperson, moreover, the shabbiest, dingiest, most verminous hospital may represent—through provision and availability of caring staff—the most consistent, reliable, and gratifying environment that some patients have ever known (see Suggested Readings—Simon).

The clinical management of this type of involuntary discharge rests on the principle of the primacy of the patient's needs, even when (on occasion) they run contrary to the patient's wishes. Hospitalization, like other treatments, outlives its usefulness and may produce "toxic" side effects, such as regression, loss of outside connections, and excessive dependency. The patient's objections to leaving are appropriate clinical material to be addressed in the usual manner, to identify subjective and objective elements, and to work through the affects around separation, loss, autonomy and growth.

In the situation where a patient is being discharged against medical advice, the clinician appropriately may attempt to use the AMA form (or its local equivalent) as a concrete focus for further exploration; the form embodies the clinician's position of disapproval of the timing of the discharge.

It is clinically valuable for an AMA discharge always to be considered as inferior to a negotiated discharge. The clinician queries, "Why must we retreat to legalistic methods to allow you to leave, instead of working together to plan the best possible discharge and aftercare for you? Why can we not work this out doctor-to-patient without dragging lawyers in?"

This approach frequently uncovers the patient's transference-based perceptions of the clinician (deriving from parental models) as inherently frustrating, opposed to autonomy, controlling, and coercive; these perceptions become thus available for exploration in the usual manner.

2. LAPSE OF INSURANCE AND ITS CLINICAL CONSEQUENCES

In order to be eligible for funding under the Hill-Burton Act, private hospitals must treat a specified percentage of nonpaying patients. The majority of hospitals rapidly fill this quota, and thus patients whose illnesses outlast their coverage are asked to leave; frequently they are transferred to state facilities. Aggressive concurrent review by third party payers may result in a refusal to pay for further hospitalization with similar results.

Since the physical plant, levels of care, and other parameters usually vary dramatically between the public and private sectors, the change experienced by the patient may be dramatic. The only study of this phenomenon, "When the Insurance Money Runs Out" (see Suggested Readings—Rivinus and Gutheil) disclosed that the effect was not entirely a negative one, since some of the subjects in the study were merely "passing time" in the private setting and felt the impact of the public setting as mobilizing; additionally, some subjects, viewing the grimmer public facility as an ominous harbinger of chronic illness and institutionalization, experienced more keenly their underlying depression. In any case, good and considerate patient care entails careful attention, both from sender and recipient hospital, to the patient's difficult adjustment in the transfer and to the often dramatic reactions by family members.

If insurance coverage has been limited by the third-party payer, clinicians may have an obligation to appeal the decision prior to discharging a patient who they believe continues to need in-patient care. Whether a hospital has a duty to retain a patient whose insurance will no longer pay for her hospitalization is unclear at this point. The answer in a given case may relate to the degree of need for in-patient care and the availability of other options.

3. EXPIRATION OF COURT-ORDERED COMMITMENTS

Occasionally, when a commitment on a patient elapses, the patient may wish to sign in voluntarily; however, the clinician may feel (for various reasons) that this is a regressive move or otherwise not in the patient's interests. Thus, the refusal of a desired voluntary continuation of hospitalization constitutes an involuntary discharge.

The patient's experience of this event is inevitably one of rejection, often resonating with past experiences. Once again, the appeal to the most autonomous and adult side of the patient constitutes the crux of the clinician's approach to this issue; the patient's long-term welfare is placed ahead of his wishes. Since a patient's voluntary admission may in other instances represent a desirable event, connoting a willingness to participate in treatment, the discharge may be difficult to explain to nonprofessionals, should that become necessary; the clinician should therefore clearly document the reasoning and the bases for the decision not to honor the request for voluntary stay.

4. INVOLUNTARY DISCHARGE FOR DANGEROUSNESS OR DISRUPTIVENESS

The inpatient clinician must constantly weigh and balance the arms of a dual responsibility: to the individual patient and to the ward population as a whole. (The latter viewpoint is usually absent from legal conceptualizations, which tend to view the patient and his care in a vacuum.) Consider this example:

Example 11: On repeated occasions a volatile, impulsive patient with a character disorder had lashed out at staff when confronted about her disruptive behavior. Staff weathered this for a time until the patient attacked another patient who refused to give her a cigarette. Since the subject patient was not psychotic, it was felt that the risk to the other patients was greater than the risk to the community (where unlike on the ward, the potential victim could leave the scene); she was discharged, protesting her wish to remain.

In understanding this example, we must note the importance of assessing the patient's "differential dangerousness" on or off the ward, a factor related to committability; the presence or absence of psychosis, as well as its treatability; and the degree of danger to other patients. Crowding on inpatient units may, itself, be a stimulus to aggression for some patients.

The staff response to the behavior in the example varies with the clinical state to which the response is addressed, according to the principles of clinical administration. For the psychotic patient whose assault is often the result of stimulus-related tension overwhelming burdened defenses, the patient is moved *in* to closer observation and decreased stimulation. For the impulsive patient, firm external controls and the setting of limits are essentials of treatment: hence the patient may be moved *out* as a limit-setting response conveying the message "You cannot do that here."

For better or worse, hospital staff are expected to accept *some* degree of risk of assault (even with attendant injury) within limits; the degree of tolerable risk is different for the patient population, who are under staff's protection.

It should also be noted that this type of involuntary discharge is at base in the *patient's* interests, since the guilt, anxiety, or criminal charges that may result from continued assaultiveness are clearly detrimental to the assaulter.

A controversial alternative to involuntary discharge for dangerousness is the use of criminal proceedings against the patient; this issue has been described in a limited literature under the rubric of prosecuting patients for assaults on staff (see Suggested Readings). In this model, the hospital staff presses charges against the patient, either by having the assaulted staff member bring the charge or by encouraging the assaulted patient to do so. This legalistic solution may have some value in dealing with personality disordered patients as a form of external limit setting; however, with more severely emotionally disordered individuals, the legal system is often quite indifferent to pursuing these cases.

An interesting compromise mechanism is for court officials (e.g., the clerk of the court) to open a folder on the case, as it were, but to take no formal legal action. The legal system explains to the patient that he is now on a kind of informal probation and that repeated offenses will result in formal prosecution. No reliable empirical data exist concerning the long-term efficacy of such an intervention; in at least one study, some patients became unmanageable or were lost to treatment as a result of these proceedings. Thus, this intervention must be considered of uncertain utility.

5. INVOLUNTARY DISCHARGE FOR INFRACTION OF RULES

Though related to the previous section, this category extends to areas that are matters of policy rather than representing danger or inherent disruptiveness.

In some hospitals and on some wards, specific actions are considered violations of the rules and may be grounds for administrative responses, including discharge. Examples might include bringing alcohol, drugs, or weapons onto the ward; engaging in sexual or other physical contact with other patients; or coming late or being absent too often for scheduled activities. Whenever possible, of course, patients should be informed, verbally or by brochure, what the rules and expectations are, and—except for blatant criminal acts like rape or drug dealing—the patient should be given the benefit of the doubt. Needless to say, all these data should be well documented and actively explored as therapeutic issues to discover the dynamic bases for the acting out.

In this consideration we should not lose sight of the specific value to the patient's treatment of an attitude of responsibility and accountability for one's actions and behavior, for hospital rules no less than societal.

6. INVOLUNTARY DISCHARGE FOR TREATMENT REFUSAL

As indicated earlier (Sec. III-D-4-a), the clinician, faced with a patient who undeviatingly refuses the prescribed treatment despite all efforts, has the recourse of discharging the patient and no longer assuming responsibility for his inpatient care. Again, this response presumes that the patient's clinical condition permits discharge with maintenance of ethical standards of practice, the grounds for this assessment being appropriately delineated in the record.

The clinician's next move, however, is fraught with ambiguity. To continue to see the patient on, say, an outpatient basis is to support the patient in a suboptimal mode of treatment; to attempt to refer the patient is problematic, since the clinician is attempting in effect to find someone who will do for the patient what the referring clinician considers bad practice; to cast the patient utterly "to the winds" does represent respect for the latter's freedom of choice but must evoke reluctance on the clinician's part to participate in so total a rejection, especially when the patient's decompensation in the not-too-distant future may be predicted.

In so complex a knot, the clinician is best guided by adherence to an "open door" policy, thus: "Should you at some future time decide to comply with my prescribed regimen, you may, of course, return to treatment here." It is a clinically validated (but ethically complex) observation that certain patients have to be hospitalized several times in succession at the onset of their illness before they fully grasp its seriousness and fully understand that it will not "go away" by itself; on occasion treatment refusal is a component in this posture of denial.

IV. PITFALLS

A. Countertransference factors in the right to treatment

The clinician is frequently subject to conflicting tropisms toward and away from the inpatient in need. The positive side of this ambivalence may be manifested by excessive treatment zeal and "rescue fantasies." The latter term describes a blind therapeutic optimism that may overlook the indispensable role in treatment of the patient's own motivation and wish to change, so that the therapist is actually more eager than the patient that delusions be given up, that suffering be faced and worked through, and that pathogenic relationships be terminated. The costs of this attitude are diminution of the patient's central responsibility in her illness and treatment; a coercive posture that, in effect, unilaterally demands recovery no matter what the patient's desires may be; and an intrusion on the development of the patient's own capacities to make responsible decisions. Coercive measures taken in the name of a right to treatment may thus eventuate in the negation of positive steps toward change.

Equally problematic is the negative side of this equation wherein the clinician withdraws from the stresses of engagement with the seriously ill patient and, in effect, discharges the patient or refuses to provide needed treatment on the basis of a wish to be rid of him rather than on clinical grounds, thus effectively depriving the patient of a right to treatment. The ideal position for the clinician is one that permits the patient maximal freedom, responsibility, and self-determination; only in those instances where the patient cannot safely function in this way is the clinician obligated to intervene authoritatively.

B. Countertransference factors in patients' rights

As noted earlier, the clinician must be attentive to the patient's needs in a context of rights. Inappropriate guilt or other conflicts may be evoked by the interventions in clinical administration, as when, for example, the clinician cannot stand to seclude the out-of-control patient because it would mean "depriving him of freedom." Here a moralistic (rather than clinical) view leaves the patient untreated, and his needs unmet.

Another countertransference issue seen in teaching settings is what may be called "legal defense as ego defense" (see Suggested Readings—Gutheil). In this instance, the clinician-trainee retreats into legalism to avoid the strains of empathic engagement with the seriously ill patient; the legal issues preoccupy the trainee to the detriment of clear perception of the patient as suffering person.

C. Countertransference factors in treatment refusal

Refusal of treatment may be experienced inappropriately by the clinician as a narcissistic injury; as one saying goes, "Telling a doctor his pills are no good is like telling a mother her baby is ugly." In addition, the clinician may feel this refusal as a personal rejection rather than as the outgrowth of factors already detailed. The pitfalls here might be of two kinds: a punitive or rejecting response that essentially abandons the patient; or, by reaction formation, an avoidance of the conflict, expressed by failure to pursue the approaches and alternatives earlier described as responses to treatment refusal.

In refusal deriving from depressive mood, where the patient feels undeserving of help and is blinded by depressive pessimism as to the hope of recovery, a pitfall may manifest itself in the clinician's succumbing to the depressive position and becoming convinced of the futility of intervention and the hopelessness of the situation. This miscarriage of empathy obscures the generally quite hopeful prognosis in depression—a prognosis the clinician must keep firmly in mind to counter contagious depressive conviction.

D. Countertransference factors in involuntary treatment, hospitalization, and discharge

Direct opposition to a patient's stated wish or intent may evoke fantasies and conflicts around aggression and sadism, no matter how thoroughly the involuntary intervention has been sanctioned by due process. Conflict in these areas, especially in regard to evoked guilt for opposing the patient's wish, may produce its effect through *inaction:* failure to petition for commitment, failure to seek guardianship, and failure to intervene decisively in an emergency. Open discussion among treatment personnel and legal counsel, and clinical consultation and supervision may mitigate these difficulties.

Factors related to involuntary commitment have been reviewed in Chapter 2; in summary, the decision to commit may be contaminated by wishes to control, keep, contain, or coerce the patient for reasons other than statutory criteria of committability; and inappropriate release (or involuntary discharge) may be fostered by decathexis of, frustration by, or hostility toward the patient, as by over-identification with the patient's wish to leave, denial of illness, or flight from engagement in treatment.

V. CASE EXAMPLE EPILOGUES

A. Case Example 1

Supervisor and resident both agree that the patient is receiving little benefit from continued hospitalization. The options appear to be: (1) continuing in the current state until the initial commitment expires, while making ongoing efforts to reengage the patient; (2) obtaining a judicial order of incompetency that would permit the patient's involuntary treatment; and (3) discharging the patient.

The supervisor points out that the reaction the patient appears to be having is not uncommon among paranoid schizophrenic patients, who often develop positive feelings for therapists of the same sex, only to panic at what they fear are signs of homosexuality. Unable to tolerate that thought, they then project those feelings on to the therapist. This patient's refusal of medication and of further contact with the resident both appear to stem from the fear that these represent attempts by the resident at control and penetration. Given such a situation, further efforts at legal coercion into treatment (e.g., guardianship)—though often necessary in other cases to resolve such an impasse—are likely to be seen by this patient as intrusive, assaultive actions that only confirm his fears and doom future long-term collaboration.

In the absence of positive benefit from hospitalization, and with clear contraindications to the more intrusive options, the therapist is asked to consider whether any indications exist for continued hospitalization. It is pointed out to him that the judicial commitment order actually allows retention of the patient for "up to" six months, but gives the psychiatrist discretion as to when the patient may be able to be released before then.

With that advice, the resident rethinks the situation and concludes that the patient is no longer imminently dangerous to anyone. Although clearly in need of treatment, he is not getting any direct help in the hospital. The resident recognizes the dynamics underlying his need to refuse treatment at this time and decides that letting his refusal stand may facilitate future cooperation. Despite the fact that the patient appears quite comfortable on the ward and has not at any point asked to leave, discharge appears to be the only means of honoring the patient's autonomy while maintaining the posture of the hospital as a place in which active treatment takes place. It has the further advantage of bringing home to the patient the need to accept responsibility for the consequences of his acts.

The resident notifies the family and informs the patient that discharge is being recommended. The family comes to the hospital for several stormy sessions in which they accuse the hospital of failing to take proper care of their son, but the resident firmly explains to them that he sees little medical value in detaining him any longer. The patient is released after he has had a chance to make plans for himself. Outpatient appointments are arranged, but the patient never appears. Six months later, the resident receives a phone call informing him that the patient has been hospitalized for several weeks in another nearby institution and is again refusing treatment.

B. Case Example 2

The consultant, herself an experienced clinician in addition to her legal expertise, ponders the dilemma, then makes the following recommendations.

She suggests that, though doing "nothing" would be a mistake, the staff should not struggle so hard, since to do so is clearly inciting such a patient to greater self-destructive activity in the service of obtaining attention. She speculates that this pattern repeats a family situation where the patient's chronically depressed, withdrawn mother could be drawn out of her apathy only by the patient's harming himself, at which the mother would feel compelled to proffer grudging attention.

The consultant recommends that all staff meet together to review and implement a treatment plan, carefully documented, as follows: the patient should be told in simple language that staff cannot intervene in these episodes without fruitless encroachment on his rights; that the patient will be observed after a swallowing or banging event, but will not be extensively worked up medically unless gross symptoms develop.

The chief resident protests, "But something could happen to him before we knew about it! That's pretty risky, it seems to me."

The consultant nods. "A calculated risk, yes, but the alternatives are more destructive to sound care over the long haul. Remember, we aren't in the business of stopping people from each and every short-term harm; we must rehabilitate the whole patient in a lasting way."

The treatment team, dubiously at first, applies the plan. Over about two weeks, indeed, the patient loses interest in the "game," settles down, and begins a vocational program.

C. Case Example 3

Finding the supervisor free, the psychology intern introduces himself. Apologizing for starting off the year with a problem, the intern describes the situation and shares his dismay at being, however inadvertently, a participant in an apparent breach of civil liberties; the patient is, indeed, not being permitted his legally mandated calls nor being allowed to sign out. He waxes resentful of being "set up" in this manner by being assigned a new case in which the patient is already probably biased against him, the intern, because of having his rights violated.

The supervisor patiently hears out the intern and invites him to sit down. She explains that the patient in question *cannot* sign out since he is here on a court commitment for evaluation of competence to stand trial. He can only be returned to court.

"Did you ask him what his charge is?" the supervisor inquires.

"Well, no," the intern admits.

"It's his umpteenth arrest for making harassing phone calls. This guy makes limitless calls to his lawyer, the superintendent, the governor, the senate, the White House; deluges them with paranoid nonsense; and turns harassing when they don't yield to his delusional demands. He has shown that he can get calls out of places you wouldn't believe—maximum security, you name it. He also gets other patients to place the calls; the victim doesn't recognize the name, then he gets on the line and harasses him. He has somehow managed to get two calls off despite the fact that we have him on *absolute phone restrictions.*"

The psychology intern rubs his forehead, abashed. "I—I guess I didn't get the whole picture."

The supervisor is reassuring. "He can get past anyone, we've seen that. Don't worry about it. Just remember: even rights have exceptions, when the rights of others are affected."

The intern nods. "My first lesson. I'll go up and talk this over with him. By the way, how did he get those scars on his mouth?"

The supervisor looks grim. "They do that in prison—when you talk too much."

VI. ACTION GUIDE

A. Right to Treatment Checklist

1. *Provide* psychiatric and medical evaluations immediately after admission and before any medications are administered.
2. *Mandate* development of individualized treatment plan within 48 hours of admission with attention to:
   a. Underlying psychiatric illness, if known;
   b. Further diagnostic procedures needed;
   c. Precipitating stresses and measures planned to ameliorate them;
   d. Proposed use of medication or other somatic treatments, based, if possible, on history of previous response;
   e. Bahavioral problems that might interfere with inpatient treatment and suggested response;
   f. Involvement of family and friends in patient's care;
   g. Assessment of social and vocational skills, with appropriate rehabilitative measures;
   h. Early attention to postdischarge planning including plans for housing, income, and follow-up care;
   i. Maximal possible participation of patient in treatment and post-discharge planning.
3. *Allocate* adequate staff to implement treatment plan.
4. *Maintain* physical facilities to implement treatment plan.
5. *Require* formal, periodic review of patient's hospital course and progress towards goals as outlined in treatment plan; *revise* treatment plan as necessary.
6. *File* model bills with legislatures to provide needed services.

B. Other Rights in Hospital Checklist

1. *Allow* visitation
   a. By family and friends subject to reasonable limitation on hours and requirements of patient's condition;
   b. Maximum possible access for *attorneys, private physicians, and members of the clergy.*
2. *Promote* communication by granting:
   a. Access to public telephone to make and to receive confidential calls, subject to limitation only if clearly contraindicated by patient's condition or by patient's abuse of the telephone (e.g., threatening calls);
   b. Uncensored mailing privileges for both sending and receiving letters;
      i. *Provide* reasonable amounts of stamps and stationery, if otherwise unavailable to patient;
      ii. *Screen* outgoing mail only if reason to believe that others are being placed at risk.
3. *Ensure privacy* by providing for:
   a. Use and secure storage of personal possessions;
   b. Private toilet and shower facilites;
   c. No access of third parties to records without patient's consent.

    4. *Foster* economic rights by allowing:
       a. Appropriate use of reasonable amounts of money;
       b. Right to manage personal affairs.
    5. *Recognize* right to be paid for work performed.
    6. *Respect* miscellaneous rights:
       a. Right to vote,
       b. Right to marry or divorce,
       c. Right to reasonable living conditions,
       d. Right to notification of all rights.
    7. *Civil Rights Officer*—Provide for one who is freely available to patients to handle complaints of abridgement of rights.

C. Responses to Medication Refusal and the Wish to Leave the Hospital. (N.B.: These are considered together since initial responses are similar.)

    1. *Identify* underlying issues, conflict, medication problem, vacation, delusional percept, milieu stress, family pressure.
    2. *Explore* identified issue as legitimate therapeutic material in usual ways (clarification, interpretation, reality testing, ventilation).
    3. *Recruit* adult, healthy side of patient into alliance, appealing to realistic perception of long-range benefits of treatment/hospitalization.
    4. *Ameliorate* contributory factors (counter medication side effects, work through crisis issues, promote staff discussion, resolve milieu disputes, obtain consultations as needed, intensify or redirect casework with families).

D. Responses to Persistent Refusal of Medication (or Other Treatment of Choice)

    1. *Consider* possibilities of alternative treatment and *decide* if alternatives, though accepted by patient, constitute negligent, suboptimal, or unethical treatment.
    2. *Offer* alternative treaters, if feasible, who may accept patient's preferred treatment and *transfer* responsibility.
    3. *Consider* discharge as possibility if clinical condition warrants this; *arrange* for appropriate aftercare and follow-up.
    4. If discharge contraindicated, *seek* appropriate authorization to permit involuntary treatment.
    5. *Prepare* for review proceedings.

E. Involuntary Treatment Checklist

    1. *Document*
       a. Need/justification for treatment;
       b. Reason alternative modes of treatment are inappropriate;
       c. Reason refusal is viewed as incompetent (delusional content, expressed reasons, muteness, characteristics of clinical state);
       d. Anticipated response to specific treatment, risks/benefits, history of previous treatment response.

2. *Inform* patient of rationale, reasons for treating against wishes, legal authorizations of treatment, legal recourses for patient.
3. *Treat* while monitoring results and *attempt* to return patient to voluntary treatment collaboration as soon as possible.

F. Response to Persistent Attempts to Leave the Hospital

1. *Assess* committability by standards proposed by local applicable statutes. If not petitionable,
2. *Assess* whether discharge should be "against medical advice" and if so respond by offering form and/or documenting this view.
3. If committability standards are met, *petition* for commitment and *await* judicial decision.
4. *Offer* aftercare plan with follow-up, provisions for return, "open door" attitude.
5. *Maintain* position of alliance as possible even during oppositional phase.

G. Countertransference Difficulties

1. *Avoid* rescue fantasies, wish to control patient, doing for patient what patient can do for self.
2. *Resist* succumbing to depressive pessimism, despair, manic insouciance, delusional world view.
3. *Work through* inapposite conflicts in areas of sadism, guilt, or anxiety around needed interventions.
4. *Obtain* consultation, both legal and supervisory, as needed.

VII. SUGGESTED READINGS

A. The Right to Treatment

1. Birnbaum, M.: The right to treatment. *American Bar Association Journal* 46: 499–505, 1960.

2. Mills, M. J.: The right to treatment: little law, but much impact, in L. Grinspoon (ed.): *Psychiatry 1982*: The American Psychiatric Association Annual Review. Washington, D.C., American Psychiatric Press, 1982.

3. Jones, L. R. & Parlour, R. R. (eds.): *Wyatt v. Stickney: Retrospect and Prospect.* New York, Grune and Stratton, 1981.

4. Santiago, J. M., Gittler, A., Beigel, A., et al.: Changing a state mental health system through litigation: the Arizona experiment. *Am. J. Psychiatry* 143:1575–1579, 1986.

5. Appelbaum, P. S.: Resurrecting the right to treatment. *Hosp. Community Psychiatry* 38: 703–704, 721, 1987.

B. Other Rights of Hospitalized Patients

1. Stone, A. A.: The myth of advocacy. *Hosp. Community Psychiatry* 30:819–822, 1979.

2. Ennis, B. J. & Emery, R. D.: *The Rights of Mental Patients.* New York, Avon Books, 1978.

3. Weiner, B. A.: Rights of institutionalized persons, in Brakel, S. J., Parry, J. & Weiner, B. A.: *The Mentally Disabled and the Law,* 3rd ed. Chicago, American Bar Foundation, 1985.

4. Sundram, C. J.: Obstacles to reducing patient abuse in public institutions. *Hosp. Community Psychiatry* 35:238–243, 1984.

5. Brakel, S. J.: Legal aid in mental hospitals. *American Bar Foundation Research Journal* 1:21–90, Winter 1981.

6. Bloom, B. L. & Asher, S. J. (eds.): *Psychiatric Patient Rights and Patient Advocacy: Issues and Evidence.* New York, Human Sciences Press, 1982.

7. Rubenstein, L. S.: Treatment of the mentally ill: legal advocacy enters the second generation. *Am. J. Psychiatry* 143:1264–1269, 1986.

8. Appelbaum, P. S.: The rising tide of patients' rights advocacy. *Hosp. Community Psychiatry* 37: 9–10, 1986.

9. Weicker, L.: Federal response to institutional abuse and neglect: The Protection and Advocacy for Mentally Ill Individuals Act. *Am. Psychol.* 42:1027–1028, 1987.

10. Cromwell, H. S., Howe, J. W. & O'Rear, G.: A citizens' coalition in mental health advocacy: the Maryland experience. *Hosp. Community Psychiatry* 39:959–962, 1988.

11. Gutheil, T. G.: Observations on the theoretical basis for seclusion of the psychiatric inpatient. *Am. J. Psychiatry* 135:325–328, 1978.

12. Tardiff, K. (ed.): *The Psychiatric Uses of Seclusion and Restraint.* Washington, D.C., American Psychiatric Press, 1984.

13. Gutheil, T. G., Appelbaum, P. S. & Wexler, D. B.: The inappropriateness of "least restrictive alternative" analysis for involuntary procedures with the institutionalized mentally ill. *J. Psychiatry Law* 11:7–17, 1983.

C. THE RIGHT TO REFUSE TREATMENT

1. Appelbaum, P. S.: The right to refuse treatment with antipsychotic medication: retrospect and prospect. *Am. J. Psychiatry* 145:413–419, 1988.

2. Rapoport, D. & Parry, J. (eds.): *The Right to Refuse Antipsychotic Medication.* Washington, D.C., American Bar Association, 1986.

3. Appelbaum, P. S., & Hoge, S. K.: The right to refuse treatment: what the research reveals. *Behav. Sci. Law* 4:279–292, 1986.

4. Hoge, S. K., Appelbaum, P. S., Lawlor, T., et al.: A prospective, multicenter study of patients' refusal of antipsychotic medication. *Arch. Gen. Psychiatry* 47:949–956, 1990.

5. Brooks, A.: The right to refuse antipsychotic medications: law and policy. *Rutgers Law Review* 39:339–376, 1987.

6. Plotkin, R.: Limiting the therapeutic orgy: mental patients' right to refuse treatment. *Northwestern University Law Review* 72:461–525, 1977.

7. Appelbaum, P. S., & Gutheil, T. G.: Clinical aspects of treatment refusal. *Compr. Psychiatry* 23:560–566, 1982.

8. Meister, R.: Psychiatrists' reactions to their patients' refusal of drugs. *Isr. Ann Psychiatry* 10:373–381, 1972.

9. Gutheil, T. G.: Drug therapy: alliance and compliance. *Psychosomatics* 19:219–225, 1978.

10. Hoge, S. K. & Gutheil, T. G.: The psychology of psychopharmacology, in: A. Lazare (ed.), *Outpatient Psychiatry*, 2nd ed. Baltimore, Williams & Wilkins, 1988.

11. Gutheil, T. G. & Appelbaum, P. S.: "Mind control," "synthetic sanity," "artificial competence," and genuine confusion: legally relevant effects of antipsychotic medications. *Hofstra Law Review* 12:77–120, 1983.

12. Gutheil, T. G. & Bursztajn, H. J.: Clinician's guidelines for assessing and presenting subtle forms of patient incompetence in legal settings. *Am. J. Psychiatry* 143:1020–1023, 1986.

13. Gutheil, T. G. & Appelbaum, P. S.: The substituted judgment approach: its difficulties and paradoxes in mental health settings. *Law, Medicine, and Health Care* 13:61–64, 1985.

14. Conrad, P.: The meaning of medications: another look at compliance. *Soc. Sci. Med.* 20:29–37, 1985.

15. Kelly, G. R., Mamon, J. A., & Scott, J. E.: Utility of the health belief model in

examining medication compliance among psychiatric outpatients. *Soc. Sci. Med.* 25:1205–1211, 1987.

16. Waller, D. A. & Altshuler, K. Z.: Perspectives on patient noncompliance. *Hosp. Community Psychiatry* 37:490–492, 1986.

D. CLINICAL AND LEGAL ASPECTS OF THE RIGHT TO LEAVE THE HOSPITAL

1. Rivinus, T. M. & Gutheil, T. G.: When the insurance money runs out. *Psychiatric Annals* 7:96–111, 1977.

2. Simon, W. B.: On reluctance to leave the public mental hospital. *Psychiatry* 28:145–156, 1965.

3. Mallard, H. C. & Feigelson, E. B.: The sign-out letter: Civil right and/or therapeutic issue. *J. Psychiatry Law* 4:265–276, 1976.

4. Miles, J. E., et al.: Discharges against medical advice from voluntary psychiatric units. *Hosp. Community Psychiatry* 27:859–864, 1976.

5. Heinssen, R. K. & McGlashan, T. H.: Predicting hospital discharge status for patients with schizophrenia, schizoaffective disorder, borderline personality disorder, and unipolar affective disorder. *Arch. Gen. Psychiatry* 45:353–360, 1988.

6. McGlashan, T. H. & Heinssen, R. K.: Hospital discharge status and long-term outcome for patients with schizophrenia, schizoaffective disorder, borderline personality disorder, and unipolar affective disorder. *Arch. Gen. Psychiatry* 45:363–368, 1988.

7. Targum, S. D., Capadanno, A. E., Hoffman, H. A., et al.: An intervention to reduce the rate of hospital discharges against medical advice. *Am. J. Psychiatry* 139:657–659, 1982.

8. Katz, R. C., & Woolley, F. R.: Criteria for releasing patients from psychiatric hospitals. *Hosp. Community Psychiatry* 26:33–36, 1975.

9. Lipsius, S. H.: Judgments of alternatives to hospitalization. *Am. J. Psychiatry* 130:892–896, 1973.

10. Washburn, S. L., et al.: Irrational determinants of the place of psychiatric treatment. *Hosp. Community Psychiatry* 27:179–182, 1976.

E. PRINCIPLES AND PROBLEMS OF INPATIENT PSYCHIATRY

1. Engel, G. L.: The clinical application of the biopsychosocial model. *Am. J. Psychiatry* 137:535–544, 1980.

2. Rothman, D. J.: *Conscience and Convenience: The Asylum and Its Alternatives in Progressive America.* Boston, Little, Brown, 1980.

3. Gutheil, T. G.: On the therapy in clinical administration. *Psychiatr. Q.* 54:3–25, 1982.

4. Gutheil, T. G.: The therapeutic milieu: changing themes and theories. *Hosp. Community Psychiatry* 36:1279–1285, 1985.

5. Sederer, L. (ed.): *Inpatient Psychiatry: Diagnosis and Treatment,* 2nd ed. Baltimore, Williams and Wilkins, 1982.

6. Hoge, S. K. & Gutheil, T. G.: The prosecution of psychiatric patients for assaults on staff: a preliminary empirical survey. *Hosp. Community Psychiatry* 38:44–49, 1987.

7. Johansen, K. H.: The impact of patients with chronic character pathology on a hospital in-patient unit. *Hosp. Community Psychiatry* 34:842–846, 1983.

8. Gunderson, J. G. Will, O. A. & Mosher, L. R.: *Principles and Practice of Milieu Therapy.* New York, Aronson, 1983.

9. Gutheil, T. G.: Legal defense as ego defense. *Psychiatr. Q.* 51:251–256, 1979.

4

Malpractice and Other Forms of Liability

4. EXCEPTIONS TO THE DOCTRINE OF INFORMED CONSENT
   a. Emergencies
   b. Therapeutic privilege
   c. Waiver
   d. Incompetence
5. SPECIAL PROBLEMS WITH INFORMED CONSENT IN PSYCHIATRY
   a. Tardive dyskinesia
   b. Psychotherapy
6. ASSESSMENT OF THE DOCTRINE OF INFORMED CONSENT
   a. Practical problems
   b. Theoretical problems
   c. A synthetic approach to informed consent

C. Other forms of liability

1. FALSE IMPRISONMENT
2. BREACH OF PRIVACY
   a. Appropriation of a likeness or name
   b. Intrusion on seclusion
   c. False light
   d. Public disclosure of embarrassing facts
   e. Breach of privacy
3. DEFAMATION
4. INTERFERENCE WITH ADVANTAGEOUS RELATIONS
5. CIVIL RIGHTS ACTIONS
6. FRAUD

D. Miscellaneous problems of liability

1. LIABILITY OF NONMEDICAL MENTAL HEALTH PROFESSIONALS
2. THE INSURANCE PROBLEM
3. THE SYSTEMS ISSUE
4. THE MOVE TOWARD STRICT LIABILITY

III. CLINICAL ISSUES

A. Prevention of negligence and malpractice

1. BEHAVIORAL APPROACHES TO PREVENTION
   a. Avoidance of exploitation
   b. Manifesting respect for the patient
   c. Avoidance of abandonment
      i. Emergencies
      ii. Patients who fail to pay
      iii. Patients who do not cooperate in their care
   d. Coverage during absences
   e. Patient selection
   f. The role of apology in liability prevention
2. TECHNICAL APPROACHES TO PREVENTION
   a. The treatment contract
   b. Acknowledging limitations versus making promises
   c. Informed consent and the sharing of uncertainty
   d. Therapeutic disinterest and the question of advice
   e. Technical handling of legalistic acting out
      i. Remaining cool
      ii. Avoiding fruitless struggle in the legal arena
      iii. Actively confronting or interpreting the clinical meaning of the acting out and/ or resistance
      iv. Extracting maximum therapeutic value from the issue for ongoing exploration
   f. The importance of clinical "outreach" in homicide and suicide
   g. The duty to protect and related matters

I. CASE EXAMPLES

A. Case Example 1

After attending a continuing education program at which the problems of neuroleptic-induced tardive dyskinesia were discussed, this hospital-based psychiatrist decides to examine her entire case load for early signs of abnormal movements and to obtain informed consent from all of her patients who are receiving psychotropes. Using one of the scales developed to identify subtle extrapyramidal effects, she notices that one of her male schizophrenic patients has a significant number of positive scores. The peculiar posturing of his hands, which she had always written off as a schizophrenic mannerism, now appears to have a distinct choreoathetoid flavor. His feet, usually concealed behind her desk during their sessions, rhythmically rotate, flex, and extend at the ankle joint. Although she is convinced that she must confront the patient with her findings and obtain informed consent to continuation of neuroleptic therapy, she is troubled by his past history.

Originally hospitalized at age 21, after a slow descent into psychosis, he was diagnosed as a catatonic schizophrenic and was begun on moderate doses of medication. Despite the efforts of his therapist and an intensive milieu, he showed little progress during his first three years of hospitalization. In fact, during that period, he made two serious suicide attempts, one of which was followed by a course of ECT. However, during his fourth year of hospitalization, placed on large doses of a different neuroleptic and treated with continued psychotherapy, he began a slow improvement. That improvement has progressed for three years until now he is subject to only occasional delusions and a mild thought disorder, and is holding a volunteer job in addition to his partial hospitalization program.

While his status was improving so dramatically, his therapists made numerous attempts to decrease the large dosage of medication he had been taking, but he resisted them all. He said that he was afraid that without the medication he would relapse and would require rehospitalization, and that if that happened, he was not sure that he would survive it. Reviewing his records, his doctor can find no evidence that he ever gave a specific consent to neuroleptic treatment, thought it is apparent by now that the patient is thoroughly familiar with the direct effects of the medications. She is concerned that raising the issue now will lead the patient to become paranoid about the medication or to become so angry at the hospital and at her that he will stop taking the medication and will require rehospitalization, perhaps even become a risk for suicide again. She seeks legal-psychiatric consultation as to how to proceed.

B. Case Example 2

Miss C, a 24-year-old woman, experiences an acute psychotic episode after breaking up with a boyfriend with whom she has had a brief realistic acquaintance and an elaborate fantasy relationship. On admission she is actively hallucinating visions of Christ calling to her, and she has the delusion that she is possessed by a devil who creates disturbing sensations in her body.

Several weeks of medication and psychotherapy result in marked remission of symptoms; the resident psychiatrist continues in psychotherapy with the patient to elucidate the precipitants to her falling ill.

Six months into outpatient work, the therapist begins to explore the patient's childhood feelings toward her father and the manner in which these feelings were recapitulated in the relationship with the lost boyfriend. The resident interprets the patient's growing discomfort as related to the sensitive nature of the material. One session, after discussing the boyfriend, the patient trails off into silence, squirms in her chair, starts to speak, turns crimson, and stares vacantly ahead into space. The resident asks quietly, "What are you feeling?" At that, the patient leaps from her chair and bolts from the office.

Early the next morning, the resident receives a call from the patient's father. In a towering rage, the father accuses the resident of sexual liberties with his daughter that have made her illness worse; warns that his attorney is on the way with a subpoena for the patient's records in preparation for a law suit; and slams down the phone. Panicked, the resident telephones his supervisor, protesting, "I didn't go near her, what's going on?" The supervisor suggests they review the case together after the resident alerts his malpractice insurer.

II. LEGAL ISSUES

A. Malpractice

The increase in litigation against physicians and other health professionals, a problem that has provoked repeated crises since the 1970s, is probably the least understood of the powerful factors shaping the face of medical care today. Although most people have heard of the difficulties physicians have had obtaining malpractice insurance coverage at affordable rates, few of them, even few of the professionals most directly affected by the situation, are familiar with the changes in the legal system that have combined with new kinds of societal pressures to provoke the crises. Psychiatrists, to be sure, continue to maintain their position as one of the least frequently sued of the medical specialties. But they, too, are feeling the pressure that the heightened sense of litigiousness has wrought, as are the other professionals in the mental health field.

Psychiatrists are the mental health professionals for whom the most data are available. They represent 5.6% of all physicians, according to a recent federal study, but accounted for only 1.8% of malpractice claims closed in the year reviewed. Yet the incidence of malpractice claims against psychiatrists has risen from 0.6 claims per 100 psychiatrists in 1980 to approximately 4 claims per 100 in the latest studies. Premiums have also risen dramatically, especially in high-risk states. A study of Florida malpractice premiums, for example, revealed annual increases of 27% to 40% for psychiatrists over a several year period, depending on county.

The effects of increases in claims and premiums include making practitioners overly wary of legal issues in their treatment of patients, sometimes to the detriment of patient care. There may also be a tendency to refuse to treat patients perceived as "high-risk." To date, the mental health professions have not seen such dramatic increases in malpractice insurance costs as to force practitioners to change locations or abandon practice—as has occurred in some surgical specialties—but that may occur in the future. The reasons for the recurrent "malpractice crises" and suggestions for ways of dealing with it will be considered after an exploration of the basic legal doctrine involved.

1. DEFINITION OF MALPRACTICE

A malpractice suit falls into the legal category of an action in "tort." A tort is a civil, that is, a noncriminal, wrong, not based on a breach of contract, committed by one person that has led to damage to a second person. An action in tort is a request for compensation for the damages that have occurred. Malpractice is a negligent tort, committed by a physician or some other professional, that leads to damage to a patient or client. As a subcategory of tort law, malpractice litigation has to conform to all the complex procedural and substantive requirements that have evolved over centuries of Anglo-American jurisprudence in this field, and also has to proceed under some rules that are peculiar to this area. There are four basic elements that must be proven to sustain a claim of malpractice.

a. Duty

Before a patient can claim that a clinician's negligent act caused him damage, he must first establish that he and the clinician entered into a relationship in which the clinician undertook to treat him in a nonnegligent way. Another way of saying this is that the clinician must have assumed a duty to care for the person. Many people are surprised to discover the restricted scope of duty in Anglo-American (as opposed to Continental) law. Ordinarily, no individual is obligated to care for another. Thus, a passerby who sees a toddler trip in a wading pool and begin to drown is subject to no legal penalty if he continues obliviously on his way. The same is true for a physician, who except in rare instances where the law specifies otherwise, is not obliged to render assistance to all the infirm he chances upon. Once the physician has agreed to provide aid, however, whether by working in an emergency room where that promise is implicit in the setting, by explicitly agreeing to treat an individual who has come to his office, or by acting in some other way such that the patient might reasonably be led to assume that a doctor-patient relationship has been established, the duty to act nonnegligently applies. When a duty to care has been initiated, it can be terminated by outright discharge (but only if medically indicated) or by the transfer of the patient to the care of another physician. The same rules apply generally to all the mental health professions.

b. Negligence

The clinician who has agreed to care for a patient cannot act negligently toward her, but since negligence is a relative concept, some external standard against which to measure care is required. A deliberately exaggerated example may clarify this. There are a large number of medical tests that a psychiatrist might order before starting a patient on lithium. Since toxic effects of lithium on the function of the brain have been reported, particularly in those patients with preexisting lesions, an electroencephalogram and perhaps a CT (computerized tomography) scan might be obtained. The kidneys are a source of concern, too, and while a serum creatinine might be sufficient as a measure of renal impairment, perhaps an intravenous pyelogram or even a renal biopsy would yield additional data. A bone marrow biopsy could rule out a preleukemic state, a possible source of concern. What determines if a physician is negligent in omitting one of these procedures if a complication that might theoretically have been avoided later develops? Malpractice law has traditionally held, with some important exceptions (see Sec. II-B-2-a), that the custom of the profession, as reflected in the standard of care common to other professionals of the practitioner's training and theoretical orientation, is to be taken as the benchmark against which negligence is to be measured. Thus, if all psychiatrists who use lithium began on reasonable grounds to order CT scans first, that would become the standard by which the defendant-physician would be judged.

All jurisdictions formerly accepted one qualification as to the nature of the peer group to which the comparison was made: only the practices of clinicians in the defendant's own locality were considered to be relevant. Now, given the existence of widely disseminated professional journals, continuing education programs, and uniform standards for peer review, the resulting homogenization of practice has led many courts to abandon the "locality rule." One is now generally judged by the standards of one's confreres of similar training and orientation throughout the country. This is true for all the clinical professions.

Even this does not always mean that if a clinician performs as well as he possibly can, given his training, he will be held to be nonnegligent. A general practitioner (GP)—or a psychiatrist—who performs major abdominal surgery will not be expected to have done only as well as his training permits; it is likely that the standard of the profession requires GPs to refer patients in need of gastrectomies to qualified abdominal surgeons. To have operated at all, under such circumstances, may have constituted negligent behavior.

c. Harm

Even a grossly negligent act—for example, a psychiatrist prescribing antipsychotic medications by telephone for a patient whom he has never seen—will not leave the clinician liable for damages unless some harm occurs. The harm can be physical—e.g., a dystonic reaction in a patient who did not require neuroleptics in the first place that causes him to lose control of his car and crash—or emotional—the anguish that the patient's wife suffers after hearing about the crash. Potential damages can be astronomical: in this example, in addition to the cost of replacing the totally ruined car, the psychiatrist can be liable for the patient's hospital bills, a lifetime of lost wages, compensation for a future filled with days of pain and suffering, and compensation to the spouse for his or her anguish and loss of the usual marital relationship (or "consortium" as the law calls it). The tendency to grant large amounts of money for pain and suffering—even $10 a day over 30 years amounts to almost $110,000—has contributed to the enormous inflation in damages awarded.

d. Causation

This is the most complicated of the four elements of malpractice. In brief, even a negligent act committed by a clinician with a duty to care for a patient-plaintiff who has suffered a permanent harm will not be held to be compensable unless the negligent act in question caused the harm. While that may sound simple or even self-evident, it is neither. A psychiatrist who hospitalizes a suicidal patient in a facility that fails to observe him closely enough to prevent his ultimate demise can, in one sense, be said to be a causative agent of his death. If the psychiatrist knew, or reasonably should have known, that the facility was likely to be negligent in observing the patient, a court might conclude both that the psychiatrist was negligent and that her negligence was so closely related to the patient's death as to constitute a "proximate cause." Some courts have defined a proximate cause to be present whenever the harm might have been or should have been predicted in advance—or in legal terms, when the harm was "foreseeable." If the patient's death, however, resulted from another patient pushing him down a flight of stairs, and that act could not have been reasonably foreseen or prevented, the psychiatrist could not be held liable; this is true despite her original negligent act in committing the patient to a facility she knew to be inadequate and despite the fact that "but for" her action, the patient would still be alive. "But for" causation is not sufficient to establish proximate cause.

2. PROBLEMS OF PROOF

The existence of each of the four elements of malpractice must be proven by the plaintiff—the patient who is suing—by a preponderance of the evidence. Certain difficulties of proof inhere in the usual therapeutic setting.

a. Lack of witnesses

Common to many medical situations, and certainly the rule in psychiatry, is the fact that the interactions in question have not been observed by anyone other than the two parties to the case: the plaintiff-patient and the defendant-clinician. Only they can give direct evidence of whether a duty of care was assumed and if the negligent act alleged was actually committed. Because the testimony of each party can be assumed to be self-serving and is often directly contradictory of the other's, what corroborative evidence exists assumes tremendous significance. This usually means that the patient's records, which represent the clinician's ongoing description of the relationship, can be determinative of the ultimate findings in the case. (See Sec. III-A-3.) The importance of complete and accurate records cannot be exaggerated.

b. *Res ipsa loquitur*

Problems of proof that seem difficult in the usual clinician-patient relationship become overwhelming when one of the two parties cannot testify directly as to what has occurred. Take, for example, the case of a patient who has suffered a respiratory arrest during the administration of ECT and who has subsequently been revived. Although the patient may have reason to suspect that the behavior of her physicians contributed to her arrest, she has no way of proving that the physicians were indeed negligent, as by administering too large a dose of barbiturate anesthesia, except by reference to the medical record of the treatment. Since the formulation of that record, however, was under the control of the same doctors who are accused of negligence in the first place, the plaintiff might suspect that it does not accurately reflect everything that occurred. The law, whose primary concern is with the compensation of those who have suffered injuries, has provided a way out of this dilemma.

The doctrine of *res ipsa loquitur*—literally, "the matter speaks for itself"—can be invoked in such a case. *Res ipsa* requires four elements to be present: (1) that the harm that has occurred rarely happens in the absence of negligence (a requirement not likely to be met in the ECT example given above, but one that could be the subject of dispute in court); (2) that the defendant (physician) had exclusive control of the instrumentality that caused the injury; (3) that the plaintiff did not contribute to the bad result; and (4) that the defendants, and not the plaintiff, are the only ones with access to the information about what actually occurred. While some commentators claim that *res ipsa* represents nothing more than a complicated codification of common sense, it does have several important technical legal functions. First, in some courts, once the four elements have been established, the burden of proof has been shifted to the defendant, who must now prove that the negligent act alleged did not occur. Second, it prevents a plaintiff's case from being thrown out of court in the absence of direct evidence of negligence. And lastly, *res ipsa* is one of the means that the courts have developed to circumvent the usual requirement for expert testimony to establish negligence; although an expert may be required to prove the first element of *res ipsa,* namely that the act in question is unlikely to have occurred without negligence on the part of the physician, one is not needed to answer the more difficult question of whether this particular physician was actually negligent in what he did.

c. Expert testimony

As just alluded to, courts generally have required that expert testimony be presented to prove at least one element of malpractice: that the performance of the defendant did not conform to the standard of care of the profession. Under the traditional rules, the expert had to be of the same theoretical school as the defendant (a particularly important requirement in psychiatry, where practices among various schools diverge widely) and practicing in the same locale or at least a similar one (a nearby small town or a comparably situated small town in a neighboring state). Combined with the natural reluctance of colleagues to testify against one another in court (deemed by frustrated plaintiffs a "conspiracy of silence"), the requirement for an expert's testimony was a formidable barrier to the successful waging of a malpractice suit (see Chap. 8, Sec. II-A).

The barrier has been substantially lowered in recent years, however, as the result of several changes in evidentiary requirements in malpractice cases. As was noted above, the locality rule has all but disappeared, in part in response to the need to broaden the pool of professionals from which potential witnesses can be drawn. Now, a physician or other mental health professional who is known to be willing to testify in malpractice cases for either the defense (although defendants had many fewer problems finding experts to support their case) or the plaintiff can travel around the country to fill that role. Trial lawyers' magazines, in fact, display many advertisements from physicians and other experts who are eager to be called upon to testify. (Ethical questions in this area are addressed in Chap. 8, Sec. II-C-1.)

In addition, and probably most significantly, the requirement for an expert's testimony has been done away with altogether in those instances in which the court determines that the alleged negligence is of such dimensions that even uninstructed lay persons could recognize it. Cases of this sort are rare in psychiatry, but an example might be a physician who, while drunk, examines a patient and prescribes medication for a condition that the patient does not have, the medication subsequently leading to an adverse reaction.

Finally, even in those cases of psychiatric malpractice in which expert testimony is still required to establish negligence, some inroads are being made in utilizing nonmedical mental health professionals, primarily psychologists, to testify to the standard of care. As psychologists expand their roles in the care of the mentally ill (and in many areas they are now permitted to testify in commitment or competency proceedings and to admit patients to mental hospitals), the increasing congruence between their activities and those of psychiatrists will make them, from the lawyer's viewpoint, an even more attractive pool of potential witnesses to be tapped.

3. COMMON FORMS OF PSYCHIATRIC MALPRACTICE

As noted above, the incidence of malpractice litigation in the mental health professions, though low, is rising, and judgments are growing in size. Knowledge of the bases on which suits are brought is thus increasingly important, both to understand trends in malpractice litigation and to develop strategies to correct underlying problems. Growing awareness of the number of allegations against mental health professionals concerning sexual contact with patients, for example, has led to concerted efforts by the professions to deter such conduct. (See Sec. II-A-3-f below.)

Despite the obvious importance of data on the frequency of particular types of malpractice claims, however, much is lacking in our ability even to rank order the most common causes of suits. There are a number of reasons for this. Only the rare malpractice suit contains a single allegation; most state several related claims against the clinician. Further, the same negligent acts might be described differently in otherwise similar suits. A patient's death by overdose with a medication that was prescribed by her psychiatrist, but was not indicated for her condition, might be characterized as misdiagnosis, negligent prescription of medication, failure properly to monitor medication, failure to assess suicidal ideation, or any combination of these.

Even if common categories could be agreed upon, getting comprehensive information about malpractice cases is a daunting task. It is estimated that only 10% of cases get to trial, and only a fraction of these result in appeals with published opinions. Insurance companies, which have records of all claims lodged against policy holders, are often reluctant to allow researchers into their files, though they may publish periodic summaries of claims lodged against them. It is on these data and the rare independent research study that our knowledge about the relative frequency of malpractice claims is based.

Since categorizations differ from company to company and are subject to the biases mentioned above, the result is little consensus on the relative importance of given types of malpractice. We make no effort here to offer a hierarchy of causes of psychiatric malpractice by frequency of allegations. Rather, the major categories of malpractice for mental health professionals will be reviewed, with special attention to those categories that raise problems unique to mental health care.

a. Misdiagnosis of psychiatric disorders

Misdiagnosis usually refers to a negligent failure to recognize the nature of the patient's condition, with subsequent harm resulting from the consequent failure to implement proper measures of care. A psychiatrist, for example, may be held liable for negligently diagnosing a patient with a personality disorder as schizophrenic but only if the misdiagnosis affects treatment in a manner that leads to subsequent harm. If as a result of the diagnosis the patient receives neuroleptic medication and later develops tardive dyskinesia, liability may well be imposed.

It is, however, important to stress that the mistaken diagnosis must have been the result of the clinician's negligence. Had the psychiatrist properly inquired about the signs and symptoms of both schizophrenia and personality disorder, only to have the patient lie about the presence of delusions, the consequent mistake could not be attributed to the psychiatrist's misfeasance. Similarly, if after conducting an evaluation that conformed to the standard of care, the psychiatrist was left with a difficult diagnostic dilemma and made a reasonable judgment that turned out to be incorrect, liability should not accrue.

The introduction of biological treatments of demonstrated efficacy has heightened the importance of proper diagnosis. If the negligent failure to consider a diagnosis—for example, the possibility that a psychotic illness represents bipolar disorder and not schizophrenia—leads to a failure to employ a potentially efficacious agent—lithium in this case—with prolonged suffering and repeated hospitalization as a result, a good case for malpractice would seem evident. If anything has prevented such cases from proliferating, it is probably (1) the condition of many of these patients, who are chronically ill and socially impaired and thus unlikely to initiate legal remedies and (2) the fact that there still is no absolute one-to-one correlation between specific illness and specific treatment with certain efficacy. Popular ignorance of potentially effective biological treatments is another limiting factor. Nonetheless, this would seem to be a ripe area for future litigation.

It should be noted that "misdiagnosis" does not always refer to the failure to make a proper diagnosis of mental disorder in the psychiatric sense. The term can also be used to refer to alleged failure to detect a patient's suicidal or homicidal propensities. (See Secs. II-A-3-d and e below for a discussion of these issues.)

b. Negligent use of somatic treatments

Most of the issues here differ little from those faced by physicians in any other medical or surgical specialty. Use of the wrong medication for a patient's condition, prescription of improper dosages (either too high, leading to toxicity, or too low, leading to delayed improvement), failure to monitor side effects, failure to take proper precautions to prevent side effects from developing (as by using insufficient amounts of muscle-relaxant in administering ECT), and prescription of medication despite contraindications can, in psychiatry, as in the rest of medicine, be construed as actionable under malpractice law.

One issue that is relatively specific to psychiatric practice is the negligent failure *not* to employ somatic treatment. Practitioners who rely entirely on psychotherapeutic approaches for all of their patients, and who do not refer patients for whom pharmacotherapy might be appropriate to more biologically-oriented colleagues, are at risk for suits of this sort. Such suits have not been common to date, in part because of the "respectable minority" rule. If a respectable minority of a profession follows certain practices, even if those practices are rejected by the majority of practitioners, the courts have been reluctant to find members of the minority to be negligent. This deference to minority opinion is a reflection of the courts' disinclination to be used to enforce orthodoxy among the professions. A recent, highly publicized case may signal a change in direction here (see Suggested Readings—Malcolm). A medical malpractice screening panel agreed with the contentions of several noted psychopharmacologists that the failure to use antidepressant medication in a patient with symptoms of severe depression was negligent, even if the psychotherapeutic approaches followed by the treating psychiatrist (whose diagnosis emphasized an underlying personality disorder) might be embraced by a significant minority of practitioners. Just how much this case, and the whirlwind of controversy it stimulated, will affect subsequent litigation is uncertain at present. But the clearer the evidence for efficacy of medications or other somatic treatments, and the less apparent the benefit from the alternative approaches employed, the greater the risk run by a clinician who fails to consider somatic treatments.

c. Negligent use of psychotherapy

The many possible permutations of negligent behavior by a psychotherapist constitute an obsessive's nightmare and a scholar's delight. While articles and books are filled with speculations about the kinds of harm that might be induced by negligent psychotherapy, such works almost always conclude with the barely noted caveat that malpractice cases alleging negligence in psychotherapy are exceedingly rare. Among the reasons advanced to explain this are the good relationship most patients have with their psychotherapists (although negative transference reactions of significant severity are hardly unusual); the patient's low index of suspicion for negligent acts, given the patient's usual unfamiliarity with technical aspects of psychotherapy; the difficulty in proving that the act was negligent, both because of the absence of witnesses and other corroborative data and because the techniques of many forms of psychotherapy have diverged so greatly from the original analytically oriented model that a professional consensus on what constitutes an adequate standard of care is almost impossible to obtain; the crucial role of the patient's own participation and, hence, responsibility; and the problems in establishing a causal link between a therapist's statements and the subsequent harms that accrue to the patient. In fact, so rare are reported cases of actual suits about the psychotherapy process itself that most discussions of this topic concentrate on cases involving nonpsychotherapeutic interactions between patients and therapists, such as sexual intercourse (see Sec. f below) or other abuses of the fiduciary relationship.

Nonetheless, it *is* possible to be negligent in conducting psychotherapy, just as it is possible to practice negligently any other form of treatment. A divergence from the standard of care for psychotherapists usually implies an intrusion of countertransference feelings into the treatment process. Thus, a therapist who, in anger at a patient's provocative behavior, berates that patient or suggests that the patient undertake some action that is not in the patient's best interest would, problems of proof aside, be liable for whatever harm occurs. Although it is possible to imagine a suit stemming from a patient's feelings that, even absent any such extraordinary events, the psychotherapy was conducted so poorly as to inhibit the patient's recovery, the problems of proof in such a case seem so overwhelming as to make a successful action extremely unlikely.

d. Negligent failure to prevent patients from harming themselves

Of the many categories of psychiatric malpractice, allegations related to patients' attempts at suicide are in many respects the most perplexing. As noted above, such allegations may be cast in a variety of forms, generally encompassing failure to detect suicidal propensities and failure to act appropriately to control them. Unlike the previously discussed categories, however, harm to the patient as a result of suicidal behavior requires the patient herself to act as a causal agent. That is, whatever errors the clinician makes in the course of treatment, harm would not accrue were it not for the ultimate actions of the patient. Generally in tort law, such behavior would be considered an intervening cause, rendering the clinician, even if negligent, free from liability, or at most apportioned some fraction of resulting damages.

Why is that often not the case where suicide is concerned? Although not usually explicated clearly by the courts, the governing assumption seems to be that psychiatric patients whose suicide attempts are motivated by their disorders lack either the ability to control their impulses or the capacity to think clearly about their options. Put somewhat differently, it might be said that they are incompetent to determine their own behavior. Thus, the legal significance of their actions as intervening causes is diminished, leaving clinicians who have committed negligent acts solely responsible for the outcome.

The difficulty of predicting suicidality was discussed in Chap. 2 (see Sec. II-E-2-b). Needless to say, clinicians are not considered negligent merely for having failed to predict suicidal acts, as long as they take the steps considered necessary by their profession. In general, patients should be asked at the time of initial evaluation about the signs and symptoms of depression and about suicidal history and current suicidal intent. Should patients falsely deny suicidal ideation, only later to act on it, the clinician can hardly be held responsible. If suicidal ideation is present, the difficult task of assessing its degree and seriousness remains. (See Chap. 2, Sec. III-B.)

Just how far a clinician must go in attempting to prevent a patient from attempting suicide is unclear, although the burden is clearly greater in an inpatient setting, where the clinician has a greater degree of control over the patient's behavior. Most experienced clinicians believe that a patient who is set on killing himself will find a way to do so regardless of the precautions taken. The task thus is to design responses to decrease the likelihood of successful suicide amongst those who are deterrable, while recognizing the limitations of the clinician's realistic capabilities and the need to balance safety concerns with other requirements for effective treatment.

If involuntary hospitalization is the only means of deterring suicide, must that be pursued? Many cases have been decided under the assumption that civil commitment of the seriously suicidal represents the standard of care. At least one recent decision, however, has challenged that standard as a matter of law. While it is safest at present to assume that commitment may be necessary if other courses of action are likely to be ineffective, this is an issue to be watched in the courts.

e. Negligent failure to prevent patients from harming others

Psychiatrists have always faced the possibility of suit as a result of negligently allowing patients to be released or to escape from inpatient facilities when those patients later cause harm to others. The California Supreme Court decision in *Tarasoff v. Regents of the University of California* in 1976 extended the duty to protect third parties to situations in which clinicians (not just psychiatrists) had never exercised physical control over their patients. The court ruled that when clinicians know or should know that their patients represent a danger to others they have a duty to take whatever steps are reasonably necessary to protect those identifiable persons. In the time since the California decision, most states have adopted some version of the *Tarasoff* rationale by case law and statute. Where no state law exists on the matter, most experts would agree that it is prudent to behave as if a duty to protect exists in that jurisdiction anyway. (See also Chap. 1, Sec. II-B-5-d.)

The *Tarasoff* decision has been subjected to a great deal of criticism from the mental health professions on two general grounds. First, it is argued that the inability of clinicians to predict future dangerousness saddles them with a responsibility that they cannot reasonably fulfill. Even when predictions of possible violence are made, clinicians have a limited range of abilities to protect potential victims, many of whom are intimates of their patients. Second, opponents of the duty to protect maintain that the harm from imposing a duty to protect outweighs whatever benefits may be obtained. Faced with the threat of breaches of confidentiality, those patients most in need of treatment may decline to seek it. Other patients, as well, may be deterred by an unfounded fear of disclosure, and maximally protective options, such as hospitalization, may be overutilized from fear of liability.

These arguments have had relatively little impact on the courts. In response to claims of inability to predict dangerous behavior, they point to assertions by many clinicians—documented repeatedly in surveys—that they *can* predict violence. The courts then note that all they are asking clinicians to do is to live up to the standard of their colleagues, that is, to do as well at prediction as would any reasonable mental health professional. Of course, this standard becomes problematic when expert witnesses testify at trial, in retrospect, that they—and therefore other reasonable clinicians—would certainly have known that the patient would be violent, and that the defendant should have as well. As for the putative negative effects of imposing a duty to protect, the courts have been willing to tolerate those (while noting that they have not been demonstrated) to avoid the harms that might result from clinicians failing to act to protect likely victims when they believe that danger may exist.

Legislatures have been somewhat more responsive to clinicians' concerns, particularly claims that court decisions often left it unclear when the duty arose and what means were sufficient to discharge it. A growing number of states are adopting roughly similar legislation to limit the duty to circumstances in which patients make overt threats against identifiable victims, thus somewhat diminishing the problems of prediction. Further, the statutes generally provide that the duty is fulfilled if one or more of a small number of options is selected, generally including warning the victim and/or the police, and hospitalizing the patient, voluntarily or involuntarily. These statutes may provide an acceptable compromise between public safety concerns and clinicians' fears of unreasonable imposition of liability.

Clinical approaches to dealing with the requirements of the duty to protect are considered below in Sec. III-A-2-g.

f. Sexual activity between patients and therapists

There has been an explosion of concern about sexual contact between patients and clinicians in the last decade. Surveys of mental health professionals have shown repeatedly that between 5 and 10% of therapists admit to sexual activity with patients, with male therapists outnumbering female therapists between 2:1 and 5:1. Other work has suggested that patients who engage in sexual activity with their therapists almost uniformly suffer adverse effects, frequently severe. The idea that sexual contact may constitute a beneficial aspect of treatment has been rejected entirely. Thus, a consensus has developed that sexual contact between patients and therapists is *never* acceptable. This view is now reflected in the codes of ethics of all the major mental health professions.

It is possible, of course, for any two people of the opposite sex who work together intimately over a prolonged period of time to develop feelings of fondness and sexual desires for each other. The special conditions of a psychotherapeutic setting and its contract, however, call for an exploration of those feelings with an eye toward helping the patient understand their genesis and their relationship to other events in his or (usually) her life. The therapist is likewise called upon to examine the origin of his own feelings about the patient and to prevent them from interfering with the treatment process. In current thinking, acting upon those feelings represents, for the therapist, a failure of self-exploration and self-restraint to such a degree as to constitute negligence. The claim that in no other setting would the physical expression of sexual longings be categorized as negligence on the part of one of the parties, though true, merely emphasizes the uniqueness of the psychotherapeutic dyad. Three factors contribute to this uniqueness: the special vulnerability of patients who seek mental health treatment; the power differential between therapists and patients, heightened by the phenomenon of transference, which makes it difficult for patients to resist therapists' sexual advances; and the strong likelihood that patients will be harmed by whatever sexual contact ensues.

Courts are unsympathetic to claims that sexual involvement was the result of overpowering passion and should therefore be excused, to allegations that the patient's freely given consent should absolve the therapist of any responsibility, and to arguments that since the sexual activity took place outside of the therapy, it is not properly considered under malpractice law. Instead, the courts are likely to stress the fiduciary relationship that exists between patient and therapist, that is, the idea that in the development of a therapeutic relationship the patient is induced to place full trust in the therapist, believing his position to be that of the patient's ally, who is committed to act unfailingly in the patient's best interests. Sexual activity is, in this view, always a betrayal of the patient's trust and an unfair capitalization on the patient's transference feelings.

As this area has been explored, additional issues have been considered. It was once considered acceptable for therapists who had "fallen in love" with their patients to discontinue treatment, refer the patient to another therapist, and then pursue romantic involvement. This is no longer the case. The American Psychiatric Association's ethical code reflects the new belief that sexual contact with former patients is almost always exploitative of them, because it is likely to be based on unresolved transference and therefore unethical. It may also be the basis for a malpractice suit.

Since sexual activity with patients is an intentional act, it may seem problematic to characterize it as malpractice, which is a negligent tort. From plaintiffs' point of view, however, this characterization is desireable, because it gives them access to clinicians' malpractice insurance policies for purposes of compensation. Though many insurers are now trying to avoid indemnifying clinicians who have been found to have engaged in sexual contact with patients, on the grounds that their actions fall outside of the negligent behavior the policies were designed to cover, plaintiffs have generally been successful in getting around these arguments. One usually successful technique is to characterize therapists' behavior as a negligent form of treatment (since therapists should know that harm is likely to result), particularly a mishandling of the transference. This allegation may even be made against practitioners who do not employ insight-oriented psychotherapy and therefore do not see themselves as dealing with transference, e.g., behavioral therapists and psychopharmacologists. In supporting these charges, the courts seem to be saying that this is one area that no clinician can ignore. Some insurers will agree to defend accused therapists in such cases but will try to avoid paying the judgment if therapists are found liable. Clinicians should be aware of their insurers' policies in this regard.

An active policy debate is ongoing as to whether malpractice policies should cover sexual misconduct. On one side of the issue are those who argue that malpractice insurance was never meant to deal with intentionally harmful behavior. To include sexual contact within the scope of the policies is to place a tax on the vast majority of therapists who do not have sexual contact with their patients, for the benefit of those who do. On the other side of the argument are people who believe that some compensation ought to be forthcoming for patients who have suffered harm at the hands of sexually abusive therapists. Without malpractice coverage, payment in many cases will not be possible, as therapists lose or dispose of their assets. Since someone must bear the cost of the harms suffered by patients, it is argued that rather than leaving the burden on the abused patients, it is fairer to spread it among all practitioners.

In response to the perception that the professions have been ineffective in sanctioning sexual activity with patients, the states have become much more aggressive. Complaints to boards of registration routinely result in therapists losing their licenses. A growing number of states are passing laws requiring the reporting of sexual activity that becomes known to other health and mental health professionals, making it easier for patients to sue (e.g., defining the cause of action, extending the statute of limitations), and even criminalizing the behavior. Therapists found to have had sex with patients, and in some cases former patients, now face long prison terms in some states.

It is clear that sexual contact with patients—and in most circumstances, ex-patients—has moved from a deplored, but tolerated status to being clearly rejected by practitioners and the public alike. To repeat, sex with patients is never justified. Following that simple rule will prevent much distress for patients and therapists alike.

g. Negligence in supervision

Negligent supervision assumed a new importance for psychiatrists with the changes in the nature of psychiatric practice that have accompanied the community psychiatry movement in recent decades. Recognizing that sufficient psychiatric manpower to meet the nation's needs did not, and probably would not, exist, the community psychiatry movement encouraged the multiplication of psychiatrists' efforts through the employment of other professionals and less fully trained paraprofessionals to conduct primary patient care under psychiatrists' supervision. The idea caught on to such an extent that many clinics are now staffed entirely by nonmedical personnel, with psychiatric involvement limited only to weekly supervisory sessions. Some private practitioners, sensing the financial opportunities available with this type of organizational structure, also began to employ other mental health professionals to treat patients under their supervision.

For psychiatrists who employ other professionals, liability problems derive from the law's assumption that those who are subject to their supervision are actually their agents—in other words, that the patient's relationship is established primarily with the physician (even if she never meets the physician), and is only mediated by the nonmedical mental health professional. As such, the physician is held responsible for the acts of his agents and for their negligence as well. The relevant legal doctrine is often known by its Latin name, *respondeat superior*—"let the master reply." The fact that the psychiatrist did not know about the act in question is no defense; the standard of care to be met is the standard of the psychiatric profession, and the failure of the psychiatrist to make reasonable efforts to ascertain that her agents were in fact living up to that standard is proof of negligence in itself.

The liability question may be less clear in clinics in which psychiatrists are themselves hired to supervise other mental health workers, rather than employing those workers directly; in some jurisdictions, a direct employer-employee relationship may be required before *respondeat superior* may be applied. In other states a psychiatrist's responsibility for the acts of others may vary depending on whether he operates in a consultative capacity, proffering advice that may be accepted or rejected, or in a supervisory capacity. In the latter case, the psychiatrist may be viewed as having ultimate responsibility for the patients' care, a responsibility that she actually exercises *through* those professionals under her supervision, but which she cannot shed completely should a negligent act occur. Psychiatrists who work in community clinics, which are often loosely supervised with only a few hours each week of psychiatric time, should clearly define the nature of their responsibilities, preferably in writing. Many clinic situations are inherently unsatisfactory from the perspective of potential liability; while endowing the part-time psychiatrist with responsibility for supervising the care of large numbers of patients, they provide too little time for a careful monitoring of the care to take place. Psychiatrists would be well advised to avoid such positions, as well as clinics in which they feel that, regardless of the amount of time spent in supervision or the extra training provided, the personnel employed cannot possibly provide an adequate level of care. While this may mean in the short run that many clinics will be left without psychiatric coverage, in the long run the problem is one for the system as a whole to solve, and perpetuating less-than-optimal levels of patient care at the risk of significant personal liability does little to facilitate that ultimate solution.

With the spread of statutes allowing independent practice for psychologists, social workers, and other therapists, issues regarding *respondeat superior* and negligent supervision are no longer the exclusive concern of psychiatrists. A psychologist supervising other non-medical mental health professionals, for example, must also take reasonable steps to ascertain that they are conforming to the standard of care.

h. Abandonment

The law's concern when the question of abandonment is raised is that the trust that the patient has presumptively lodged in a mental health professional should not be abused by the sudden termination of the patient's care. Because of the "trusting"—or fiduciary—nature of the relationship, this means in practice that the clinician must frequently do more than an average person would in comparable circumstances. At the least, this means that before a clinician unilaterally stops seeing the patient, a proper locus of referral should be identified. Ideally, the clinician will have already contacted the practitioner or agency to which the referral is being made and will have obtained agreement for the transfer of care.

Patients who threaten their therapists.   The law, of course, recognizes that there will be instances in which this orderly approach to termination will be untenable, for example, when the patient has seriously threatened the physical safety of the therapist. Yet, even here a clinician cannot simply refuse to see the patient and leave it at that. An effort at referral to an appropriate source of care must be attempted. While one can argue that this requires an extraordinary amount of devotion on the part of a therapist whose life has just been threatened, the law tends to see it merely as a quid pro quo for the benefits that the clinician obtains from the relationship: money, status, and a certain measure of power over patients who depose their trust in him.

Patients who fail to pay.   For reasons that probably have a great deal to do with interprofessional rivalries, courts are likely to look least favorably upon therapists who have stopped seeing patients for failure to pay their bills than those who have terminated patients for any other cause. Though the realities of the situation are quite different, the popular, and this includes the legal, view of psychiatrists and other mental health professionals is that they not only charge extortionate fees, but are unmerciful in dropping patients who cannot afford to pay them. Clinicians, therefore, who find that they have exhausted the usual recourse of extensively discussing the situation with the patient and who desire to terminate treatment with a patient who has not paid a bill over a substantial period of time would do well to document the repeated discussions carefully, to make clear to the patient that if the bill is paid she can return, and to offer referral to a public clinic or other available source of care. (See also Secs. III-A-1-c-ii and III-A-2-h.)

Patients who do not cooperate in their care.   As with a failure to pay one's bills, the failure to comply with a clinician's instructions may remain resistant to exploration and interpretation and may thus eventuate in the therapist's desire to terminate therapy. This is a tricky matter. To the clinician it may make perfect sense to reason that if the patient does not follow advice, such as to abstain from alcohol or to avoid hallucinogens, there is little point in continuing with treatment. The lay mind—and it is laypeople who sit on juries—sometimes sees things differently. Mere contact is often viewed as being therapeutic, as captured in the phrase, "I am being seen by a doctor." Even in the face of no progress whatsoever in treatment, a jury might—perhaps correctly—perceive a valuable supportive function of continuing therapy. A similar problem arises when a patient is being denied admission to the hospital, another thing that laymen have difficulty in not seeing as antitherapeutic in itself.

This is not to say that a decision to terminate treatment for compliance failure should never be made, only that, given these popular biases against such a move, the grounds for the decision should be recorded carefully. Frequently this will come down to the clinician's judgment that his approval of the patient's conduct implicit in continuing treatment is actually more destructive to the patient than would be terminating treatment altogether, with an option for reentry should the patient's behavior change. The reasoning should be explained to the patient and the patient should be given a chance to respond. If the decision is made to go ahead, the patient should also be given sufficient time to make alternate arrangements for care.

Disliked patients.   Psychiatrists and other psychotherapists, unlike orthopedists, may find it impossible to continue to work effectively with a patient whom they dislike. This goes, of course, to the core of the psychotherapeutic process, which is built on a mutually accepting and trusting relationship. Nonetheless, to discharge a patient from care because she is disliked sounds to the lawyer like the paradigm case of abandonment. If it is clear that, because of personality differences, the psychotherapeutic work is stalled, then the situation should be explained to the patient, and noted in the record, in these terms. A good faith referral to another caretaker should complete both the clinical and legal aspects of the termination.

Coverage during absences.   Abandonment, to result in liability, need not be manifested by a permanent withdrawal of services to a patient. The negligent nonavailability of a therapist, even for a brief period of time, is equally culpable. Clinicians who work with patients for whom emergencies are likely to arise are, when they assume the patient's clinical care, committing themselves in the eyes of the law to more than just one hour per week. They must be reachable in an emergency and able to provide care or referral as needed. It is not as clear that this obligation applies equally to nonmedical caregivers, although it is likely that as they assume roles more comparable to those of psychiatrists, they will be held to have assumed similar obligations.

As no therapist is ever continuously available, the law permits the delegation of this responsibility to another professional. Clinicians who will be unavailable for a prolonged period, for example, if they are leaving town for the weekend, ought to arrange in advance for coverage for their practice and ought to notify their patients of how the covering clinician can be contacted. Although the primary clinician will not be held responsible for the negligent acts of the covering clinician, she will be held liable for negligence in the selection of coverage; that is, if coverage is arranged with someone whom the primary clinician knows or ought to know not to be capable of performing properly, the primary clinician will share liability for her acts. Whether coverage is needed for shorter periods of time is strictly a function of the clinician's practice and of how likely it is that an urgent situation will develop in the interval in question. A psychiatrist with an active inpatient practice may want to have continuous coverage, or may elect to rent a beeper to ensure her availability at all times.

B. Informed consent

1. EVOLUTION OF THE DOCTRINE

Under common law, any unconsented touching constitutes a battery, even if that touching takes place for the purpose of rendering medical care. Because of this, physicians, particularly surgeons, have long operated under the obligation to obtain the patient's consent before proceeding with treatment. Obtaining a valid consent, however, was a simple matter, requiring only that the physician disclose the nature and purpose of what he proposed to do. The patient's assent to this proposition was sufficient to protect the physician from liability.

The rationale for the law's approach to liability for unconsented touchings was to protect patients' rights to bodily autonomy, an interest highly valued in our society. By the late 1950s and early 1960s, however, many courts had concluded that the existing requirements for consent were insufficient to accomplish that end. With the growth of multiple approaches to most medical problems, each with its own balance of risks and benefits, protection of the right to determine what is done with one's body seemed to require that patients be told more than just the nature and purpose of the one procedure selected by the physician. In place of this limited duty, the courts began to require an "informed consent" and began to create a body of decisions that defined what that phrase entailed. Although it was unclear at first whether treatment, especially surgery, that took place in the absence of an informed consent constituted a battery or an act of malpractice, that issue has been substantially resolved: treatment *without* any consent or over a patient's objections may constitute a battery, but treatment following an *inadequate* consent is properly considered as a form of malpractice.

The application of informed consent to treatment in psychiatry is less clear than in general medicine. In the latter, it is widely agreed that invasive surgical and diagnostic procedures, as well as treatment with medication, require patients' informed consent. This requirement applies to psychiatric treatment in which medication is used and to other psychiatric treatments directly affecting the body, such as ECT. Whether informed consent is required for non-somatic psychiatric therapies, such as psychotherapy, is unclear at present. (See further discussion of this issue in Sec. II-B-5-b below.)

2. ELEMENTS OF INFORMED CONSENT

Since the doctrine evolved from a series of court decisions over a period of time, it may differ from jurisdiction to jurisdiction. Despite this, the general outlines of the doctrine are fairly well agreed upon. There are three components: information, voluntariness, and competency, all considered below. (See also Sec. II-B-3-b below, where the relationship of these components to malpractice is explored and Sec. II-B-6 below, where difficulties in the doctrine of informed consent are explored.)

a. Information

This marks the greatest departure from the previous legal standards. Consent given in the absence of sufficient information to make a decision is no longer considered to be an adequate consent. Of course, the question immediately arises as to how much information is enough. Physicians argued that the standard of care of the profession should be the measure applied here: the sufficiency of information should be judged by how much most doctors reveal to their patients.

Many courts agreed, adopting a "professional standard" of disclosure that is still the law in almost half the states. This was one instance, however, in which a large number of courts rejected the right of the profession to set its own standard of care. These judges argued that to permit this essentially would be to maintain the status quo and that the current situation was insufficiently respectful of the rights of the individual to control what happened to her person. The alternative standard that has evolved requires the physician to disclose all the information that a reasonable person might want before deciding to accept or to reject treatment: this includes precisely what the treatment consists of, the potential benefits of the treatment, its potential risks, any alternatives that exist and their benefits and risks, and the benefits and risks of no treatment at all. An opportunity should also be offered for the patient to ask questions.

It should be noted that the "reasonable person" standard is a halfway step between allowing physicians to disclose whatever they think to be material and the radical position of requiring disclosure of everything that might be important for the decision of the individual in question. If a patient is fearful of being in tall buildings, for example, the information that after the operation she will be cared for on the fifteenth floor of the hospital might be quite material to her decision whether or not to have the operation; under the "reasonable person" standard, however, such disclosure would not be required because most people would not find it material to their decision making. Therefore, although the informed consent standard goes a long way in the direction of ensuring individual autonomy and allowing for idiosyncratic opinions, it pulls back in almost all states from the ultimate step. This does not stop the clinician, however, in the interest of having an optimally informed patient, from inquiring about the particular concerns of his patient and individualizing disclosure accordingly.

b. Voluntariness

In conformance with previous common law notions, a consent, to be adequate, must be freely given. Voluntariness (or its converse, coercion) can be a gross or a subtle matter. Obviously, a patient who is threatened by the hospital staff that they will not feed him or give him his clothes back until he agrees to surgery, is being coerced in a significant manner and in a way that undermines the autonomy of his decision. But there can be more subtle forms of coercion, as well. It might, for example, be suggested to a patient that a letter she needs to obtain welfare benefits might not be attended to very promptly unless she goes along with the recommended course of treatment. This is clearly illegitimate.

Even more subtle, and controversial, forms of coercion might be called "situational coercion." There are some who believe that residents of total institutions, whether psychiatric, penal, rehabilitative, or other, cannot be presumed to be giving a voluntary consent to *any* procedure desired by the institution. The reasoning here is that these individuals are so dependent upon the institution for their every need, and in some cases for the opportunity to return to the outside world, that they are facing subtle coercion to agree with the institution's recommendations. While there may be cases in which this is true, the result of applying the theory broadly—namely, depriving all inhabitants of total institutions of the right to make any decisions on matters of importance—hardly seems in accord with the desire to maximize autonomy, a desire that underlies the whole concept of informed consent. Coercion, in its subtlest forms, exists in all interpersonal relationships and, at this level, should probably be excluded from consideration by the legal system. This formulation is in keeping with the usual legal and philosophical approaches to the analysis of coercion, which emphasize that in order for pressure to constitute proscribed coercion it must be illegitimate. This means that the justified exhortation of a care-giver to a patient to accept a recommended treatment, or the equally acceptable pressure from family members to consent to or refuse care does not render the patient's decision void. Only illegitimate forms of pressure, such as those described above, have this effect.

c. Competence

The law of informed consent requires that the patient be competent to offer a consent. The intricacies of competence will be discussed in detail in Chap. 5 (Sec. II-A). For our purposes here, we shall say that although the legal system has yet to define competence in a consistent and clinically useful way, the goal is to ensure that the individual has sufficient mental abilities to be able to engage in the informed consent process. Types of patients who may have an impairment of their competence include the mentally retarded, the organically impaired, psychotic patients, and children. (See Chap. 5, Sec. II-A for a more complete discussion).

Children are by law deemed incompetent until they attain the age of majority, regardless of their actual capacity at any given time. It should be noted that state laws vary widely with regard to the age at which an individual is no longer a minor for the purpose of consent to mental health treatment. Exceptions often exist as well for "emancipated minors"—those who have lived on their own for a period of time—or for certain kinds of diagnosis and treatment—of venereal disease, for example, or consent to abortion. Every practitioner should be aware of the laws in his particular state.

3. LACK OF INFORMED CONSENT AS MALPRACTICE

Informed consent may now be required before the treatment of psychiatric patients can proceed, but the simple failure to obtain an adequate informed consent does not, in itself, constitute malpractice.

a. Elements required

The elements required to establish malpractice on the basis of improper informed consent resemble those required in malpractice cases generally (see Sec. II-A-1 above). The existence of a clinician-patient relationship and therefore a duty of care is usually self-evident from the fact that the clinician did something to or with the patient. The clinician's negligence would here consist in not obtaining a proper informed consent for what was done; most cases revolve around the specific issue of whether the patient was adequately informed prior to the procedure or treatment. Even if a proper consent was *not* obtained, the patient must still establish that some harm occurred as a result of the procedure. And finally, a link must be drawn between the failure to obtain an adequate informed consent and the resulting harm. This last goal is usually attained by requiring the patient to prove, to a preponderance of the evidence, that had a reasonable person been given the information that was omitted, she would have chosen not to go ahead with the procedure or treatment. Some courts will allow the patient merely to prove that he himself would not have consented had the information been available. It is important to note that even in the absence of demonstrable negligence in the actual procedure or treatment, should a bad result occur the physician may be liable if a proper informed consent was not obtained, because that in itself is evidence of negligence.

b. Problems of proof

The difficulties of establishing that a duty of care existed and that a harm occurred are no different in the informed consent case than in malpractice cases generally (see Sec. II-A-2 above). What is special about these cases is determining the adequacy of the consent and establishing causation. (See also Secs. II-B-2 above and II-B-6 below.)

Information.   The patient-plaintiff will usually be in the position of alleging that certain key information was not presented to her prior to her rendering a decision about the treatment. If no records exist, it is a matter of the jury choosing between believing the patient and believing the clinician, assuming the latter alleges otherwise. Most clinicians, who are naturally enough uncomfortable with this situation, would like to have some documentary evidence with which to counter the patient's allegations.

Two options are generally used. Some practitioners and facilities prefer to have a patient sign a written consent form that outlines the relevant material. While this is useful in some cases, other clinicians avoid written forms because of the possible implication that this material and only this material on the form was communicated to the patient. Additional discussions between the doctor and the patient, or between the patient and other personnel, are not recorded on the form and might tend to be ignored in court. In addition, routine use of consent forms often has the effect of turning what should be a free and spontaneous interaction between clinician and patient into a rigid procedure in which the clinician allows the form—often loaded with jargon—to substitute for a clear presentation of the facts to the patient, rather than simply serving as a documentation of such presentation.

The second option is for the clinician to record in the patient's chart that a consent interview has taken place, enumerating the topics covered in general terms, and noting specifically whether the patient had particular concerns. The patient need not sign the note. Courts are usually quite willing to accept such notes as evidence of the consent discussion and, since they are not exhaustive, there is scope for the clinician to elaborate on the contents of the discussion in court. The good faith demonstrated by placing the note in the chart is generally supportive of the clinician's supplementary testimony.

There are of course, more imaginative options. Reports exist of practitioners who audiotape or videotape consent interviews; that seems like an unnecessarily conservative step and one that might backfire on a competent clinician who comes across poorly on tape or on a video screen. In any event, some record of the consent transaction is important. Several studies have demonstrated that patients often forget much of what was discussed in such sessions or forget that the session took place at all. Patients can, in good faith, argue that they were not informed about potential risks, when the information definitely was conveyed.

Naturally, the same applies for clinicians: it can be acutely embarassing to be asked to reconstruct in court several years after the date in question the exact contents of a consent interview without any record to rely upon.

Voluntariness.   Depending upon the type of undue influence alleged, it may be quite difficult in retrospect to determine the level of voluntariness of a given consent. This is, in fact, usually a policy issue (i.e., should a given class of patients be presumed to have been subject to coercion) rather than one that affects the individual patient. Nonetheless, if some special circumstance (for example, the threats of staff members to beat up a patient unless he consents to ECT) might be construed as impairing voluntariness, the reasoning as to why that is or is not the case should be recorded carefully along with the record of the consent interview.

Competence.   The prime difficulty of establishing a patient's status in regard to competence is the lack of clear-cut standards to be used (see Chap. 5, Sec. II-A). Again, the rule of thumb is that if there might be any reason to doubt the patient's competence in retrospect, a careful examination for competence should be conducted (see Chap. 5, Sec. III-A) and its results recorded. One technique for measuring competence to consent to a specific procedure is the two-part consent form: this consists of a written information form, supplemented by oral discussion, that is followed by a series of questions to elucidate the degree of understanding that the patient has of the information that has been conveyed. While understanding is only one component of competence, it is the element that the courts focus upon most closely. The two-part consent form has, until now, served mostly as a research technique. Its adoption for routine clinical use, however, has much to recommend it, both as a record of the understanding of the patient at the time of the consent, and as a guide to the clinician as to the specific deficits in the patient's understanding that may be remedied by further education.

Causation.   Drawing the causal link between the deficiencies in the informed consent process and the ultimate harm is very difficult. What it requires, as noted above, is the patient's demonstration that—had the information been supplied—his choice, or the choice of a reasonable person, would have been different. The subjectivity of this assessment is demonstrated by the numerous court decisions that have varied greatly in the kind of risks that they deem to be material enough to have been disclosed. Cases range from risks of 3% chance of death and 1% chance of loss of hearing where disclosure *was* required to 1.5% chance of loss of eye and 1/8,000,000 chance of aplastic anemia where disclosure was *not* required. (See also section II-D-4, where it is suggested that the courts may be influenced by a desire to award compensation in setting these standards.) Some legal commentators look more closely at the statistical probabilities, while others are more inclined to say that any risk that might deter the patient, no matter how unlikely it is to occur, should be disclosed. The latter seems too extreme a view to be implemented in practice, but there are two rules of thumb: (1) the more severe the potential harm, the lower the threshold should be for disclosure; (2) the most common risks of most treatments or procedures should probably be disclosed, even if they are relatively minor. Unfortunately, no more definitive guidelines are available for the practitioner.

4. EXCEPTIONS TO THE DOCTRINE OF INFORMED CONSENT

The objections of many psychiatrists to the doctrine of informed consent are rooted in the supposed rigidity of the doctrine and its inapplicability to clinical psychiatric practice. Some of the difficulties with informed consent will be considered below (see Sec. II-B-6), but we will begin the discussion here by noting that the law itself recognizes some of the difficulties and provides for four situations in which the requirements of informed consent do not apply.

a. Emergencies

Informed consent need not be obtained in emergency situations. The key to this exception, of course, is how one chooses to define an emergency. Clinical medicine generally has an easier time of this than does psychiatry. For a near comatose patient in diabetic ketoacidosis, a severely traumatized patient with internal bleeding, or a patient in a hypertensive crisis, it is apparent to all that the time required to obtain an informed consent, or a substituted consent if the patient is not herself competent to offer a consent (see Chap. 5, Sec. II-C), would so delay the needed treatment as to pose a direct danger to the patient's life. In such circumstances, the physician may treat without a formal consent. The law, to make its balance sheets come out even, creates the fiction of an "implied consent" in these cases; since almost any rational person facing an acute, life-threatening crisis would elect to proceed with treatment, the law allows the physician to read the consent as being implicit in the situation.

Genuine emergencies do, of course, exist in psychiatry. A violent, excited, or self-mutilating psychotic patient in the emergency room or on the inpatient ward may require immediate restraint and/or medication to prevent physical harm to self or others. This is perhaps the most clear-cut case and the only exception to the informed consent requirement that has been granted consistently in court decisions concerning the right to refuse treatment. Other situations are a bit more ambiguous from the legal standpoint. Acutely psychotic, nonviolent patients, though suffering great distress, may not, in some jurisdictions, present a sufficiently emergent situation (from the legal viewpoint) to justify complete disregard for obtaining informed or substituted consent. The same appears to hold true for severely depressed patients, even if food and fluid intake are minimal to nonexistent, as long as their physical status (i.e., electrolytes, blood pressure, cardiac function) is stable. In both these cases, in some jurisdictions, an attempt must be made to obtain an informed consent prior to treatment or, if the patient is incompetent, to obtain a substituted consent.

Many psychiatrists argue that psychiatric emergencies should be defined more broadly (see Chap. 3, Sec. II-C-4 on the right to refuse treatment) to encompass a variety of acute situations in which the potential for great suffering or for rapid decompensation exists. Some courts have agreed, and in other states psychiatrists continue to hew to a more clinically oriented standard, awaiting a definitive court ruling in their jurisdiction.

b. Therapeutic privilege

Even before the time that the requirement for consent became the mandate for informed consent, there were situations in which it was recognized that the normal procedure for informing the patient about the nature of her condition and the proposed treatment could be suspended, if it were in the patient's best interest to do so. This exception, called "therapeutic privilege," applied whenever the physician felt that the information to be conveyed would in itself be so damaging to the patient that disclosure would be antitherapeutic. Whether or not a patient was told that she had cancer often revolved around this issue.

Some doctors are delighted with the idea of therapeutic privilege, both because it reinforces their status as someone who is allowed to decide what is or is not in the patient's best interest and because it seems to provide an "out" as far as informed consent is concerned. "If I tell any of my paranoid schizophrenic patients about the side effects of their medication," a psychiatrist who falls into this group might say, "of course they'll refuse to take it. Then they'll decompensate and require rehospitalization. So it's clearly not in their best interest for me to get an informed consent from them." Naturally, if the court accepted this construction of the therapeutic privilege, it would all but vitiate whatever impact informed consent has had. More alert courts, realizing this, have drawn the privilege much more narrowly: if the information itself might be directly damaging to the patient, it can be withheld (e.g., a fragile schizophrenic patient need not be told her diagnosis), but not if the damage would be mediated by the decision of a well-informed patient to refuse treatment. Judicial decisions have emphasized strongly that this option to refuse is precisely what the informed consent doctrine was designed to allow. In theory, if the disclosure would interfere with the patient's powers of rational decision making, it could be withheld, but that, too, is likely to be construed narrowly where the nondisclosure of risks is involved. So construed, the situations in psychiatry in which therapeutic privilege can be involved are relatively circumscribed.

c. Waiver

The right to an informed consent, insofar as it belongs to the patient, can be waived by a patient who chooses to do so. No clinician is required to reveal information to an unwilling patient. In sensitive situations, waiver can be a subtle phenomenon. A physician who begins to explain the risks of a procedure to a patient, only to have the latter say, "That's okay, Doc, I trust you. Just go ahead and do whatever you have to," has just received a waiver that, if properly recorded, would probably stand up in any court. Waivers of basic rights are usually required to be "knowing waivers"; e.g., in a criminal setting, a suspect must be told that he *has* a right to speak with a lawyer before he can be said to have waived that right. Although it is not clear whether such a strict interpretation applies to the informed consent process, in situations in which it is uncertain if a patient who is apparently waiving his rights is actually aware that he has a right to the information, a comment such as, "I'd be glad to tell you whatever you'd like to know about the treatment, but, of course, we don't have to go through it if you'd rather not," might ensure that the waiver is truly knowing. Patients may waive either their right to information or the right to consent, or both.

d. Incompetence

(See Chap. 5, where this issue is discussed at length.) An incompetent patient is, by definition, not capable of giving an informed consent regardless of the category of incompetence, whether legal (e.g., she is a minor) or functional (e.g., she is psychotic). The exception to the informed consent requirement here differs from the other three discussed above in that the requirement is not negated altogether: rather, its form is changed. Although consent cannot be obtained from the incompetent patient, it must be obtained from a substitute decision-maker, the identity of whom will vary across jurisdictions. (See Chap. 5, Sec. II-C.)

5. SPECIAL PROBLEMS WITH INFORMED CONSENT IN PSYCHIATRY

a. Tardive dyskinesia

Perhaps the most complicated and controversial issue of informed consent in psychiatry concerns how much psychotic patients who require neuroleptic medication should be told about the long-term risk of tardive dyskinesia (see also Chap. 3, Sec. III-C-2-e-iv). There is no satisfactory answer that applies in all situations nor is there much guidance from the courts on the subject. One opinion that seems to exist among clinicians is that acutely psychotic patients should not be told about the risk of tardive dyskinesia when treatment is initiated because, given their psychotic state, they can neither comprehend the information nor balance the risk with possible benefits, and might thus be led to refuse treatment. This opinion, however, appears to be based on a combination of the common misconception about therapeutic privilege (see Sec. II-B-4-b above)—that if information will lead a patient to reject needed treatment, it can be withheld—and the feeling that acutely psychotic patients are incompetent to consent to treatment anyway—which is certainly true in many cases, is not true in others, and may call for a substitute decisionmaker or special consent procedure in any event.

Another common rationale for withholding information from psychotic patients about tardive dyskinesia is that the risk of TD does not accrue until several months after treatment begins, thus allowing disclosure to be deferred until that time. This rationale, however, does not apply to a previously treated patient, whose putative grace period may have expired long ago. Nor, given evidence suggesting that TD is in part a function of total lifetime dose of neuroleptic medication, is it true that any period of administration is without risk. Finally, it seems unfair to patients to neglect to mention an important long-term side effect of a treatment they may come to rely upon, only to reveal it to them at some later time.

Thus, there is good reason to reject approaches that fail to provide some information to patients about tardive dyskinesia, even at the beginning of treatment. An acceptable practice may be to titrate the amount of information disclosed to the patient's ability to assimilate it (assuming that the patient is consenting to treatment on her own behalf). This would mean some mention of the risk of TD at the initiation of treatment, with more details provided as the patient improves. This sensitive process should be documented in the patient's chart, but would seem difficult to incorporate into a procedure that required the use of written consent forms.

b. Psychotherapy

As indicated above, it has never been clear whether the requirements of informed consent apply to procedures—such as psychotherapy—that do not involve direct intrusion into the patient's body. It has been argued in favor of requiring informed consent to psychotherapy that: 1) many patients are unaware of what is involved in psychotherapy and need to know something about the process prior to becoming involved in it; 2) there are risks attached to the process, including the risks that the patient will get worse or regress in therapy and that confidential information may fall into the hands of others (see Chap. 1, Sec. II-B-4); and 3) alternative treatments exist for most conditions, including other forms of psychotherapy, as well as medications, of which patients have the right to know before committing themselves to a particular therapeutic approach.

Opposition to obtaining informed consent to psychotherapy comes in part from therapists trained in psychoanalytic approaches who believe that discussions of the sorts of issues mentioned above would both contaminate the transference and foster non-constructive intellectualization and therefore undermine the therapy. Therapists of other schools may minimize the risks associated with psychotherapy, maintain that patients know what they are getting into, and in the case of non-medical therapists, be reluctant to assume a burden that traditionally has been associated largely with the medical profession. Yet others note the paradox of the patient's giving "consent" to what are essentially her own productions, psychotherapy being almost entirely the patient's own procedure.

There is no clear guidance here from either case law or statutes. It does seem reasonable, however, for patients to be told something of what they might expect in psychotherapy at the initiation of treatment. An exception might be made for psychoanalysis here, on the grounds that most analytic patients come to the analyst with a fairly good idea of what the process entails. It is difficult to believe that discussion of this sort would undermine most non-analytic therapies; many psychotherapists, supported by literature on the therapeutic alliance, already orient their patients to the process in precisely this way. When medication would be a reasonable alternative to psychotherapy, some discussion of this option may well be indicated. (Non-medical therapists should probably offer to refer patients to a consulting psychiatrist for this purpose.) And when some particular threat to a patient's confidentiality is likely to arise (e.g., for patients involved in custody disputes with current or former spouses), some comment on the likelihood of this being a problem should be offered. On the other hand, formal consent forms and detailed notes would seem to be excessive precautions at the present time.

6. ASSESSMENT OF THE DOCTRINE OF INFORMED CONSENT

The construction of the doctrine of informed consent is an ambitious effort by the legal profession to alter the nature of medical and psychiatric care; by attempting to change the elements of the clinician-patient interaction, it appears to hold the potential for what many would deem a radical redistribution of power in the therapeutic relationship. Such a conclusion, however, may be excessively optimistic. In addition to the practical problems of the doctrine, many of which have been discussed above, there are significant theoretical difficulties with informed consent law as it now stands.

a. Practical problems

When courts began to require that doctors provide patients with all the information material to their decision, they were operating with a model that rested on several implicit assumptions: that patients would pay attention to the information, that they would understand it, and that they would use the information in reaching their decisions. Empirical studies (though most suffer from methodologic problems) have cast serious doubt on all these propositions. Patient attention and understanding, as measured by tests of recall, has almost always been found to be poor. While there are suggestions that this might be a result of the way in which the information was presented (i.e., use of technical language, complicated sentence structure), it is also possible that simplification of much medical information to a lay level is either impossible or is so difficult to achieve as to be practically impossible in everyday clinical work. Even given the requisite simplification, it is unclear if, in many cases, an individual without a medical education has the context in which to analyze the information. Further, to the extent that illness induces a state of regression in which patients seek a reliable authority figure on whom to depend, they may ignore the information altogether, preferring to ask the doctor at the end of the recitation, "What do you think I should do?"

Also implicit in the model of informed consent is the idea that the revealed information, assuming it is assimilated and understood, will have some bearing on the patient's decision. This has been challenged from several directions. If we examine the situation temporally, it is clear that many patients make up their mind to accept or to refuse a given treatment well before the formal consent interview, perhaps even as early as the time they decide to seek medical attention. Nor is the kind of information that is transmitted by the physician necessarily the kind that most influences a patient's decision. Social factors such as family pressures, the financial burden of entering a hospital or of refusing to, the attitude toward this form of treatment in the patient's social milieu, and the nature of the setting in which treatment takes place—all may be more influential than a description of potential side effects with unpronounceable names and remote statistical probabilities. Yet the informed consent doctrine implicitly assumes that these social factors are relatively unimportant determinants.

b. Theoretical problems

In so far as the doctrine of informed consent was intended as a mechanism to force clinicians to share information with patients, many legal commentators charge that the ways in which the doctrine has evolved have short-circuited that objective. These critics point to such factors as the use of a professional standard of disclosure, the classification of failure to reveal adequate information as a matter of malpractice rather than battery, and the difficult problems of proof confronting plaintiffs who allege failure to obtain informed consent as substantially limiting the impact of the doctrine. Taken together, they make it unlikely that clinicians will be sued for failure to obtain consent (an allegation validated by the data on the frequency of such cases), and even more unlikely that such suits will be successful. This, it is argued, in turn limits the degree of compliance with the mandates of informed consent law, which is consistent with empirical studies of informed consent in psychiatry and general medicine.

c. A synthetic approach to informed consent

If the realities of dealing with patients make it unlikely that disclosure of information will alter their decisionmaking, and if the law itself is a relatively weak means of enforcing this requirement in the first place, what is the point of the doctrine of informed consent? Would clinicians' lives not be simpler without it? Perhaps. But the practical and theoretical objections to the current shape of consent law are, in many ways, beside the point. Even granting their legitimacy, there are strong reasons to value informed consent in psychiatric practice.

Some patients may reject attempts to inform them, but many patients desire such information, even if they do not intend to use it to make their own treatment decisions. Ironically, most physicians and other caregivers probably fall into this latter category when they themselves assume the patient role. Given the high value our society places on the right of persons to make knowledgeable choices about important issues, it does not seem unreasonable to respect the right of patients to receive this information. Even more importantly, the process of informed consent can be used to strengthen the therapeutic relationship by enhancing trust and understanding between clinician and patient. (See Sec. III-A-2-c below.) Thus, it may have positive therapeutic benefits, when properly employed, that go well beyond those that were envisioned for it by even its most ardent legal advocates.

C. Other forms of liability

Malpractice is not the only form of liability that the mental health professional faces. In addition to the kinds of suits to which everyone is susceptible (e.g., the patient who sues after slipping on an unsecured rug), there are several other categories of liability that are especially relevant to the clinician-patient relationship. Most of these fall under the general heading of torts—non-contractual civil wrongs—but, as we shall see, there are also civil rights actions and criminal actions that can be brought. Some of these types of actions have been discussed in previous sections and will therefore be discussed only briefly here. The most important aspect they have in common is that they are *not* covered under the usual malpractice insurance policy.

1. FALSE IMPRISONMENT

This tort arises when one individual deprives another of his freedom in an unjustified manner. In psychiatry, such a situation is most likely to occur when a patient is involuntarily committed to a hospital. Unlike malpractice, which is a negligent tort, false imprisonment is classified as an intentional tort; to be liable, the clinician must willfully have deprived a person of his freedom, even though she was aware that the person did not meet the legally mandated criteria for commitment. False imprisonment does not require the use of force. If a patient is simply told that she cannot leave and she believes that to be true, that is sufficient to demonstrate that she was held against her will.

Willful acts of this sort by a clinician are the stuff that lurid movies are made of, but they are undoubtedly rare in practice. More common are acts of negligence that lead to involuntary confinement. A clinician who fails to examine the patient carefully or who is negligently mistaken about the scope of the commitment laws can be sued for malpractice. In most jurisdictions, practitioners who examine patients for the court (e.g., in a court clinic) are considered to be acting as officers of the court and are thus immune from suit for negligent (but not willful) acts. Some states provide statutory immunity for all clinicians who participate in commitment proceedings, as long as their actions were neither grossly negligent nor intentionally harmful to the patient.

2. BREACH OF PRIVACY

The law has traditionally pointed to four ways in which an individual's privacy may be invaded. Her likeness or name may be appropriated for commercial purposes; there may be intrusion on her state of seclusion; her activities or condition may be cast publicly in a false light; or public disclosure of facts that she considers embarrassing may take place. These may constitute either negligent or intentional torts. In theory, any of these injuries to the individual's privacy can occur in psychiatric practice. More recently, as noted in Chapter 1 (see Sec. II-B-3), breach of privacy per se, in a relationship in which an expectation of privacy exists, has been recognized by the courts as a legitimate cause of action. Although remedies for violations of patients' confidentiality will usually be pursued as malpractice actions alleging departures from the standard of care, they can result in complaints under any of the following categories.

a. Appropriation of a likeness or name

This tort requires that a person's likeness or name be appropriated without his consent for the pecuniary benefit of a third party. Thus, the potential for this tort arises, for example, when an illustrated case history or chapter is published in a book or lay periodical and the pictures used have not been sufficiently disguised so as to render the patient unidentifiable. The remedy is obvious. All published or publicly presented pictures of patients should be altered enough to make identification unlikely. If that is not possible, either because to do so would obscure the significant clinical details, or because the case is so well known as to be immediately identifiable, the patient's consent should be obtained before publication. Needless to say, patient's actual names should never be used.

b. Intrusion on seclusion

It is not uncommon for emergency room or walk-in service clinicians to be approached by concerned friends, neighbors, or relatives of someone whom they claim is behaving strangely and is mentally ill. They may report that the person in question has cut off all his ties to the outside world and has retreated into his house. They will usually ask the clinician to "do something."

Whether the clinician does something or not should depend on whether she believes that she has sufficient evidence that the person in question is both mentally ill and meets one of the criteria for involuntary emergency commitment. An action taken in the absence of such evidence might leave the clinician open to a suit for invading the seclusion of someone who may turn out to be an eccentric, but hardly committable, person. In general, people have the right to be left alone. Clinicians faced with such a situation, who do not believe that they have sufficient data upon which to act, or who, even more wisely, refuse as a matter of principle to write commitment orders for patients they have never personally examined, would do well to refer the informants to the police, who are empowered to conduct further investigations, or to the courts, which can issue warrants of apprehension, permitting detention for evaluation.

c. False light

This is related to the tort of defamation, which will be considered below, and represents an alternative cause of action in situations in which a person has been publicly portrayed in an offensive and incorrect manner by someone who knew or recklessly disregarded the fact that the information was false. Publications and presentations containing identifiable data again place one at risk.

d. Public disclosure of embarrassing facts

The situation here is usually similar to the problem of appropriation of a person's name or picture discussed in Section a above. Again, we must stress the need to disguise the identity of the individual or, alternatively, to obtain the patient's permission.

e. Breach of privacy

As noted, this is becoming a tort in its own right. A mental health professional who discloses information obtained in confidence leaves himself open to suit on these grounds. An example might include a psychiatrist who informs a patient's employer of his diagnosis and prognosis without the patient's permission. Some states, in addition to a common law cause of action, have enacted statutory protections for patients' privacy, which can constitute alternative grounds for recovery of damages. At least one recent case has held the person soliciting the confidential information—in this case the employer—to be equally liable with the psychiatrist who revealed the data.

3. DEFAMATION

Defamation is defined as a communication that "tends so to harm the reputation of another as to lower him in the estimation of the community or to deter third persons from associating or dealing with him." There are two types: libel—in which the communication takes a written form—and slander—in which the communication is oral. The defamatory communication will usually be false, although it may be possible to allege defamation if true, but compromising, information is revealed solely for the purpose of causing harm to the person in question. In some circumstances (for example, when public figures are concerned), the U.S. Supreme Court has ruled that the defendant must have acted in malicious disregard of the fact that the information is false.

The precautions previously referred to concerning disguising published material should be extended here to include ascertaining carefully the veracity of any material to be published. A clinician should refrain from public discussion of a patient's case whether or not the statements made are accurate, but if they are inaccurate, liability may accrue for slander as well as for breach of privacy. The rules dealing with a plaintiff's recovery for acts of slander are more stringent than those for libel: the plaintiff must usually prove pecuniary loss. Unfortunately for the therapist, actions for slander are also allowed if the plaintiff has been imputed to have a "loathsome disease" or if aspersions have been cast on his ability to perform in his business, trade, office, or profession. Many statements about patients in psychiatric treatment, and sometimes even the statement that someone is *in* psychiatric treatment, could conceivably be construed as falling into one of these two categories. Thus, there are good legal as well as ethical reasons for not speaking of one's patients abroad, except insofar as the communication is necessary for their care (see Chap. 1, Sec. II-B-5).

4. INTERFERENCE WITH ADVANTAGEOUS RELATIONS

This class of tort covers intentional behavior that results in a financial or personal loss to the plaintiff. An example is interference with contractual relations. In the psychiatric context, an allegation of this sort might arise if the therapist persuaded a patient not to complete contractual obligations the patient owed to a third party. The therapist might then be liable to suit by that person and recovery of damages. Another example comes under the category of alienation of affections, with which a therapist might be charged if he persuaded his patient to leave her husband or a child to leave his parents' home. Some jurisdictions may require a finding of adultery to establish alienation of the affections of a spouse.

The traditional analytic stance of refusing to advise patients to perform any act, while remaining ready to explore all the possibilities open to them, should effectively preclude charges of interference (see Section III-A-2-d below). Suspicions are certainly heightened when the therapist is a direct beneficiary of the act in question, as when the patient leaves her husband only to move in with her therapist. Ethics aside, this does not constitute a conservative approach to loss-prevention.

5. CIVIL RIGHTS ACTIONS

A long-neglected nineteenth-century law, Section 1983 of Title 42 of the U.S. Code, has been resurrected in the last several decades to provide one of the most potent litigatory weapons for plaintiffs who feel that their civil rights have been infringed. Section 1983 provides that "every person who, under color of any statute, ordinance, regulation, custom, or usage of any State or Territory, subjects or causes to be subjected, any citizen of the United States . . . to the deprivation of any rights, privileges or immunities secured by Constitution and laws, shall be liable to the person injured in an action of law. . . ."

Civil rights actions have become popular means for members of the mental health bar to attempt to effect systemwide changes. They provide for both injunctive relief (the halting of the practices in question) and the possibility of compensation to those who are found to have been deprived of their rights. In addition, successful plaintiffs' attorneys can have their legal fees paid by the defendants, usually state governments, even in cases (unlike the situation in a malpractice case) in which no monetary awards are made. While suits for deprivation of rights can be directed against those in charge of the system (for example, the commissioner of mental health in a given state), they can also be targeted against the line personnel who deliver psychiatric care. This puts the psychiatrist who has merely followed state regulations—for example, in administering medication to refusing patients—at risk for being sued for violating patients' constitutional rights. Since the existence of these rights is usually not clearly defined before the final court ruling, clinicians are left with little guidance as to how to proceed with patient care while minimizing the risk of suit.

The courts are not totally unsympathetic to this awkward position of the person responsible for direct patient care. They have ruled, in general, that good faith actions on the part of the individual, as opposed to the governmental agency for whom he works, provide immunity from liability for damages. Nonetheless, the individual clinician often has had to undergo a traumatic and prolonged legal process before his immunity is proclaimed, and he may have to withstand appeals, as well. What complicates the matter is that malpractice insurers may refuse to provide either legal assistance or coverage for damages for Section 1983 actions, because they do not come within the scope of traditional malpractice. This can mean astronomical legal bills for the unlucky practitioner. So far, most Section 1983 suits have been targeted against state facilities, probably because conditions there have tended to be the poorest; whether psychiatrists or other clinicians in private facilities can be said to be acting "under color of statute, ordinance, (or) regulation" and thus to be subject to suit as well is, at present, unsettled.

Civil rights suits under Section 1983 are one of the most powerful stimuli to the pervasive sense of paranoia about the legal profession that exists in psychiatry today. (See Sec. II-D-3 below.) Clinicians interpret the use of such actions, directed against them as individuals, but actually intended to effect systemic changes, as personal assaults. Lawyers, on the other hand, see Section 1983 as one of the only handles they have on the states' power to run institutions as they see fit. Given this fact, their prevalence is not likely to diminish.

6. Fraud

Fraud can be either a criminal or a civil action. Therapists need to be concerned about its occurrence in two modes. To the extent that a therapist advertises falsely, that is, when she promises a patient a certain result that she knows she cannot deliver, the therapist is liable for a charge of fraud. The "advertising" need not be in a public forum: the promise of a good result to a prospective patient is sufficient. (In those circumstances in which the therapist did not knowingly deceive the patient, but nonetheless promised a result that was not obtained, a civil suit for breach of contract can be filed.) The take-home lesson should be obvious. It is unwise to promise any results other than that the therapeutic process will take place: the therapist will try to work with the patient to understand the problems involved (in a psychotherapeutic model), to help the patient alter the behaviors involved (in a behavioral model) or to control the patient's symptoms (medical model). Patients' inquiries as to the likelihood of success can be answered frankly with statistical data, answered with acknowledgement of ignorance of the future, used for interpretative purposes, or ignored, as best fits the model of the practitioner's school, but no guarantees should be made. (See section III-A-2-b below, as well.)

Unfortunately, another reference needs to be made to the problem of fraud. A tight set of rules has developed to govern the interactions between third-party payers and the therapist, especially when the third party is the government. Clinicians who provide false diagnoses, even if done to maintain patients' privacy, who bill for sessions that have never taken place, or who otherwise falsify the information on the billing forms are subject to prosecution for criminal fraud. The same is true, although the practice is reported to be widespread, for psychiatrists and psychologists who certify that they have personally attended to patients who, in fact, are being treated by other mental health workers under their employ. Such practices should be shunned. One potential source of fraudulent claims, the problem of billing for missed appointments, can be avoided if it is worked out in advance with the patient. On both clinical and legal grounds it seems more advantageous to hold patients who miss appointments directly responsible for the payment for the missed session, rather than to be in the position of attempting to bill the third party for nonexistent sessions.

D. Miscellaneous problems of liability

1. LIABILITY OF NONMEDICAL MENTAL HEALTH PROFESSIONALS

Although the bulk of the literature and case law on malpractice deals with the medical profession, it should be clear from the discussion in this chapter that many of the same problems exist for the other core mental health disciplines. As clinical psychology, clinical social work, and the independent practice of psychiatric nursing have become professionalized, they, too, have become liable to suits for malpractice. The standard of care to which each of these disciplines is expected to conform is that established by the discipline itself. Further, to the extent that psychologists, social workers, and nurses assume primary responsibility for patient care, they can be said to establish the same duty of care, within the context of a fiduciary relationship, that exists for psychiatrists.

Although few cases in which the other disciplines are involved have attracted attention (there have been some cases concerning treatment administered by behaviorally oriented psychologists, who seem to be at particular risk and a large number of cases concerning sexual involvement), the potential for liability has not gone unnoticed. Many of the professional organizations and some private insurance companies sponsor malpractice insurance for these other disciplines. Nonmedical professionals who are supervised by psychiatrists or by other physicians are not free from liability simply because of that supervisory relationship; though the doctrines of *respondeat superior* and negligent supervision may force the psychiatrist to assume responsibility for their acts, these nonmedical professionals share liability for the consequences of their actions.

2. THE INSURANCE PROBLEM

What makes any kind of medical or mental health practice possible in the face of potentially enormous damage judgments is the availability of malpractice insurance. Such was not always the case. Until the 1800s, insurance for negligent acts was not permitted as a matter of public policy; it was thought that enabling individuals to insure against their negligence would encourage recklessness. The temper of the times changed as the pace of industrialization increased and negligent acts came to be recognized as statistically inevitable occurrences: if enough people are performing a given act frequently enough, someone is bound to make a negligent mistake. The moral opprobrium that once attached itself to negligence disappeared. Remnants of that approach remain today, however, in that most policies will not cover "intentional" torts ("intentional" is used in the sense here of any voluntary, nonnegligent act) or other "intentional" acts, such as civil rights violations.

We have witnessed two distinct "crises" in the malpractice insurance industry in the last two decades. The rising tide of malpractice suits in the early 1970s made insurers reluctant to continue to issue malpractice policies. In the climate of aggressive litigiousness and large awards that characterized the period and that continues today, it became difficult for the companies to predict actuarially the extent of the damages for which they would be responsible and thus to set their charges so as to guarantee a fixed rate of profit. Those companies that remained in the business increased their rates dramatically to compensate themselves both for the higher level of damage payments and for the greater risk that they were incurring. The combination of skyrocketing insurance premiums and total unavailability in some areas led to the first much-publicized "crisis" in malpractice insurance.

Several solutions to the crisis were proposed and implemented. In some areas in which the medical profession was completely abandoned by the insurers, the profession itself organized insurance companies to fill the gap. Professional associations in mental health, including the American Psychiatric Association and the American Psychological Association, similarly offer insurance policies to their members. Statutory changes in laws governing malpractice suits made it more difficult for actions to be brought; these included measures that shortened the period during which suit could be brought after discovery of the harm (the statute of limitations), tinkered with the burden of proof traditionally left to the court to allocate, and provided for the screening of all malpractice suits by multidisciplinary panels. Actions taken to reduce the overall size of judgments, including caps on awards and the offset of any compensation received by patients from their own insurance policies, were also implemented. The effect of these changes remains controversial and some have been overturned on constitutional grounds. Whatever the reason, however, the rate of malpractice cases declined somewhat following this period of tort reform, and the crisis passed.

In contrast to the "crisis of availability" that characterized the 1970s, the 1980s were marked by a "crisis of affordability." Insurers appeared better able to project losses, but with judgments continuing to soar (the size of judgments being a more important factor than the number of cases filed), rates rose steadily. The astronomical sums paid by obstetricians and neurosurgeons are well known. So far, however, the mental health professions have been relatively spared.

Psychiatrists tend to be placed in the lowest risk category of medical professionals (unless they perform ECT, in which case their risk category rises somewhat). Their premiums have increased greatly in recent years, but remain relatively modest in comparison with those of most of their medical colleagues. Psychologists and other mental health professionals pay even more modest premiums. Nonetheless, there is no guarantee that this situation will continue, particularly as issues such as patient-therapist sex become frequent targets of malpractice litigation. In the absence of further effective tort reform, mental health professionals too may look forward to having their practices increasingly impacted by rising malpractice insurance rates.

3. THE SYSTEMS ISSUE

Health care professionals in general, and mental health professionals, especially psychiatrists, in particular have borne the brunt of a desire for certain kinds of social change that has been prevalent in the land. The inertia inherent in legislative bodies and their general conservatism have led reformers of all stripes to seek alternative means of providing new rights or creating new systems of care. What they have found has been a way to achieve their goals by using the personal liability system, originally erected to permit those who had suffered harm to obtain compensation.

The desire of reformers to promote individual autonomy has been advanced by the promulgation of the doctrine of informed consent, enforced through the tort law. The goal of improving the performance of psychiatric care systems has been pressed by widening the possible grounds for malpractice and for civil rights actions. The fact that individuals will bear the burden of the resulting suits and the damage judgments, when it is the system or the society as a whole that is in fact responsible, is ignored in this rush to achieve social change. Professionals, who are thrown on the defensive by what they perceive as direct and personal assaults, are then often forced into the position of opposing generally desirable changes in society (e.g., improved care for the mentally ill and mentally retarded) because of the fear that they will be asked as individuals to pay the price of this progress.

That is not to say that genuine abuses—negligent medical care, deprivation of civil rights, and the like—have not taken place and that some individual practitioners might not be responsible for them. But in general professions that are probably better trained and more highly skilled today than they were forty years ago are subject to an enormously magnified legal burden compared with those days.

It is hard to know what to do about this tendency to use individuals in the professions as the battering rams of change. It would be ingenuous to expect reformers to give up what appears to be a highly useful tool. The legislatures, whose hyporesponsivity was often the cause of the problem in the first place, are unlikely to provide a basis for relief. Perhaps all that this analysis can accomplish is to decrease the tendency for the professions to respond to these trends with wildly directed anger, sulking hurt, or withdrawal from the political system as a whole. A sustained effort to educate the public at large about the root causes of this aspect of the malpractice crisis in the professions might ease the way for the development of means of accomplishing social ends that are less personally traumatic. But it also might not; to the extent that someone must bear the burdens of change in every period of societal reorganization, the health care professions seem to have been chosen for the role today.

4. THE MOVE TOWARD STRICT LIABILITY

As one element of the process described above, court rulings in a number of areas have sought to prevent the wealthy from benefiting at the expense of the poor by altering the rules that govern liability actions. In place of a system in which a finding of liability requires proof of negligence, a system of strict liability is developing. Strict liability means that whoever performed the act or produced the product is liable for whatever harm results, even if every possible precaution was taken to prevent that harm. The justifications for such a change are socioeconomic ones: (1) the producers or providers tend to be wealthier than the consumers or clients; (2) the producers or providers are in a better position to defray the cost of damages, either by insurance or by raising their price or fee sufficiently to provide self-insurance; (3) the cost of damages is in reality a cost of producing the good or service and thus, for reasons of efficiency ought to be borne by the producer or provider; (4) in an increasingly complex society in which one is likely to become a victim without any forewarning or any action of one's own, it is only fair to provide compensation for victims, since society as a whole benefits from the product or activities that have led to the injury.

Strict liability has not yet been adopted in malpractice law, although it has been suggested as a standard. As the review above notes, negligence is still ostensibly required to obtain a damage judgment. But professionals are also not incorrect when they sense that the rules of evidence and of proof and legal reasoning in general tend to be twisted in such a way as to provide compensation whenever possible if some harm—*any* harm—has taken place. Though professionals, especially doctors, often take this tendency as evidence of an attack upon their profession by the courts, it is in fact part of a wider change in the nature of tort law that is designed to redistribute some measure of wealth in our society.

Whether it is just thus to use law to foster a particular economic viewpoint is a matter of controversy, although legal scholars maintain that every legal system advances one or another economic philosophy. If the trend continues, it is likely that, when the new system settles out, a mechanism will evolve for preventing the professional from bearing too large a part of the cost of that redistribution. In the meantime, there appears to be little that can be done, and some would argue little that ought to be done, to stop it.

III. CLINICAL ISSUES

A. Prevention of negligence and malpractice

Section II above has addressed the legal and technical definitions of the elements of malpractice. The real world roots of malpractice litigation are usually a malignant synergy between a bad clinical outcome for any reason and what might be called "bad feelings." Proof of this assertion is found both in empirical studies demonstrating that only a small percentage of bad outcomes result in litigation and in the common observation that top-level care may trigger litigation, while remarkably low-level care may not evoke a lawsuit. While bad clinical outcomes are only to a limited degree under clinicians' control, the bad feelings may offer some opportunity for clinicians' tactful and empathic interventions.

The "bad feelings" in question encompass a wide variety of human reactions to bad outcomes, but the most common ones seen in the litigative arena are guilt, particularly the kind that survivors of a suicide may feel; rage, particularly the outrage that is triggered by a clinician's insensitivity, unavailability, and arrogance; surprise, particularly when the patient experiences a side effect of treatment against which he had not been forewarned; a basic feeling of betrayal, such as might be evoked by the sense that the clinician was practicing entirely defensively and did not make the patient's interests the prime issue; and psychological abandonment, or the patient's feeling that—after a bad outcome has supervened—the clinician's unavailability, lack of outreach, lack of responsiveness, and—at times—active avoidance of the patient leaves the latter experiencing the feeling of being "out in the cold" to cope with the bad outcome entirely alone.

All these reactions may trigger a fundamental adversarialization of attitude about the doctor-patient relationship which may be expressed in its ultimate form, the malpractice suit.

At the beginning of any discussion of preventive measures directed against negligence or malpractice, some caveats are in order to establish a frame of reference: (1) anyone can initiate a lawsuit against anyone for (almost) anything; (2) suit may occur for perfectly valid reasons or utterly irrational (even psychotic) ones; (3) given the complexity of the field, the relative absence of hard standards, and the variability of juries, being free of blame *in fact* does not necessarily lead to one's being *found* to be free of blame.

These points, however realistic, justify neither despair nor nihilism. The approaches that are addressed below can effectively tip the balance in favor of avoiding charges of malpractice or of prevailing if suit for malpractice is actually brought. These approaches may be organized around four rubrics: behavioral approaches to prevention; technical approaches to prevention; and the "twin pillars" of malpractice prevention, documentation and consultation. Each of these will be reviewed in some detail below.

1. Behavioral Approaches to Prevention

A dominant principle of the medicolegal field has always been that good clinical practice and careful attention to the work have represented fundamental elements of malpractice prevention. This timeless principle might be modified to the effect that the therapeutic alliance—conceived as a fundamentally collaborative attitude on the part of both clinician and patient—represents the best antidote to the adversarial posture whose extreme version is the malpractice suit. Therefore, the best behavioral preventive to malpractice litigation is maintenance of the therapeutic alliance. Some particular examples of this basic approach are described below.

a. Avoidance of exploitation

The clinician should avoid any manner of exploitation of the patient. To do otherwise would violate the clinician's fundamental ethical principle, *primum non nocere*, "first, do no harm." This approach should include avoiding financial exploitation (e.g., charging for services not rendered, charging extortionate fees, or seeing the patient at a needlessly high frequency); sexual exploitation (see Sec. II-3-f above and further discussion below); or more subtle exploitation of the patient's feelings (e.g., using the patient to express one's dependency needs, one's wish to be liked or one's wish to control others). The clinician must behave as a professional in the employ of the patient who is dedicated to that patient's interests, well-being, and health.

In today's litigious climate, particularly with the greater attention by boards of registration, courts, and the media to clinician-patient sexual misconduct, clinicians should avoid even the *appearance* of exploitive interactions with patients. This notion of remaining "above suspicion" flows from several phenomena revealed by empirical investigation of sexual misconduct cases.

One of the most important concepts for the clinician to grasp is that of "boundary violations." The boundaries in question are the boundaries of the professional role and of the nature of the clinician-patient relationship, including the fact that this relationship represents a power asymmetry (the clinician has the power to do certain things to and with the patient that the patient does not have). Empirical evidence further suggests (see Suggested Readings—Simon) that many sexual misconduct situations begin with minor boundary violations that gradually become more and more egregious until actual sexual relations occur—an extreme form of boundary violation in themselves. In a related manner, fact finders in such matters—courts in malpractice suits brought for sexual misconduct, ethics committees of clinical societies, and boards of registration—find accusations of sexual misconduct more credible when an acknowledged history of boundary violations exists. Indeed, some malpractice suits alleging sexual misconduct are settled, not necessarily because the clinician is in fact culpable of this behavior, but because those non-sexual boundary violations acknowledged to have occurred are so pervasive that the defense attorney despairs of convincing a jury that the clinician—who crossed so many boundaries—drew the line at the last one, as it were.

Some common boundary violations include: having sessions outside of the office (such as in cars, in restaurants, over meals, or—under certain circumstances—in patients' domiciles); non-therapeutic interactions between doctor and patient (e.g., asking the patient to bring in food, pick up laundry, clean the office, and the like); and shifts in the relationship, such that some ambiguity intrudes as to who is therapist and who is patient (e.g., clinicians' self-disclosing of significant personal details, including those about their personal, social, financial, and sexual difficulties—presumably disclosed in the interest of having the patient console them, or at least listen sympathetically).

Other forms of physical contact—some would say, regrettably—have also become ill-advised in the new stringent atmosphere militating against boundary violations. While handshakes and occasional pats on the shoulder may be the limits of acceptable contact within the therapeutic envelope, kissing the patient and any form of hugging (including quick squeezes around the shoulder, even if performed in the most asexual and sympathetic manner) have probably come to represent unacceptable boundary violations with adult patients. The issue here derives not only from the fact mentioned earlier about even minor physical boundary violations lending credence to a later accusation of sexual misconduct; an even more relevant factor, unfortunately misunderstood by many clinicians, is that the clinician's non-erotic intent in, say, hugging may bear no correspondence to the patient's potentially highly erotic response.

While none of the above-described boundary violations by itself necessarily constitutes malpractice in mental health, and while each may indeed serve innocent purposes, the intensified ambiguity about such interventions and the present more suspicious climate (created, in part, by the real and appalling extent of sexual misconduct) may have a serious implication: that such contacts should, on principle, be forsworn. Such restraint by clinicians may actually reassure many patients, especially those with previous histories of boundaries having been violated by family members and others; in addition, such clarity may strengthen the clinician's capacity to challenge specious charges of misconduct if such are brought.

The problem is a particularly complex one for clinicians who practice according to the behaviorist school of mental health intervention. Going on trips with patients to confront fear of flying, or even going along in certain circumstances on rather personal errands, are part of the legitimate treatment regimen within a behaviorist framework despite the fact that such acts would be considered significant boundary violations (and hence, anathema) in an analytic context (see Suggested Readings—Goisman and Gutheil). This problem has not been addressed extensively either in the literature or in case law, but represents an area of potential ambiguity of a dangerous sort.

To deal with this and related phenomena, clinicians may need to begin to consider the use of a medical technique widely employed in other branches of medicine, namely, chaperoning. While the presence of a chaperone (such as a nurse or office assistant) may represent a significant and perhaps prohibitive intrusion into some clinical work, the climate of the times may make this a valuable investment in defense against future litigation. Normal clinical procedures particularly meriting consideration for the use of chaperoning include amytal interviews; hypnosis; home visits; and the use of behaviorally-based sexual dysfunction interventions, such as the use of dilators in treatment of vaginismus.

Clinical experience also suggests that borderline patients pose special difficulties for clinicians, not only in the area of boundary violations but also in the area of sexual misconduct. In one survey, borderline patients accounted for more than 90% of the litigation cases of true sexual misconduct; and, more disturbingly, accounted for 99% of the false accusations of sexual misconduct. The latter appear to represent broad expressions of borderline rage and the wish to punish the object, in this case, the therapist. In the present climate, which reflects an appropriately growing impatience with sexual misconduct and its widespread occurrence, even a false accusation can have a significantly destructive effect on the clinician. To make matters even more complex, borderline patients, while often having difficulty themselves with maintaining boundaries, call for the clearest of boundaries to be maintained by the clinician. With these points in mind, clinicians are well advised to adhere strictly to boundaries and to keep the clinical work unambiguously in the forefront.

In addition, clinicians dealing with patients of any diagnosis might do well—when the transference becomes erotized or when direct statements or requests concerning sexual contact arise in treatment—to begin presenting the case to a clinical supervisor, peer, consultant, or specialist in this area; such consultation may be anonymous to protect the patient's privacy. Such presentation not only offers an opportunity for valuable consultative input but may also decrease the isolation of the clinician and patient in an emotionally intense dyadic island, often steeped in feelings of mutual admiration and idealization—a "magic bubble" of insularity, which consultative experience demonstrates to be proof against later influence by advice or supervision. Such presentation, in addition, renders appropriately more dubious a false accusation of sexual misconduct, should such arise.

b. Manifesting respect for the patient

Patients are entitled to be treated with the respect afforded all human beings, and with the compassion deserved by all individuals in distress. Untold numbers of malpractice suits are filed as indicated earlier, not primarily because the patient has suffered egregious harm, but because he has felt himself to be the object of outrageous conduct on the part of the therapist. The clinician who—in the presence of a receptionist and a family waiting to be seen—yells after a departing patient, "Mr. Jones, you are the most *impossible* patient that it has ever been my misfortune to treat!" is guilty of such outrage. The preventive approach here is, of course, to maintain reasonable social manners throughout and, for example, should yelling at a patient be necessary as a therapeutic approach (as it occasionally is), to maintain the same privacy about it as about other communications in the treatment. The patient is deserving of no less.

In this regard, clinicians may well want to reconsider the tendency to use first names in therapeutic work, rather than the last name with an appropriate honorific. While use of last names might seem excessively formal and hence likely to promote an atmosphere of distance and coldness, we would do well to recall that the use of a last name is also a sign of interpersonal respect. What is more, it may clarify those very boundaries addressed above and may help both parties maintain a clear focus on the fact that the therapy is serious work and not an affectionate relationship between chums.

c. Avoidance of abandonment

As a contractual relationship between consenting adults, one might expect that the usual outpatient therapy could be terminated at any time by either party; however, there is an asymmetry that must be acknowledged. The patient may stop without prejudice, with or without notice to, or agreement of, the therapist; for good reason, bad reason, or "no reason"; with the work finished, unfinished, or partly finished. The therapist is not free, however, to stop treatment in a similarly arbitrary manner; the risk of so doing is the charge of abandonment, as outlined above, Section II-A-3-h. But in addition to this legalistic form of abandonment there is another, more psychological form of abandonment, in which the patient feels deprived of the therapist's support even if no technical legal rule has been violated. Such feelings may be productive of litigation and should be foreclosed by careful attention to avoiding psychological abandonment.

The preventive approach here might be styled the open-door policy (see Chap. 3, Sec. III-G-6), which means in practice that a patient, once in treatment, may almost always return.

> ***Example 1:*** A highly entitled patient dropped out of treatment and was unreachable by phone or letter. The therapist made note of each phone call and kept a copy of each letter of inquiry. After the third letter, the therapist wrote that he could no longer keep the time open and scheduled another patient for that time. Six weeks later the patient, who had gone impulsively to California, reappeared and demanded her time. The therapist scheduled the patient for a new time, answering her objections about its inconvenience by showing her the record of his attempts to contact her after she had left. The patient settled down and began work on understanding the entire episode.

By sending serial letters (with copies) and by offering an alternative time for the patient, the therapist avoids any semblance of abandonment, legal or psychological.

A similar "Approach of Three Letters" (the precise number is not sacred) should be actively considered for patients who disappear from treatment. The patient who attends two sessions of an evaluation sequence and then disappears represents a potentially risky ambiguity in the medicolegal arena: is that patient still one's patient? In certain cases of injury by patients to third parties (further discussed below) courts have claimed that the duty that the clinician once owed the patient during treatment continued to exist, long after the clinician has forgotten the patient and closed the case.

The content of such a letter, sent after several attempts to reach the patient, might read as follows:

Example 2:
Dear Patient,

I have not heard from you in (TIME) [this should be a reasonable amount of time to permit patients who are uncertain or ambivalent to have adequate time to consider whether they wish to continue]. I assume you no longer wish treatment (extended diagnostic evaluation, etc.) at this time. I am closing your case [at this point the duty may be presumed to end, but the question of abandonment still remains]. Should you at any future time wish to employ mental health services, please do not hesitate to call me (the clinic, the center) for an *evaluation* [Note: treatment should never be offered, only an evaluation; the offer of treatment might be construed as the offer of *continuing* treatment, implying that the duty persisted. Actual phone numbers of the local clinic, clinician's answering service, and so on, should be provided in the letter].

Such an approach remains respectful of patients' potential autonomous decisions to drop out of treatment without notice but exerts some control over plaintiffs' attorneys claiming potentially limitless extension of duties to patients who later go on to injure others.

Emergencies. There are, of course, situations in which rational approaches to avoiding abandonment are untenable. If a patient has seriously threatened the physical safety of the therapist or of his family, immediate steps are warranted to protect the potential victims; this may include immediate cessation of sessions with the patient, civil commitment, filing of a criminal complaint, or notification of the police. Even here, however, a documented referral to an appropriate alternate source of care, for example the local community mental health center, is good practice, not only to prevent the charge of abandonment but to acknowledge that a treated patient is liable to be less dangerous in the long run than an untreated one.

Patients who fail to pay. The problem of dealing with patients who do not pay their bills is hardly limited to therapists. Nonetheless, delinquent payments often take a different form in psychiatric practice. A patient's failure to pay may be a manifestation of the very difficulties for which he is presenting for care: narcissistic entitlement, counterdependent acting out, or the desire to provoke a rejecting response from an authority figure. The psychiatrist's or other therapist's response should take these dynamic considerations into account by seeking to bring the issue of payment into the therapy. It is not uncommon for patients to refuse to pay for months, only to begin payment again when the underlying issue has been explored. There are, however, limits to what is expected even from a therapist. If, after exploration of the issues over a period of time, it appears that the patient still has no intention of paying his bill, a clinician who refers the patient to a public clinic or other available source of care can hardly be faulted. Such a referral should not be made if the patient is acutely ill and requires immediate care, with no other source of care available; the original treating clinician has an obligation to continue to shepherd the patient through the acute episode until termination can be accomplished safely. An extremely important clinical issue here is the need for the clinician to begin discussions of delinquent fees *before* she becomes too angry at the patient to explore the matter with the requisite cool dispassion.

> **Example 3:** A patient was derelict in paying a bill and the back balance mounted up to the point where the therapist could no longer afford to treat the patient. Treatment then stopped and the therapist sent the patient a letter (with a copy for her own records) stating that, as discussed, they could no longer continue in therapy at that time. If the patient wished to continue at some future time, he could do so (the "door is open") provided he paid the back balance (or 50% or 75% of it) and perhaps something in earnest of future good faith (e.g., paying each session in advance or paying some part of the back bill each month).

Needless to say, the therapist should explore the therapeutic implications of nonpayment as a clinical issue; see also Sec. II-A-3-h-ii, and compare section III-A-2-h, concerning management of defaulted payment.

Patients who do not cooperate in their care. Like a failure to pay ones bills, the failure to comply with a therapist's instructions may derive from the patient's underlying psychopathology and should be considered as a therapeutic issue. In addition, the patient should be given every benefit of a doubt that he is exercising an autonomous choice; the clinician's position should be extremely flexible. Once again, though, the utility of continued treatment may be dubious if, even after exploration, the patient cannot conform to the recommended procedures, whether these be ingestion of medication or abstinence from alcohol. If, because of the patient's actions, the therapist finally decides he cannot provide adequate care, it does not constitute abandonment to terminate the relationship with the patient. (This may not be true if the patient is incompetent to understand what is taking place.) Whether less than optimal care is better than no care at all is a more difficult question. In any case, referral should, of course, be attempted (see Sec. II-A-3-h-iii).

d. Coverage during absences

Related to abandonment is the question of clinical coverage during such events as vacations, illnesses, or other absences of the clinician for educational, recreational, or personal reasons. The issue proves divisive (even acrimonious) at times among the disciplines. Many clinicians have others cover for them routinely, even for weekends when they are unavailable; others see their responsibility for given patients ending with the working day (or work week) (see Sec. II-A-3-h-v). Others leave nothing but an answering machine for all coverage situations.

Not only malpractice prevention, but conscientious practice, requires all clinicians who work with patients or clients to provide some form of backup for emergency situations. Optimally, a trusted colleague agrees to cover, receives necessary information about urgent or pending matters (a "sign-out"), and makes herself available in some way, e.g., by providing a phone number. At a minimum, patients can be given the number of a clinic, hospital, mental health center, or similar agency to call as needed.

The role of covering clinician is a difficult one because the substitute must act with all the authority and responsibility of the original therapist but without the alliance with, or knowledge of, the patient. The person covering, in practice, is often torn between the wish to temporize until the absent clinician returns, and the wish to provide a definitive resolution to the crisis or problem. Ideally, the covering clinician should deal with the patient as her own and should see the goal of the evaluation or intervention as resolution of the acute crisis. If the matter is not critical (e.g., an optional prescription refill), it may be postponed until the absentee's return.

In those cases where the covering clinician is a stranger to the patient, the clinician should probably make greater-than-usual efforts at availability, personal interviews, data gathering, documentation, and conservative practice, since the therapist-patient bond cannot be invoked in the usual manner. The absence of this bond not only dilutes the positive interpersonal component of the intervention, thus making it more difficult for the covering clinician to accomplish the therapeutic goal, but also increases the risk of malpractice suit should something go awry. The patient, already resentful of his therapist's absence and suspicious of the interloper who is covering, may choose to express his anger at his therapist in a displaced, and therefore psychologically "safer," manner by suing the covering clinician. Covering clinicians may also be named as defendants to increase the award pool.

e. Patient selection

In general, as a preventive measure to charges of malpractice, clinicians should only treat patients within their capabilities; patients, for example, with medical problems or with a clear need of medication should probably be treated by physicians or—if treated by nonphysicians—should have close medical backup, consultation, or supervision (see Sec. III-A-4 below).

f. The role of apology in liability prevention

A remarkable number of plaintiffs comment during interviews in connection with litigation, "If that clinician had only admitted he was wrong and had apologized, I wouldn't have sued." Clinicians vary in their willingness to take such comments at face value, but experts agree that the improvement in the feeling tone of a relationship under stress and restoration of the therapeutic alliance can be fostered to a remarkable degree by an appropriate apology.

What constitutes such an appropriate apology? If a clinician were to say, "I apologize for deviating from the standard of care so as to proximately cause you these harms," her insurer would doubtless consider that remark infelicitously phrased, since that is the technical definition of malpractice! But short of such statements, there is significant room for expressions of apology. First, clinicians should maintain a low threshold for admission of simple or minor errors, such as misplaced lab slips or misscheduled appointments. A rigid policy of refusal to apologize, based on some distorted psychodynamic rationalization, is ultimately destructive to the alliance. Similarly, all clinicians should feel—and express—regret, sympathy, or condolences for bad outcomes of any kind. Under narrow circumstances clinicians might apologize for more serious error: "I'm truly sorry that I missed that side effect (medical problem, diagnosis, choice of medication type), but I will continue to do my best to treat you appropriately."

Clinicians may worry about placing a weapon in the hands of the plaintiff's attorney. Is saying, "I'm sorry" tantamount to saying, "I did wrong, so sue me"? This understandable fear can be considerably decreased by enactment of an "apology statute" that ensures freedom to say one is sorry. Massachusetts law provides one version of such a statute:

> Statements, writings or benevolent gestures expressing sympathy or a general sense of benevolence relating to the pain, suffering or death of a person involved in an accident [defined as a non-willful occurrence resulting in injury or death, hence including malpractice contexts] and made to such a person or to the family of such a person *shall be inadmissible as evidence of an admission of liability in a civil action.* (Mass. General Laws, C.233, s. 23D, emphasis added)

In those areas where comparable statutes do not exist, regional professional societies could attempt to promote their enactment. Such protection for saying one is sorry has the potential to avert litigation by resolving the "bad feeling" component.

2. TECHNICAL APPROACHES TO PREVENTION

Certain approaches directed toward preventing charges of negligence and malpractice fall under the rubric of technique, not in the sense of the technique of therapy itself, but in the sense of technical handling of the administrative transactions surrounding the treatment.

a. The treatment contract

With surprising frequency, this essential component of treatment (and an important factor in malpractice prevention) is omitted, largely by being inappropriately taken for granted. Steiner (see Suggested Readings) describes how this occurs in practice, paraphrased as follows:

PATIENT: My wife's been after me because of my drinking.
DOCTOR: Fine, I'll see you Mondays at eleven o'clock.

In this interchange, of course, there is the illusion of a contract being formed, but there is no actual statement by either party of their intentions, their wishes, or what they are agreeing to; that is, there is in actuality no contract at all. While the example represents an heuristic exaggeration, one can readily imagine milder versions occurring with distressing frequency in daily practice.

The significance of the absence of a true contract is that, without one, it is impossible for therapy to succeed or fail since the goals or problems to be solved are not agreed on; however, it is not impossible to be *sued,* since the absence of clear agreement allows the patient's wishes and fantasies about the results of treatment to burgeon unchecked and allows the disappointment at their nonfulfillment to be equally unbounded.

The technical remedy for this problem is to begin any treatment with a clear understanding of the agreed-on goals. It is for the same reasons equally important to spell out policies for fees, billing, handling of missed versus canceled appointments, and the like at the earliest appropriate opportunity.

b. Acknowledging limitations versus making promises

Related to the notion of contract is the clinician's acknowledgment of the limitations of treatment, so as not to make promises impossible of fulfillment. This matter is especially charged in connection with prognosis; a prognosis is a statistical/epidemiological prediction, yet may readily be experienced by patient, family, or attorney as a promise to deliver certain results. Among familiar "promises" therapists are asked to keep are keeping someone alive, stopping someone from drinking, getting back the departed spouse, getting someone married, getting someone through examinations, and so on. While therapy may be quite helpful with all these goals, their actual realization does not lie in any therapist's power, and this limitation must be candidly acknowledged, perhaps even in the case record.

For similar reasons, excessive therapeutic optimism is inappropriate for the written record, again because it may be seen as a contractual promise. Attorneys are occasionally prone to seeing clinical forecasts as contracts, as in the following example.

> *Example 4:* A patient's attorney decided not to file a writ of habeas corpus when told by the patient's physician that the patient would probably be sufficiently recovered by the next Monday. Over the intervening weekend, however, the patient's clinical state worsened markedly and commitment had to be petitioned for.
>
> At the hearing, the attorney maintained that a Monday discharge had been "promised" (in the sense of a contractual agreement); he thus failed to realize the significance of a clinical estimate and to understand that the patient's actual state must, from the clinician's viewpoint, govern what happens. The patient, not the calendar, is being treated.

The clinician is urged to bear in mind, especially when speaking to attorneys, this possible misperception of clinical forecasting and to attempt to avoid making statements that can be construed as "promises" (see also Sec. II-C-6 above).

c. Informed consent and the sharing of uncertainty

Offering a realistic view of future possibilities may be viewed as an aspect of the concept of informed consent. This topic was extensively reviewed in Sec. II of this chapter and will be further explored in Chapter Five. Certain clinical dimensions are expanded on here.

For a regrettably large number of clinicians in all specialities of medicine, informed consent represents little more than obtaining the patient's signature on a lengthy, occasionally multi-page document, whose use of court-tested "boilerplate" language may do far more to confuse and obfuscate the matter for the patient than to inform, as it is ostensibly intended to do. More significantly, the patient's mere signature on a form provides empirically a very feeble defense against the malpractice claim of failure to obtain informed consent: when read aloud in court, the consent form is as baffling to the jury as it was to the patient. Predictably, the result is the jury's identification with the patient, a process inimical to the clinician's hoped-for outcome.

Informed consent, appropriately conceptualized, represents an atmosphere of openness and honesty, nurtured by an ongoing dialogue between clinician and patient that begins from the first encounter and lasts for the duration of the relationship. It is not a brief conversation, capped by the patient's signature on a form, which renders the issue closed. The model used here has been described as a "process model" of informed consent (see Suggested Readings—Lidz, Appelbaum and Meisel) where differing perceptions of illness, values, and expectations are shared in a manner termed "mutual monitoring" by patient and clinician.

Envisioned in this manner, an informed consent dialogue can represent an effective preventive to the kinds of bad feelings earlier noted that lead to litigation.

Specific cases at law have faulted clinicians for saying both too little and (rarely) too much in informing the patient; it appears that the ideal degree of information appears to be "just enough. . . ," titrated, as it were, to the patient's capacity to integrate the information. We suggest that this focus on the information in question may be too limited to exploit fully the benefits of the informed consent model. The outcome of the informed consent process should be a sharing between clinician and patient of the fundamental uncertainty of both the patient's condition, the clinician's proposed treatment regimen, and, indeed, of the future itself. When clinician and patient conjointly confront, within a therapeutic alliance, the inherent uncertainties of the course on which they are about to embark, the relationship becomes less susceptible to those bad outcomes that may supervene (see Suggested Readings—Gutheil, Bursztajn, and Brodsky).

To understand the operation of this approach, we must begin by appreciating that individuals who are ill experience, as part of the normal process of illness, a regression to more magical stages of mental development. Magical wishes, deriving from infantile feelings of omnipotence, lead patients unconsciously to seek out clinicians for magical cures, even though their conscious assessment of the situation may be quite realistic. The clinician who offers "only" reasonable clinical care is thus in danger of disappointing the patient's unconscious magical expectations, a result leading to potential bad feelings in the context of a bad outcome.

The appropriate intervention for this dilemma is an effective, albeit counter-intuitive one. The clinician begins by empathizing with the patient's unrealistic wishes, in a manner that brings them into the open, yet permits a gradual disillusionment (one might even call it "weaning") of the patient from these magical fantasies. Several examples of how this might sound in practice may be more illuminating than the concept in the abstract.

Example 5

"I sure wish the good Lord had invented a medication that was guaranteed to be entirely free of side-effects."

"I sure wish I had a written guarantee that this course of psychotherapy would be guaranteed to keep you alive despite your suicidal preoccupations."

"I wish I could assure you that the couple's work that we are about to embark on would be certain to save your marriage."

"I wish I could promise you that with this treatment regimen you would be guaranteed to lose this crippling phobia of yours."

Note that these interventions (which represent, of course, short forms of an entire spectrum of interventions, depending upon the particular clinical situation) have in common the clinician's overt acknowledgement of the fact that he or she, too, wishes for magical solutions to life's problems, yet the tone of rueful regret in which these communications are couched begins the process of tactfully bringing forward the uncertainty of all clinical work. The desired outcome of this intervention is to render the alliance strong enough to tolerate a bad outcome *without* bad feelings, since the uncertainty of the intervention has been faced squarely by clinician and patient and thus made available for integration, processing, and joint discussion.

Two particular problem areas will now be explored. In psychiatric practice, medications and ECT are the most significant areas to which informed consent applies. Each presents its own difficulties.

For ECT, as noted in Chap. 3, Sec. III-C-2-d, complex issues concerning the treatment and the illnesses for which the treatment is used render informed consent problematic (see also Chap. 5, Sec. II-B-2-b). The problem is further compounded by the common side effect of memory loss for the time period surrounding the treatment. Even when optimally applied (unilaterally, on the nondominant side), ECT tends to produce some loss of memory; since the forgotten period usually contains one of the most painful human experiences (severe depression), the loss is usually viewed by patients (and clinicians) as benign. However, the act of consenting is not uncommonly included in the memory blank, a fact that places a significant burden on the documentation process.

With medication a slightly different problem presents itself. For functioning outpatients being started on medications one usually (but not always) has the leisure to negotiate a reasonably informed consent with presumption of reasonable competence in the outpatient. The newly admitted inpatient, on the other hand, presents with far more equivocal competence to consent to medication as treatment.

Furthermore, reading a package insert to the acutely psychotic patient would clearly be as futile as it is self-defeating. Yet to fail to alert the patient to some of the direct effects and side effects to be expected from the medication is to risk further distressing the patient who may have delusional ideas about what is happening to her—a situation that may readily induce panic, rage, increase in psychosis, or flight, as well as straining both alliance with, and trust in, the physician.

In clinical terms, a compromise is indicated. As earlier noted, information is titrated to the patient's needs and condition and is individualized to the patient's fears, concerns, vocation, life-style, and similar considerations.

Needless to say, all such informing transactions and the patient's responses should be documented in the record.

d. Therapeutic disinterest and the question of advice

The technical point at issue in this section is both complex and controversial, in part because there are so many different forms, modes, and styles of therapy. Under most circumstances the psychoanalytically oriented psychotherapist eschews giving advice; the supportive or behavioral therapist, on the other hand, may use directive instruction or advice as the main currency of the interaction. Clinicians whose practices emphasize the pharmacotherapies are dealing extensively with a form of advice-prescription: "You should take this medication." Yet there is one forensic issue related to advice giving, the problem of litigation for undue influence (including alienation of affections, see section II-C-4 above), that is of concern to all therapeutic orientations.

This problem may arise clinically when one member of a couple is being treated and the result of treatment is an actual or threatened breakup of the relationship. In this context, the therapist must make clear from the outset (and repeatedly during treatment, if the issue arises again) that the therapist works for the individual's interests, which, under therapeutic scrutiny, may not turn out to be identical with the interests of the couple or the marriage.

For example, the husband may recognize through therapy that his wife represents another in the line of maternal figures on whom he has been hostilely dependent all his life; or a wife may realize that her marriage represents another of the self-defeating, masochistic relationships she has unconsciously sought time and again. These realizations may or may not prompt these individuals to try to change their situation, but that is up to the individual, and ought not to be the thrust of the therapist's directives. (In couples therapy, of course, the contract differs and may legitimately include attempts to save a marriage.)

The most useful posture for the therapist in such cases is that of a neutral and disinterested consultant, one who has no particular stake in the patient's remaining in (or leaving) a marriage, a job, a school, a career, or a relationship. The therapist is there to explore, not to advise and certainly not to influence. While a therapist's opinions inevitably will be conveyed to the patient, even if only by unconscious cues, such subtle influences are not the stuff of which suits are made.

The indications for this dispassionate stance are not entirely forensic, of course. Because the therapist learns more and more about the question at hand as time passes, and the relationship deepens in candor, his evolving understanding of the issue may alter its clinical significance; an apparently gratifying relationship, for example, may emerge as fundamentally frustrating on closer inspection over time. This universal clinical experience must serve as a powerful caveat against advice or other directive interventions based on early impressions of the status quo.

e. Technical handling of legalistic acting out

The forms, papers, and other paraphernalia of the legal aspects of psychiatric practice are not uncommonly put to use by some patients in acting out against authority figures; these legal paraphernalia represent embodiments of a judgmental, authoritarian attitude attributed by the patient to treatment personnel or to the institution against which the patient rebels. Adolescents, borderline or psychopathic patients, and manic patients are particularly prone to use these legal concretizations to provoke or to test the interpersonal field, or as a signal of some distress not communicable in other modalities.

> ***Example 6:*** A borderline adolescent girl discovered several days into her voluntary admission that the desire to leave could be conveyed by a form giving three days' notice of this wish (a "three-day paper"); she

further discovered that the paper could be revoked by another form. She then launched a veritable paper blizzard of three-day papers and last-minute retractions. Because by law the patient had to be given the papers on demand, the staff felt helpless, manipulated, and furious at the patient.

Example 7: A man with bipolar disorder, beginning the manic upswing, became obsessed with the delusional idea that a previous commitment to the facility had been illegal; he launched a two-month campaign (culminating in another admission) of vituperative phone calls and letters to many state officials (some completely uninvolved in mental health), attempting to gain acknowledgement of this claim. He called the hospital as well, the calls escalating to dawn-to-midnight harangues, interfering with hospital routine.

In the first example, staff were tempted to refuse to give the patient the forms since "she's just playing games"; such a move would have been both illegal and ineffectual since the behavior would have simply escalated. The legal-psychiatric consultant suggested giving the patient the forms without hesitation, but asking each time about what the patient could not put into words. The therapist also led a virtual chorus of staff members in pointing out to the patient that the "paper blizzard" was keeping everyone—patient, staff, and therapist—from taking her problems seriously and from being of any use. Faced with this unified front, the patient became first angry, then bored with the "game," then eventually ready to talk instead.

In the second case, hospital officials designated one of their number, Dr. X, to be the "pipeline" for the legal issue. All other personnel referred calls and letters to Dr. X; Dr. X's invariant and ceaselessly repeated response was, "Of course, your record can be checked, just have your lawyer call me." Even when the storm abated because of the patient's admission, the invitation was proferred and eventually accepted. The lawyer reassured the patient about the record; the patient's therapist meanwhile continued to explore how the desire to "see the crime" related to primal scene material from the patient's childhood.

In both these examples, the clinical approach followed certain basic principles:

Remaining cool. Being swept up into the passion of the encounter is useless and self-defeating. Obtaining consultation, if needed, may help to restore perspective.

Avoiding fruitless struggle in the legal arena. Even if the transaction transparently represents symptomatic acting out, the patient's legal rights must be respected. If it is what the law requires, the clinician should give the paper, let the lawyer see the record, etc. Note that abstaining from struggle in this way does not rule out, say, going to court to contest a habeas corpus writ on clinical grounds, when the clinician believes discharge may be dangerous to the patient.

Actively confronting or interpreting the clinical meaning of the acting out and/or resistance. It is in the therapeutic sphere that the intervention should occur, preferably in a unified manner with team, staff, or institutional support as needed, as indicated in the examples above.

Extracting maximum therapeutic value from the issue for ongoing explora-

tion.   The resolution of the issue does not close, by any means, the possibility of further work in the treatment. The patient's behavior can be considered as a symptomatic act that requires exploration.

f. The importance of clinical "outreach" in homicide and suicide

Families or parties involved with patients who commit suicide or homicide experience major personal disasters. The catastrophic reaction for the living (which includes the patient who has killed someone else) takes precedence for the clinician over all other issues. It matters not if the clinician believes that the wife drove the husband or the family, the son, to suicide; at the moment of crisis the living require the best, nonjudgmental efforts of the clinician.

In practice, of course, the matter is emotionally enormously complex; every clinician who has lost a patient by suicide experiences feelings of grief, guilt, anger, regret, or a sense of failure. These and other feelings are powerful and preoccupying, making it difficult at such a time to think of solace to others, but there are two major reasons to make this considerable effort.

First, this subject is discussed under the heading of technical approaches to prevention of suit because, in fact, clinical outreach often defuses the guilt, shock, and rage of the afflicted family so that the common reaction does not occur, namely, translation of these painful feelings into blame fixed, not on the original object (the patient), but now on hospital and treatment staff. It would be unduly cynical, however, to present this as the sole motivation for outreach. The second major reason to reach out with clinical skills is that it is the humane response to profound need. Because the clinical staff essentially have shared the catastrophe with the family, they are in an ideal position to be of help, for there exists a potential alliance based on shared loss.

The treating therapist and the clinician working with the family, as well as staff members who worked closely with the patient, should consider attending funeral services for a patient who has committed suicide. While those who attend such an event invariably experience great conflict about it initially, they invariably report afterward that they found it helpful in dealing with the loss and in terminating with the memory of the patient. Families of the deceased are usually grateful for the respect thus shown by the treatment staff; one bereaved mother later told her social worker that it meant so much to her to see staff members there because, of all persons present, they alone fully understood the horror of the experience and the meaning of the loss to her. At a minimum, personal condolences should be sent by individual staff members who worked with that patient.

A psychiatric patient who commits homicide presents a different problem. Treatment staff are usually fearful of a murderer and do not always realize that they are not important enough to the patient to be at risk in most cases; i.e., the feelings toward them are not intense enough for murder. Nevertheless, the patient needs clinical aid, and clinicians must labor to leave the legal aspects of the case to the criminal justice system; the patient is their object for a clinical reaching out. Though inexperienced staff members are often ethically confused by this issue, it is not condoning murder to treat the patient for an illness. Individuals who have committed murder or crimes of violence while psychotic, for example, need clinical aid to recover from, and "get over," such experiences, not unlike trauma victims in other contexts.

Another form of outreach here that again serves the dual role of malpractice prevention and humane clinical response to need focuses on the relatives of the victim (who may, of course, be in the patient's own family) who have suffered an acute bereavement under shocking circumstances. To avoid a conflicted and charged situation, the outreach to the relatives should be undertaken by clinical personnel not directly involved with the patient-murderer.

In all the foregoing intense matters, the value of documentation with appropriate consultation, both forensic and clinical, cannot be overestimated.

g. The duty to protect and related matters

The "duty to protect" citizens from danger from a patient one is treating is a thorny and controversial issue (see Sec. II-A-3-e of this chapter). In clinical terms, the possibility of imminent danger to third parties has always called for action, such as emergency commitment (according to the requisite criteria, if mental illness is involved) or notification of the police. As earlier noted, the California Supreme Court added the concept of protecting the potential victim, obviously with careful documentation thereof. Many clinicians in other jurisdictions where the matter has never been judicially decided or statutorily enacted are acting in an anticipatory way as if that were already the controlling doctrine.

> **Example 8:** A manic-depressive male with a recent history of death threats to his girlfriend was voluntarily admitted in psychotic decompensation. He was told that hospital staff would have to inform his girlfriend if he escaped or left prematurely; staff members posted the girlfriend's number in the ward nursing station. After some weeks, the patient signed a three-day paper (notice of intent to leave from a voluntary admission). He was evaluated and found not to fit criteria for committability at that time. However, he was told that his girlfriend would be notified of his leaving on the grounds that it was clinically premature (though legally not preventable).

For the clinician the task posed by the threatening patient is assessment of risk, much as in other emergent or preemergent situations. Laypersons are surprised to hear of the frequency with which powerful feelings, including murderous ones, are unleashed in intensive psychiatric treatment; these feelings are a recognized part of the process. The clinician faces the burden of (1) deciding when the feelings and/or statements portend actions (rather than pure feelings, fantasy, or wish) and (2) markedly shifting the agency away from alliance with the patient and toward protection of society, at the cost of no longer keeping confidential the material itself and at other costs to the treatment as well.

The clinician is best advised to use an approach similar to that mentioned earlier in relation to suicide/homicide: careful assessment matched by equally careful documentation of the decision-making process either to take action to protect the hypothetical victim or not to do so. Ethical practice prompts informing the patient of the intention when it crystallizes. Clinicians should employ the intervention which, while effective, occasions the least disruption of the therapeutic relationship. On some occasions, this may mean hospitalization, on others, police notification may serve.

Under this added burden some clinicians have taken a pseudopreventive approach, saying to their patients (literally or in effect), "Don't tell me about any past crimes or crimes you may intend to commit, because I can't keep that confidential." This appears ill-advised from several viewpoints.

First, the clinician is under no legal obligation to take action in regard to past events, felonious or not, since almost no citizen is obligated to report a crime; merely not reporting a crime does not make one an accessory (see Chap. 1, Sec. II-B-5-d). In addition, the clinician has no evidence (other than "hearsay" in many cases) that these reported events are not fantasies. (Consider the number of people who confess to publicized crimes in large cities.) The prohibition thus serves only to close off potentially usable material from the therapeutic work: under the umbrella of "possible felony," much highly charged germane material may take refuge in therapeutic resistance. That is, the patient may independently (and erroneously) decide that a whole list of things are under the heading, "Don't tell me."

Second, the clinician thus potentially cuts herself off from helping the patient overcome the conflicts leading to the dangerous situation, that is, from treating the causes of the potential crime. This is, of course, the clinical crux of the dilemma. The clinician is torn between wanting to treat the patient for the problem versus protecting the potential victim (as legally indicated), possibly losing the patient in the process. As earlier noted (Sec. II-A-3-e), it is unclear whether this benefits the potential victim *or* society. (See also Chap. 1, Sec. II-B-5-d.)

Unexpected benefits may accrue from the duty to protect or warn potential victims in regard to the therapeutic alliance with either the patient or the family. As one author has noted (see Suggested Readings—Wexler), the threat of harm often involves members of the patient's immediate family who, by virtue of the duty to warn, may be brought into the therapeutic purview. Thus it might even be said that the *Tarasoff* decision forces a family systems approach on the clinician. Clinical experience confirms that attention to the possibilities of forming (or repairing) an alliance with family members through the "warning" itself may yield valuable therapeutic advantages for the patient; a liability threat is thus transformed into potential clinical leverage.

As earlier noted in Chapter 1 (see Suggested Readings—Wulsin et al.), further clinical benefits can accrue from having the patient herself warn the potential victim, since such intervention may defuse the actual dangerousness of the situation as well as serving the purpose of refuting the charge of negligence. Such a warning by a patient most typically occurs from the clinician's office by telephone with the clinician as witness, but other approaches may also be useful.

Clinical aspects of liability for patients' driving.   A growing number of cases have imposed liability on clinicians for injuries caused by negligent driving of their patients. These cases range from allegations that the clinician failed to warn the patient of the impact of medication on alertness, to claims that the clinician knew or should have known that the patient represented a danger behind the wheel. In this latter formulation, driving cases represent an extension of the *Tarasoff*-like duty to protect (see Sec. II-A-3-e above). They are particularly troubling because clinicians rarely observe their patients' driving, are not trained to ask about it routinely, would in any event have to rely on patients' own reports, and generally lack the skills to determine which patients ought not to be behind the wheel. Most clinicians can recall examples of seriously disturbed, even psychotic, patients whose driving remained unimpaired.

How ought clinicians to respond to these cases? They could modify their practices to ask routinely about driving history. For the reasons noted above, this is unlikely to be a useful move, and it may paradoxically increase the risk of liability for the clinicians who follow this practice and for the mental health professions at large. If a clinician takes a driving history, she will be expected to do so accurately, probe appropriately, and follow up with interventions if necessary. If the practice becomes widespread enough, it may be taken as a standard of care and imposed wholesale on the professions.

Until the courts in most jurisdictions take such a drastic step, more moderate measures seem called for. Clinicians sometimes learn of patients' actions behind the wheel that raise significant questions as to their safety. In such cases, clinicians may want to consider implementing a hierarchy of interventions. If the patient's driving is suicidal in intent, the appropriate interventions for that condition should be invoked. If other factors appear to account for the dangerous driving, the clinician should first counsel the patient about the relevant dangers: e.g., the risks of driving while mixing even a small amount of alcohol with prescribed medication. The effects of such advice should be monitored with later inquiries. If no change in the dangerous behavior occurs, the clinician should recommend in increasingly strong terms that a constructive change take place. Family members can be involved to restrict the patient's driving. If this is to no avail, the clinician may consider threatening to inform the motor vehicle bureau. Before this occurs, the patient should be asked for permission to inform the agency. If such permission is refused, the clinician must note this and then decide if the dangerous behavior constitutes an emergency. If not, the other efforts should continue. If so, the motor vehicle bureau should be informed by letter, with a copy to the clinician's chart. The letter should be limited to noting the relevant behavior, and the clinician should make no claim as to having knowledge of the behavior (when this is the case) other than from the patient's report. Thus, the letter constitutes notification of a situation to be investigated by the agency, rather than the clinician's own conclusions.

Clinicians should also be aware of a factor that appears to influence the resolution of driving cases once they reach the courts. Observers note that the clinical care rendered to the patient in their cases often appears to exude an "odor of negligence"; generally sloppy or substandard care appears to have been given, independent of the driving issues. We might speculate that the courts' findings—an ostensible failure of the clinician to prevent a driving injury by the patient—may be serving as a vehicle for the court or jury to punish clinicians for care seen as broadly deficient. This hypothesis may help to explain why courts seem willing to stretch the realistic limits of clinical predictability in order to hold clinicians to duties to patients weeks or even months after patients' last contacts. These speculative insights, of course, merely reinforce the value of attentive clinical management in even difficult cases.

h. Managing defaulted payment

The clinician who has responsibly performed services according to the treatment contract is entitled to the agreed-on fee (see Sec. II-A-3-h-ii and III-

A-1-c-ii). When a patient has been terminated from treatment for failure to pay, clinicians vary in their approach to soliciting the unpaid balance.

Some clinicians request payment but do not pursue the matter if there is no response (and, perhaps, if the amount is not excessive), reasoning that the effort is not worthwhile and the loss should be written off. This conservative approach makes the fewest litigational waves, but is clinically controversial since it appears to deny the reality—or worth—of the services rendered.

Other clinicians treat the matter in strict business terms, employing collection agencies or filing lawsuits to obtain the unpaid balance. This is accepted practice but requires one caveat: overintrusive or harassing behavior by the collecting agency or attorney can render the clinician liable for countersuit. One remedy is a choice of reputable agents who are persistent, but controlled.

Clinicians pursuing this route should be aware of the fact that some patients, reacting to collection efforts, may attempt to fabricate specious liability claims in order to reverse the flow of currency, as it were, or may manifest other kinds of reactions to the antagonism created by the clinician's collection efforts. Recall that any litigation in this context occurs against the societal perception of clinicians (physicians in particular) as excessively wealthy; thus egregiously harassing efforts to collect fees may be seen as particularly sordid and hence, compensable in a harassment action.

In either case, the clinician who becomes emotionally caught up in the matter does his work a disservice and becomes more likely to act in legally compromising ways. A clinical perspective should prevail (see Sec. III-A-1-c-ii).

i. Dispensing dangerous medications

It is commonly the case that a physician will prescribe medications that can be abused for a patient whose condition predisposes to that abuse. The most serious (and familiar) example is the depressed (and thus potentially suicidal) patient who is being treated with tricyclic antidepressants, among the most toxic of the psychotropic drugs, yet proven effective and appropriate for treating depression.

Many clinicians deal with the tension inherent in giving potentially lethal medications to patients in potentially lethal clinical states by prescribing limited amounts of medication at any one time, e.g., one week's worth of medication at each weekly appointment or one prescription with no refills for a limited amount. For a variety of reasons, clinical and legal, this may be a somewhat empty gesture:

- A patient seriously intending suicide can simply hoard or save up the pills, or obtain more from other sources.
- Similarly, life virtually bristles with alternative methods for committing suicide (even *within* hospitals), rendering *absolute* suicide prevention a fantasy.
- The focus on the psychiatrist's dispensing end, rather than the patient's taking end, of the prescribing relationship inappropriately shifts the focus of ultimate responsibility from patient to doctor.
- The practice, if widely followed, creates the illusion of control over something not truly controllable; this illusion may either lull the clinician into a false sense of security or convey to lawyers the equally false sense that outpatient

suicide is preventable and, consequently, that *not* to prescribe in this "small amount" way is automatically negligent.

- All too often clinicians employing this method do not employ open and free discussion of the issue. If this approach is used, it should take place within an alliance-based, collaborative assessment of the patient's history of impulsivity and a joint agreement that having only small amounts of medication on hand will, indeed, be helpful.
- It could readily be argued on clinical grounds that a patient so fragile as to be swayed by the size of the prescription should be in a hospital and/or receiving ECT.

Some clinicians would maintain that prescribing in this controlled fashion conveys to the patient a sense of the clinician's concern and wish to take the patient seriously. Impulsive patients, or those not well known to the clinician, may also benefit from this practice. Whether these benefits outweigh the foregoing problems must be evaluated on a case by case basis.

j. Clinical "clearance"

On occasion clinicians are requested to provide clearance for patients' abilities to perform certain life tasks—abilities thought to be potentially compromised by a history of mental illness or hospitalization; examples include owning firearms, taking a job, earning a security clearance, driving a car and the like. As a risk management technique clinicians should avoid attesting that the patient *has* certain abilities, since this position may portray the clinician as seeming to endorse the patient's performance of the task. For many of these tasks the clinician may not have the requisite knowledge (e.g., may not have seen the patient actually work). Such ostensible "endorsement" may create a claim of liability if the patient misuses the firearm, drives dangerously, etc.

The wisest course is for the clinician to address only what she knows—that patient's condition—in the form of a double negative, thus:

> "Based on my evaluation of the patient on _____, it is my professional opinion that there are *no clinical contraindications* to Mr. X's (going back to work, owning a gun, etc.)"

This double negative clarifies the fact that the evaluator can only state the absence of a clinical condition, based on an evaluation, that would bar the activity in question. Any semblance of endorsement or of prediction of future success in the activity is also avoided.

k. Psychiatrists as "medical back-ups"

Psychiatrists are sometimes asked to serve as "medical back-ups" for the patients of non-medical clinicians. In this role, they are usually expected to assess the patients' needs for medication, prescribe appropriately, and follow the patient periodically. Unfortunately, there are several liability issues that complicate the medical back-up role.

First, law lags somewhat behind practice in this area. It has long been assumed that when a physician and non-physician collaborate in a patient's care, the physician is in charge and bears ultimate responsibility for all treatment decisions. This assumption may bear little relationship, however, to the realities of collaborative care today. A psychiatrist who serves as medical back-up may assume no clinical responsibility for a patient's psychotherapy (indeed, the non-physician psychotherapist may be by far the more experienced member of the team), seeing the patient monthly or even less frequently to reassess her status relative to medications. Decisions concerning hospitalization and the need to respond to potential suicidal or homicidal emergencies may lie outside the scope of his "back-up" role.

If the psychiatrist is to avoid undue risk of liability in these cases—a risk heightened by the fact that physicians' malpractice insurance coverage is usually more extensive than that of other professions—clarification of the collaborative relationship should be made explicitly at its inception. A letter from the psychiatrist to the referring non-medical clinician should make clear the responsibilities assumed and not assumed in the back-up role. In particular, the psychiatrist's function as a medical back-up should be distinguished from a supervisory role, since the latter leaves the psychiatrist open to vicarious liability for the non-medical therapist's actions.

A second problem that must be addressed is the common practice of clinics and community mental health centers hiring part-time psychiatrists to fill the medical back-up position for a large number of non-medical clinicians. Anecdotes abound of cases in which psychiatrists are asked to prescribe medications for scores or even hundreds of patients, when their limited hours at the agency make it impossible for them to follow so many patients with any reasonable degree of care. At its worst, this system leads to psychiatrists leaving signed blank prescription forms for non-medical therapists to complete or mechanically signing dozens of prescriptions for patients they have never seen. Needless to say, both these practices represent an abdication of the psychiatrist's clinical, ethical, and legal responsibilities.

Physicians should not work in settings in which they are being asked to provide substandard care. If they cannot negotiate reasonable case loads that permit them adequate time to meet with patients and discuss them with other care-givers, they should get out. Facilities' efforts to save money by forcing psychiatrists into situations in which the standard of care cannot be met are reprehensible.

There may also be occasions when the medical back-up role is stretched beyond mere prescription of medications. Psychiatrists may be asked to sign treatment plans, team summaries, and insurance forms on a routine basis. A useful axiom for such cases is: "If you sign, the case is thine." It is likely that psychiatrists will be held responsible as the supervisor of the care for patients in these cases. Psychiatrists should familiarize themselves with published guidelines concerning the implications of their signatures. (See Suggested Readings—American Psychiatric Association.)

l. The ethical approach to problem solving

Certain exceedingly complex or novel situations—such as, at present, the multiple dilemmas around AIDS—occur in an area where relevant, unambiguous legal rulings have not yet occurred, and where clinical wisdom provides no easy answers (as with any untreatable condition). Faced with such a situation requiring action, clinicians may wish to attempt an ethical analysis as a solution to a clinical and legal impasse; that is, an ethical analysis—an extensive and documented discussion of the goods and harms to be expected from different approaches to a problem—may appropriately portray the clinician as non-negligent in areas where the standard of care is impossible to determine with confidence. Clinicians should reserve this technique for clinical situations susceptible of no other resolution.

3. DOCUMENTATIONAL APPROACHES TO PREVENTION

Second in importance to "do no evil" (previous sections) is "write no evil," and it is a close second, indeed; documentation has represented the "make or break" determinant in countless acts of litigation. While Chapter 1 addressed some important considerations in areas of record keeping, we here review and expand on this important topic from the specific aspect of the prevention of negligence and malpractice.

Clinicians should consider by way of overview that simply writing "more" in the chart is not in any sense a liability preventive strategy. Documentation is most effective when the clinician writes more efficiently, which may indeed mean writing less—a viewpoint inspiring relief in many clinicians experiencing themselves as drowned in paperwork.

Documentation for both clinical and risk management reasons should focus on three realms of discourse which often represent linchpins of both clinical decision making and subsequent second-guessing of such decisions in a litigation context.

The first realm represents the risk-benefit analysis—explicit or implicit—of the intervention proposed. Recall that decisions often involve at least two alternatives—"do it or don't do it"—although many more than two, of course, may be involved. Each of these forks in the path, moreover, has its own separate risks and benefits. Thus, when a patient is being considered for a pass, both going out on the pass *and* remaining in the hospital without a pass have demonstrable risks and benefits. Clinicians tend to focus more on the riskier side of the decision—in this case, going out on pass. The clinician who has performed a careful, documented risk-benefit analysis may be proven by later events (and indeed, by hindsight) to have been wrong in the decision, but the care in the risk-benefit analysis refutes the claim of negligence. It should go without saying that the risk-benefit analytic approach is a highly acceptable method of general clinical decision making in any case.

The second important realm for documentation is the exercise of the clinician's judgment at key decision points in the work. What was the clinician's assessment? Based on that assessment, what was the clinician's response? Clinicians are often in danger of recording only the conclusory final steps of the decisionmaking process without allowing subsequent caretakers (and subsequent juries) to share the training, experience, and thoughtfulness that may have gone into the decision in question. Here the "thinking out loud for the record" discussed below becomes particularly important.

Finally, the third realm is an assessment and record of the patient's capacity to participate in treatment planning. This ability resembles the competencies addressed in the next chapter. One could indeed speak meaningfully of the patient's competence or capacity to weigh the risks and benefits of giving or withholding information to or from the treating caretakers. In dealing with the suicidal patient in particular, the information in question might include the status of the patient's suicidal intent or impulsivity, as well as the nature of internal controls and the ability to resist such lethal inclinations. In the more general sense, careful assessment of the patient's ability to manage her own care and make reasonable decisions therein may well exonerate the clinician from an obligation to intervene in a highly parentalistic or protective manner.

Accurate evaluation of the patient as having the capacity to share this sort of information may play a significant role in capturing the patient's ability—and actual responsibility—to inform the clinician about a change for the worse in his suicidal condition. This may free the clinician from the apparent requirement of reading the patient's mind during particular interventions, e.g., passes or discharge from the hospital. In addition, the image of the patient as a competent decision maker refutes the common image of the patient, favored by plaintiff's attorneys in such litigation, as an incompetent child who is incapable—because of being "too sick" or "too crazy"—of letting the clinician know what is going on in his mind. Since competent patients universally can reject or refuse life saving treatment, a suicidal patient competent to weigh the risks and benefits of giving or withholding information may elect not to call or notify caretakers when suicidal feelings reach the dangerous point—but this is not the clinician's problem.

Note further that this view of the patient rests upon a rock-solid clinical foundation. That is, a patient whose illness *does* render him incapable of sharing information about his inner state with the clinician should, indeed, be treated in a much more conservative or protective manner. The next example reveals a way in which this assessment might take place:

> **Example 9:** A borderline patient admitted for suicidal preoccupations is about to be given her first pass. In exploring the issue, the clinician asks, "You realize that I can't help you if you don't level with me? The only way I'll know what's on your mind is if you tell me." The patient acknowledged awareness of this fact. The clinician then began an inquiry as to whether the patient was aware of the interventions available to her, should her suicidal preoccupations return or increase. The patient was able to articulate the responses: making phone calls to the ward or to the hospital's emergency room; premature termination of the pass; or at worst, having her family or an ambulance bring her on an emergency basis back to the hospital. The results of this assessment, appropriately recorded in the chart, capture the nature of the patient's autonomous adult capacities to participate in the treatment planning, to the degree of being able to share her internal state with the clinician who is in a position to make the appropriate interventions.

From the standpoint of these general principles, areas of particular relevance are addressed below.

a. Facts

The major use of the record, of course, is as a durable statement of what has happened or what has been done. So forensically powerful is this function that it commonly operates in its converse: if an event is not recorded it "did not happen." At times even eyewitnesses are less convincing than a statement in a record or chart that something occurred.

The record of certain aspects of the patient's care is crucial. For inpatients, the neurological examination is essential, since it serves not only to detect illnesses with neurological components but also to establish baseline readings against which injuries in the hospital (falls, assaults), medication side effects, and tardive dyskinesia may be measured—all matters of great significance in court.

For all patients, medication allergies and sensitivities are particularly important items for recording, as are concomitant medical conditions and other medications taken (e.g., nonpsychiatric drugs).

Another recording function of the chart or record is describing the impact of interventions made by the therapist (or by the inpatient treatment team). Effects of space restrictions, medications (changes in dosages, additional or different medications, etc.), psychotherapeutic approaches, trial passes, and the like all have some result, even if that result is "no change." These should be noted not only for forensic purposes, of course, but to ensure the quality of patient care.

Emergencies should evoke particular scrupulousness in recording details, both because emergencies are critical points in care where details are required to assess the meaning of the events, and because emergencies are disproportionately charged with potential liability.

b. Judgments

The clinician's problem in many a malpractice suit is the fact that the clinician's judgment is assessed post facto (after the crucial event that catalyzed the suit has occurred) with all the specious clarity and certainty peculiar to a retrospective view. Thus it is essential that the bases for the clinician's judgment in general, and certainly in crises, be articulated for the record, as noted earlier.

Example 10: A patient voiced suicidal ideation and, after careful exploration of the subject, the clinician elected not to hospitalize the patient. The record of that session contained specific assessment of risk factors (see Chap. 2, Sec. III-A-2) and resources, especially those that the clinician knew from familiarity with the patient and her history. It is just this material that is often taken for granted since it is so well known to the clinician that she fails to spell it out in the record. The record articulated the bases for the decision in terms of disadvantages of hospitalization and factors making continued outpatient status desirable (i.e., preservation of autonomy). Finally, specific mention was made of pathways by which the patient could report any change of status, especially for the worse (i.e., giving therapist's phone number, covering clinician's number, and the number of the local emergency ward).

The data suggested for recording in the example may seem excessive as a response to so ubiquitous a clinical event, yet one must weigh such material, not in terms of the patient's successfully weathering a difficult period and going on to improve, but in terms of the patient unexpectedly committing suicide and the family bringing suit. The clinician faces the possibility of the jury reasoning that, "since the patient *did* kill herself, the decision not to hospitalize must have been negligent." To counter this "retrospective certainty," the clinician must have evidence of care in judgment, care in thinking through the issue, care in meticulous weighing of the pros and cons, and care in consulting with other clinicians when warranted—evidence that can be supplied only by the word written at the time of the actual assessment (see also Section c below). The clinician, terrified by tales of the whimsicality of judges and juries, may take heart from the knowledge that her clinical skills and unique knowledge of the patient *do* count for something—but only if recorded in the chart.

A particular form of recording judgments relates to the question of indications for treatment, especially novel, experimental, or atypical applications of known treatments; for example, the use of lithium for bipolar illness is well accepted, but lithium has proved effective in selected cases of impulsive violence—an atypical usage that would require more documentation of indications and risks/benefits. While all treatments sometimes fail, failures of atypical applications of known treatments or of experimental treatments tend to be more forensically sensitive, for obvious reasons.

c. Reflections

While the average record entry should be crisp, detailed, specific, and objective, there are certain exceptions (hinted at in Section b above) where a more narrative, first-person mode of recording may be indicated—an approach best termed "thinking out loud for the record." This approach should be invoked whenever the clinician is about to take a calculated risk (as in Example 3 above) or to do the "less conservative" thing (e.g., *not* hospitalize the patient). The "thinking out loud" should represent a record of the clinician's assessments, reflections, standards, and indices of decision making, reports of supervisory or consultative insights, and the like. The justification for this kind of "thinking out loud" is based on the fact that *not* thinking (or not leaving a record of one's thinking, which may amount to the same thing) may be seen as negligent. (See also Suggested Readings for Chapter One.)

d. Anticipating evidentiary use of the record

While, as a field, psychiatry does not do well in the prediction of future behavior, a certain degree of anticipation of future events forms a legitimate part of record keeping.

The clearest example of this function occurs when it appears that the clinician may petition for involuntary commitment at some future point. This possibility places a premium on recording signs of dangerousness (or, for that matter, lack of dangerousness) so as to have available the data for the eventual hearing.

If a patient injures another patient, one may anticipate possible future litigation; thus, detailed descriptions of the event from all observers, as well as recording all the findings of examinations and the clinical responses of the staff, fulfill the anticipatory role.

In this regard, it is useful to review one's records from the viewpoint that the "eyes of the future are upon you"; that is, one must ask, "What ambiguity or misperceptions may arise from this note if read in the future by a stranger?"

(Needless to say the most infelicitous such occasion would be a reading by the plaintiff's attorney.) With this in mind, it is advisable for trainees learning to write progress notes to imagine the note being read aloud to a jury by a hostile counsel, a fantasy that aids perspective in note writing!

> *Example 11:* A resident reviewed a progress note that said, in part, "Patient was asking repetitive questions, so he was secluded." The resident realized that this would appear illogical and illegal to future readers (since in that jurisdiction seclusion was permitted only for dangerous behavior or threat of same); he then included the datum (so familiar to him that he took it for granted), "The patient's history gives numerous examples of repetitive questioning in a compulsive manner being the prelude to assaultiveness."

While dramatic, this example clearly illustrates the value and purpose of reviewing documentation "with the future's eyes."

e. Professionalism in record keeping

As in other aspects of the treatment relationship, a professional attitude should prevail in the records (See Chap. 1, Sec. III-G, concerning the distinction between progress and process notes and related matters; see also Suggested Readings for that chapter and see Sec. III-A-1-b above.) This means that an objective, descriptive tone should govern the recorded material. There is no place in a professional record for derogatory, judgmental, value-laden, abusive, sarcastic, mocking, or ridiculing remarks; even mild facetiousness or witticisms are potentially destructive, not only because they are rarely quite so funny when read aloud in court, but because they may convey disrespect or an unsympathetic attitude toward the patient—a serious problem for the clinician attempting to counter a charge of negligence by avowing that he had the best interests of the patient at heart. Even more significantly, the difference between a written description or a psychodynamic formulation and libel or liability may turn upon just such matters of professional intent conveyed by the tone of the material.

f. Correcting the record

A detected omission can most appropriately be corrected in a review of the record by making clear the retrospective nature of the emendation:

> *Example 12:* July 20, 1994, 5:00 P.M. Review of note of July 14, 1994, reveals inadvertent omission of notation of patient's parent's visit, which contributed to the upset of the next day; currently, . . ."

Under no circumstances should corrective notes be interpolated unlabeled into the body of the chart; done even with the best of intentions, such interpolations may seem duplicitous in the light of subsequent review, especially in the context of litigation. The difference between the conscientious remedy of an oversight and a venal attempt at "fudging" the record may lie in the transparent depiction of the time frame and context of the inserted note. A "flag note," dated and signed, is acceptable, as in the next example:

Example 13: For the situation in Example 5 above, one might place in the margin of the earlier note (July 14, 1994) the following:

July 20, 1989, marginal note: "See progress note of July 20, 1994, for additional data." (signed)

Especially to be avoided is any attempt to squeeze emendations, interpolations, or corrections into existing chart notes. Clinicians should be aware that forensic document experts are extremely skilled at identifying the relative timing of written material. Document experts aside, the word "suicide precautions" squeezed between two closely-set lines of a written progress note, so that the insert clearly overlaps existing letters beneath it, requires no document expert to detect its post facto nature. Recall that in the process of litigation, such tiny handwritten inserts appear on four-foot by six-foot foam-backed displays that sit on easels in front of juries. At those frequent moments in the trial where the material gets boring, the eyes of jurors will wander to your inept emendation, with its inescapable aura of retrospective cover-up, no matter how contemporaneously and honestly the correction was made. Clinicians should sacrifice the wish to save paper and use the retrospective annotation noted earlier.

Finally, attempting to go back to "correct" data after a suit has been filed is not only futile but self-defeating. Instead, for forensically sensitive events (assaults, suicides, etc.), a clinical review of the entire situation (perhaps presided over by a senior clinician) often proves valuable, not only in unearthing data that might be lost in the tumult of the emergency, but also in maintaining and demonstrating ongoing attention to and review of clinical problems in the service of high standards of care; such reviews are often helpful as well in providing data useful in countering charges of negligence brought at some subsequent date (see also Sec. III-A-4-e below and Chap. 3, Sec. III-A-2).

g. Hospital policies and related documents

Clinicians may be subliminally aware of the existence of large volumes of documents entitled "Hospital Policies or Regulations"; such documents are often an important part of the accreditation process for hospitals. As a practical matter, it is unusual for those clinicians not involved in the direct design of hospital policies ever to have a close familiarity with them, though they may have read them as part of the initial credentialing process.

For good or ill, such policies represent the institution's own self-set standards; thus these documents bear directly upon the question of the standard of practice of the clinicians at that institution. Clinicians on treatment units should have at least some general familiarity with policies involving clinical-administrative decision points, for example, what does it mean in this institution to be on suicide precautions? How often are such patients checked? What are the official procedures regarding the assignment of a pass? How are various kinds of medications handled? And the like.

In complementary fashion, those clinicians involved in designing hospital policies should design them with significant flexibility and with an eye toward providing a great deal of discretion for the treating clinician on the scene. Despite their often functionally negligible role in the actual running of the hospital, such policy documents provide an easy target for attorneys attempting to point out that clinicians violated the policies of their own institution and thus were more likely to have been negligent.

h. The question of old records

Most clinicians would agree that the old clinical record is of great importance to the clinician for treatment. The same clinicians would easily agree that obtaining those old records—in particular, obtaining them before the patient's hospitalization is over and the patient, long discharged—is often difficult, given the problems of under-staffing and high work volume in many institutional record rooms throughout the country.

The clinician faced with this reality of institutional life should not, however, assume the ostrich position and either fail to send for previous records or send off the request and assume that the records will be a long time coming. Instead, especially where the patient's history contains elements of suicide or violence to others, clinicians should consider calling up previous institutions or arranging for such data gathering, and obtaining at least the highlights of clinical care. If the patient cannot or will not give permission, or if the previous institution will not release such information, one makes the best of the situation, but in many cases, certain key points constituting emergency information may be transmittable in this informal fashion. A discouragingly common element in litigation involves the imputation that the clinician failed to obtain significant old records that allegedly would have altered the treatment plan.

i. The limits of documentation

Both clinicians on the scene, as well as forensic experts reviewing records subsequently in the context of litigation, should keep in mind the limits of documentation itself. Everything that transpires cannot be recorded, for the simple reason that—if attempted—no time would remain for the care of patients. Core documentation addressed to the three principles mentioned above would be more than adequate for clinical and risk management purposes.

There are two areas that are clinically meaningful, but that almost never appear in formal fashion in the records: subjective data and inter-staff communication. Subjective data refers to those impressions gained by the clinician from direct observation of the patient's tone of voice, body language, facial expression, sounds, and even smells—and to the clinician's internal subjective responses to these data—that are not transmissible to individuals not on the scene. While such sensory observations may be determinative of clinical decision making in a given case, they are rarely conveyed directly in the record in a form that permits their perception by later observers.

The second area rarely captured in record keeping is the astonishing amount of inter-staff communication that goes on at all times, among staff members at the nursing station, in the halls and cafeterias, and the like. Such informal sharing of information may also powerfully influence decision making, but rarely appears explicitly in the record.

The comments above do not imply that this material must necessarily be recorded in exactly these forms. Clinicians should remain aware, however, of the fact that documentation possesses inherent limits and should not be confused with the totality of the care delivered: the menu is not identical to the meal.

4. CONSULTATIVE APPROACHES TO PREVENTION

As indicated in Sec. II-A-1-b of this chapter, the usual benchmark employed in the assessment of negligence in malpractice is the prevailing standard of practice of the profession. It is this point that adds a preventive dimension to the generally laudable use of clinical consultation. Consultation—the second "pillar of liability prevention"—may be utilized in a number of ways.

a. Consultation vs. supervision

Consultation implies an arrangement in which an outside clinician is invited to provide information to the clinician with responsibility for the patient's care without assuming any clinical responsibility for the case. The information offered by the consultant may be primarily educational in nature, for example when a clinician hires a more experienced psychotherapist to review his treatment of one or more patients, so as to enhance the consultee's psychotherapy skills. (Note that in some areas this person is referred to—confusingly—as a "supervisor.") Or the consultant may be asked to make suggestions relative to the treatment of a particular patient, with broader educational goals secondary to the immediate problems of patient management. In either case, the hallmark of a consultative relationship is that the consultee is free to accept or refuse any suggestions made by the consultant.

In contrast, in a supervisory relationship the supervisor shares some degree of responsibility for the patient's care flowing from the structure of the situation rather than from an invitation. This is generally the case in formal training programs, such as psychiatry residencies, psychology internships, or social work placements. It may also be the case when one clinician, usually a psychiatrist or psychologist, allows another clinician to bill third-party payers under the first clinician's name; this widespread practice results in the first clinician—knowingly or not—assuming supervisory responsibility for the conduct of the case. When a true supervisory relationship exists, the treating clinician is not free to disregard the supervisor's views of how the case should be managed. Legal aspects of the supervisory relationship were discussed in Sec. II-A-3-g above. Here we consider pure consultative situations.

b. Occasional consultation

In this form, a consultant is invited to review at a specific point in the treatment an inpatient or outpatient case; this is the mode most familiar in teaching settings, but it is employed in the private sector as well, typically when a clinician seeks out a senior colleague for help with a treatment impasse. This represents perhaps the most common form of obtaining a "second opinion," as in general medicine. More importantly, even a very brief and informal consultation represents a "biopsy of the standard of care."

c. Ongoing consultation

Here a clinician hires (either privately or through an institutional arrangement) a senior colleague to review her work on a regular basis (e.g., weekly or monthly). The consultation may cover a single difficult case, the consultee's entire caseload, or anything in between.

d. Peer consultation

This approach may be formal or informal, individual or group, where clinicians at comparable levels of age, training, or professional development give ongoing suggestions to each other about patient care and clinical work.

e. Retrospective review

This form of consultation represents an attempt post facto to understand more about why a particular event occurred. Examples of such events are a flight from therapy, a suicide or serious attempt, an adverse treatment reaction, an escape from a hospital, an admission to a hospital, and a severe assault. Many utilization and peer review procedures fall into this category. Such reviews are aimed at monitoring and improving professional care through education and better understanding of critical events in treatment.

Depending on state laws and the mechanisms by which such reviews are accomplished, some retrospective reviews will be subject to discovery in subsequent litigation, whereas others will enjoy immunities from such exposure. Regulations on this charged subject reflect the tension between the value of clinicians' candid peer-scrutiny and peer-criticism on one hand, and the appropriateness of the plaintiff in a lawsuit gathering hindsight evidence for his case on the other. Regional and institutional policies vary on this subject; many forms of quality assurance activity are not discoverable, for example. Clinicians should clarify these issues before settling down to review case materials retrospectively.

All the four foregoing consultative approaches serve the purposes (among others) of malpractice prevention by bringing the individual practitioner into touch with representatives of the prevailing standard of practice (i.e., her colleagues in the field). In fact, in all but the most egregious forms of dereliction, a second opinion exerts a powerful counterforce to the accusation of negligence; the clinician who seeks professional advice thus gives evidence of scrupulousness of practice and so stands to present the disputed action as an honest error in judgment rather than negligence—an error shared, moreover, by more than one party in the profession. (See also Sec. III-A-3-c above, and Chap. 3, Sec. III-A-3.)

B. Responding to charges of negligence and malpractice

1. OPENING GAMBITS

Any practitioner, regardless of experience, training, unimpeachable standards of practice, or success in the field, may be charged with malpractice, as noted earlier in Sec. III-A. While clinicians may take heart from having followed the preventive measures earlier outlined to aid in the outcome, the actual experience of being charged is always demoralizing and distressing. To maintain perspective one must keep in mind certain fundamentals of the experience.

The announcement can come from a variety of sources and in various forms: from one's institutional superiors, when the suit names and includes a facility head; from a letter from the plaintiff's attorneys or directly from the plaintiff-patient; or from a face-to-face confrontation with patient and/or attorney. One of the most disconcerting aspects of attorneys' letters, calls, or statements is the style of many attorneys in such matters of entering "with guns blazing"; that is, their tactical approach to the inexperienced clinician (and, fortunately, most clinicians *are* inexperienced in these events) often appears to involve accusing everybody involved with the patient of having done everything not merely wrong, but willfully and maliciously wrong. The average practitioner has never heard such accusations outside of psychotic transferences, but these are often part of the routine. The clinician's own attorney may respond with threats and accusations of libel against the charges, and so on.

Recognizing that these are standard opening maneuvers may aid the clinician in retaining composure under this assault; none of the accusations is meaningful until proved in court. But clinicians who overreact with panic or rage on receipt of these terms may act rashly and self-defeatingly.

The clinician must also remember that at the point of initiation of litigation it is only a distraction—albeit a comforting one—to interpret what is occurring in dynamic terms. That is, it may well be the case that the charge represents the patient's transparent acting out of the transference, of psychotic fantasies, or of entitlement or rage at the patient's parents, all being expressed by the patient filing suit; such insight into the patient's behavior, no matter how perspicacious, should have no influence on a serious, businesslike, and realistic approach to the matter at hand.

The first reaction, of course, should be to contact one's insurer immediately with the news of even a possible suit; it is almost always the insurer's lawyer who will be responsible for the defense should a suit be filed. In addition, clinicians working in institutions should notify the institution's risk manager. One should, in addition, never respond in any manner to the plaintiff's lawyer's communication; a response should be left to one's own lawyer. Statements made in haste at such times are often repented at leisure.

2. WORKING WITH A LAWYER

Few experiences are as reassuring as working with a skilled and experienced attorney during the Sturm und Drang of malpractice litigation; success in this crisis often depends on how well the collaboration between lawyer and clinician operates. Certain principles should guide the clinician in this undertaking.

a. A collaborative approach

There are numerous ways in which the nuances, unique issues, and approaches to psychiatric malpractice litigation differ even from general medical malpractice suits, and these differences may be pivotal. The defendant clinician should recognize that his attorney may not always be possessed of the familiarity with psychiatric (or general medical) issues that the clinician himself enjoys. His most useful role in his own defense may be to fill in those gaps in his lawyer's knowledge that are evident to him. Psychiatrist and lawyer should work as a team.

Example 14: A malpractice suit hinged on the testimony of opposing psychiatric expert witnesses. At the defendant psychiatrist's prompting, his attorney asked whether the opposing expert witness was board certified. He was not, as it turned out; plaintiff's attorney had not ascertained this datum, being ignorant of its significance. This revelation severely weakened the impact of the testimony of that witness.

b. Absolute candor

The courtroom is the arena in which the attorney will make tactical decisions about which evidence is best introduced; in the lawyer's office "admissibility" should be total. Questions, uncertainties, subjective assessments of the situation, acknowledgments of omission or wrongdoing, impressions and self-assessments are all legitimate subject matter for communication to the attorney; self-effacement, grandiosity, entitlement, and any form of concealment of these data are utterly inappropriate to the transaction.

c. Expert witness selection

The clinician can be further helpful to the attorney by making recommendations for selection of expert witnesses, since—unless the attorney has acquired a "stable" of capable clinicians from previous cases—the clinician may be better acquainted with members of the field who have special expertise on the disputed subject. Important qualities of a desirable witness include:

1 *Experience,* not only in the subject matter, but in being on the stand, being cross-examined, and thinking quickly under stress.
2 *Renown* in the subject area, perhaps as conveyed by an extensive curriculum vitae, many books and publications, high academic rank, or wide reputation.
3 *Personal knowledge of the clinician* and reasonably good opinion of the latter.
4 If possible, *personal knowledge of the patient,* e.g., from having consulted on the case, given a conference on the patient, etc. (Of course, the witness should not be in the line of clinical responsibility for that patient.)
5 Most critically, the witness should have an opinion about the case parallel to the clinician's. (See Chapter 8 for further discussion of expert witnesses.)

d. Role of the records

Under most circumstances of a suit an attempt will be made by the plaintiff's attorney to obtain the patient's records, sometimes under subpoena, sometimes merely with the patient's release; here, of course, the impact of the preventive measures of Sec. III-A is most keenly felt. The experienced lawyer will request "all records," which includes private (process) notes (see Chap. 1). If an attorney requests "a record" or "the official record," the front record or progress record is indicated; the clinician is under no obligation to volunteer his private notes unless specifically asked to do so. All requests for records should be channeled to the clinician's attorney and acted on only with her advice. The clinician should retain the originals, providing clear photostatic copies as needed.

As an addendum, we may note that the clinician's candor should be reserved for his *own* attorney. Not volunteering gratuitous information to the "other side" of the case is a good general rule for all communications; blurting "I didn't mean any harm!" when interviewed by the patient's attorney would be considered a notable gaucherie. Whenever possible, communication should take place via the attorneys.

Attorney and clinician are well advised to go over the records carefully together to clarify ambiguities, technical jargon, unsuspected omissions, latent implications, or possible misinterpretations. Under certain circumstances, a given patient's record or chart may contain material irrelevant to the subject of the suit but potentially damaging, embarrassing, or otherwise harmful to the patient. The clinician cannot legally or ethically withhold such material; however, through his attorney a request to the judge may be made to review that material in chambers to decide if it is indeed irrelevant and may thus be excluded from public revelation at trial. If the judge refuses the request, there is little to be done except to attempt to prepare the patient (preferably by lawyer-to-lawyer communication) for the possible impact of disclosure. (See Chap. 8, Sec. III-B-1, concerning use of records by the expert witness.)

C. Treating patients during malpractice proceedings

This section confronts two aspects of a complex subject: the treatment of patients in general by the sued clinician and the treatment specifically of the suing patient.

1. EFFECTS OF BEING SUED ON THE CLINICIAN'S GENERAL PATIENT TREATMENT

Clinicians in the regrettable position of being sued describe the enormous power of the suit to preoccupy them, not just at odd moments during the day, but even during work with other patients. Like a raw nerve, the issue of the suit resonates painfully with similar material from the treatment session, serving as a distraction from concentration on the work at hand. In addition, clinicians describe having flashes of association to some important issue or question in the suit while seeing a patient, wanting to "stay with" the patient before them, yet feeling terror that they will lose or forget the crucial datum.

Empirical data relatively recently available (see Suggested Readings—Charles et al.) has revealed that clinicians experiencing malpractice litigation may stop seeing certain types of patients (perhaps resembling those referred to above); consider early retirement from the practice of medicine; and seriously discourage their children and others from entering the field. More significantly, physicians experiencing litigation clearly indicated that it caused suffering to them and to their families. It is of interest to note that later work by Charles and associates revealed that physicians for whom being sued was the most significant catastrophic event in their lives were coping far less effectively than those physicians who had had an earlier catastrophe in another context—a result suggesting that the experience of trauma provides either armor or practice with a set of coping skills.

For the foregoing reasons, clinicians must weigh heavily the impact of litigation in the short run on their capacities to do good work and should consider taking on no new patients or responsibilities, even perhaps cutting back on those they are carrying. Certain aspects of this difficulty may be unavoidable. For example, consider the clinician sued for negligence by the family of a patient who commits suicide. It may happen that another patient expresses suicidal feelings—a not unusual experience in psychiatric practice, but always stressful in its own way. Clearly the clinician in this example, being human, cannot bring to bear the same dispassionate assessment as would be possible were there no suit. Ethically, however, the clinician's duty is to be as useful as possible to the patient then before him. In this exceptionally charged situation, the most appropriate approaches would involve active use of consultations, strong efforts at introspection and consciousness raising, and—as a last resort, if the conflicts become unmanageable—conscientious referral of the patient to another clinician, with appropriate explanations. Responsible referral in this manner avoids the further charge of abandonment of the patient.

The danger especially to be guarded against is avoidance or turning away from patients' distress since patients, sensing this withdrawal, may become increasingly desperate, the more so because they would have no way of correctly interpreting the basis for the clinician's reaction.

2. TREATING THE PATIENT SUING THE TREATER

This rather *outré* situation requires some explanation at the outset. Modern attorneys sophisticated in the mediolegal sphere openly recommend continued contact (and even treatment) by the clinician of the plaintiff. They reason that the fact that the patient stayed with that clinician will make a positive impression on the jury: the clinician can't have been all that bad. For psychiatry, however, this model is far less applicable because of the requirement that the relationship be free of encumbrances. This has several implications. First, when there is a choice, the clinician should not elect to treat the patient suing her, legally because there is a danger of adding fuel to the forensic fire and clinically because of the countertransference problem described in Section 1 and above. The reason the question can be discussed at all is threefold:

- The fact that the patient (or others) is suing the clinician does not necessarily eliminate the patient's need for care.
- The existence of the suit does not automatically imply that the patient no longer wishes to see that clinician; as suggested earlier, the patient's filing of the suit may reflect, in curious form, the intensity of the patient's involvement with that clinician. Thus, wanting to continue seeing the clinician you are suing is a logical contradiction, but not a clinical one.
- In the public sector, especially, other choices may not be available. For example, the head of a ward at an overcrowded, understaffed state hospital may be the target of a suit by a patient in that catchment area; should the patient require readmission during (or, conceivably, because of) the litigation, there may be simply no other bed space, facility, or clinician available. Thus, it may happen that a clinician, as in this example, may find herself in the position of being clinically responsible to treat a patient by whom she is being sued.

This extraordinary dilemma admits of no easy approach, but the patient's transfer to another facility (perhaps under an exchange agreement) is the only acceptable course. The reality that the clinician must look to defense of his case totally contaminates the work; not only is the clinician's purpose slanted toward proving himself correct, but his interventions must of necessity be suspect as attempts to convince the patient to change her mind. Ethical treatment is probably impossible under these circumstances.

IV. PITFALLS

A. "Defensive" practice

In earlier discussions, we have intentionally avoided the concept of "defensive" practice or "defensive" psychiatry in favor of focusing on negligence prevention. This terminological distinction highlights the pitfall at issue here—seeing the patient as "the enemy" even before any litigation arises. Such a view is enormously destructive to the treatment alliance, to empathic receptivity, and to one's ability to listen perceptively. The preventive approaches outlined in Sec. III-A enhance patient care as well as provide insurance against possible litigation. Ironically, defensive practice may actually *provoke* the very result it purports to avoid. Feeling antagonized, alienated, and "defended against," the patient may well feel that the clinician is not placing his interests foremost and may express this view in litigation.

B. Remaining the clinician

Staying in the "therapeutic chair" is one of the most difficult tasks of the clinician facing or fearing suit; the temptation is strong to become a lawyer (or lawyer-like) under the stresses of litigation. Since the patient has a lawyer, the clinician should have a lawyer; he, himself, however, should retain his dedication to treatment of the patient.

C. "Political" use of the record

The record should at all times be used for its documentational and communicative purposes. Clinicians should actively resist the temptation to fight out ward battles through the chart; to admonish (or for that matter, inspire) other clinicians; or to demonstrate one's skill, intellect, baroque verbal facility and the like. No amount of staff amusement or improved morale can repay the destructive impact on this legal document of such approaches in a liability context.

V. CASE EXAMPLE EPILOGUES

A. Case Example 1

The consultant reviews with the therapist recent court rulings on informed consent, especially those concerning the extent of the therapeutic privilege—the right of the doctor to withhold information that might damage the patient. He notes that this privilege is usually invoked only when the information might be harmful in itself and not when the information might provoke the patient to refuse treatment, which might then lead to harmful results. In addition, he cites the writings of leading psychiatrists who feel that information about the potential for tardive dyskinesia need not be exhaustively disclosed to acutely psychotic patients, but that after a period of several weeks to months, whether the patient had improved significantly or not, the matter has to be discussed fully.

Reluctantly, the clinician decides to raise the issue with her patient. She notes that she is not sure if all the risks, benefits, and alternatives to medication have been explained previously and that she wants to go over them with him now. She further notes that her concern has been evoked by some movements of his hands and legs that she thinks represent a side effect of the medication.

After she explains the long-term risks of continuing neuroleptics in a patient who already has signs of tardive dyskinesia, the patient asks what the alternatives are. The doctor says frankly that while discontinuation of the medication is usually recommended, at least on a trial basis, it does produce a risk of relapse and does not guarantee the resolution of the movements. The patient responds that he is aware of his movements, since his family points them out to him whenever they are angry with him, and, though he does not like them and certainly would not want them to get worse, he is more afraid of relapsing and being readmitted. Consequently, he wants to continue taking the medication and is not interested in being referred to a neurologist for a definitive diagnosis of his abnormal movements. Since he would continue with the medication in any event, he says, there is no point in further work-up of the condition.

The feared paranoid reaction does not develop nor does the patient become overtly angry. When the psychiatrist asks him to share his feelings about the discussion they have just had, he says that he appreciates the way she has brought him into the decisionmaking process and interprets that as a sign that she respects the progress he has made toward becoming "normal" again.

B. Case Example 2

After alerting his malpractice insurer, the resident hurries to the supervisor's office and presents the entire case in review. The supervisor nods. "Sounds like you needed to pay more attention to her transference to you; she may have become psychotic as a defense against those feelings, just as she did with the boyfriend. I suggest you try to get the family together to discuss this. Meanwhile, call the lawyer who issued the subpoena and try to get him into the meeting, together with our hospital counsel."

The supervisor goes on to explain that the intensity of therapeutic exploration can mobilize powerful earlier feelings that—ideally—become available for necessary therapeutic work. These feelings, he cautions, may also burgeon undetected, with the result that the ideas that accompany these feelings may become delusional when the patient's defenses can no longer contain the affect. The supervisor's session is interrupted by a call that the patient has been readmitted.

Energetic efforts by the social worker to have the father come in to discuss the issue are successful. A group conference with patient, resident, supervisor, social worker, father, and both lawyers aids in clarifying the issue. The father dubiously agrees to hold the suit in abeyance; though confused by the whole matter, he is influenced by his daughter's willingness to continue work with the resident. Months later, the patient describes the earlier office incident: "I was flooded with the strongest sexual feeling; I sort of blanked out, and I thought we'd made love—you know, through the air." More months of therapeutic work permit the patient's greater acceptance of her sexual feelings.

VI. ACTION GUIDE

A. Checklist for Preventing Negligence/Malpractice

1. *Behavioral approaches*
   a. *Refrain* from unprofessional behavior
   b. *Avoid* exploitation of patient (sexual, financial, dependent).
   c. *Maintain* "open door" policy to avoid abandonment; send letters (with carbons) signaling cessation of treatment, cancellation of time slot.
   d. *Treat* patients within area of competence; *refer* others.
2. *Technical approaches*
   a. *Establish* a clear treatment contract.
   b. *Acknowledge* limitations and *avoid* statements implying promises.
   c. *Exercise* care regarding informed consent and its documentation; *remember* memory loss from ECT as factor and *renegotiate* information about medication at point of clinical stabilization or discharge from hospital (see section E below).
   d. *Maintain* a position of therapeutic disinterested impartiality; *resist* giving premature advice.
   e. For legalistic acting out
      i. *Remain* calm.
      ii. *Avoid* struggle in the legal arena.
      iii. Actively *confront* and *interpret* clinically.
      iv. *Extract* maximum therapeutic benefit from the event.
   f. *Outreach* to victims and affected parties in suicide or homicide; *consider* attending funeral.
3. *Documentational approaches*
   a. *Record* factual details, especially forensically sensitive events, e.g., emergencies.
   b. *Describe* in detail the bases for clinical judgment, especially in sensitive areas.
   c. *"Think out loud"* for the record, especially for calculated risks and indications for nonroutine interventions.
   d. *Anticipate* forensically significant events (e.g., commitments, possible suits) and *write* record with clarity from viewpoint of future readers.
   e. *Maintain* a professional tone throughout record.
   f. *Correct* errors and omissions in transparent, present-time manner.
4. *Consultative approaches*
   a. *Participate* in peer review, private review, private supervision, retrospective review; *seek* specific colleagues' advice in complex, risky, or unusual areas.

B. Checklist for Responding to Charges of Negligence/Malpractice

1. *Maintain* calm and perspective under "blazing guns" approach of attorneys; *resist* dynamic formulation of suit at outset.
2. *Obtain* legal advice.
   a. *Use* collaborative approach with attorney.

    b. *Inform* attorney with absolute candor of all data relevant, including uncertainties, ambiguities, and omissions.

    c. *Assist* attorney in selection of expert witnesses; *weigh* witnesses' renown and experience, personal knowledge of patient and/or clinician, similar viewpoint.

    d. *Surrender* only requested records and only through your attorney.

    e. *Avoid* discussions with plaintiff's attorney; *refer* to your attorney.

C. Checklist for Treating Patients During Litigation

1. *Avoid* increasing caseload or administrative responsibilities, if possible.
2. *Avoid* electively treating patient suing you.
3. If inevitable
    i. *Obtain* consultation actively.
    ii. *Attempt* transfer to alternative facility.
    iii. *Remain* alert for inevitable countertransference difficulties.

D. General

1. *Avoid* seeing the patient as enemy.
2. *Remain* the clinician.
3. *Use* record for clinical purposes only.

E. Checklist for Obtaining Informed Consent

1. *Provide sufficient information concerning*
    a. Nature of procedure/treatment,
    b. Risks and benefits of procedure/treatment,
    c. Risks and benefits of alternatives,
    d. Risks and benefits of no treatment.
2. *Simplify* language so that laypersons can understand.
3. *Offer* opportunity to ask questions.
4. *Test* patient's understanding after process is completed.
5. *Reeducate* as needed according to gaps in knowledge detected by testing.
6. *Consider* presence of factors that might impair voluntariness of consent.
7. *Assess* patient's competence to offer consent (see Chap. 5, Action Guide).
8. *Document* all relevant factors:
    a. Patient's consent, either by patient's signature or clinician's note in chart,
    b. Material disclosed,
    c. Patient's understanding,
    d. Voluntariness and competence.

VII. SUGGESTED READINGS.

A. MALPRACTICE AND OTHER FORMS OF LIABILITY

1. Wettstein, R. M.: Psychiatric malpractice, in Tasman, A., Hales, R. E. & Frances, A. J. (eds.): *American Psychiatric Press Review of Psychiatry,* Vol. 8. Washington, DC, American Psychiatric Press Inc., 1989.

2. Tancredi, L. R.: Psychiatric malpractice, in Michels, R., et al. (eds.): *Psychiatry.* Philadelphia, J. B. Lippincott, 1989.

3. Klein, J. L., & Glover, S. I.: Psychiatric malpractice. *Int. J. Law Psychiatry* 6:131–158, 1983.

4. Danzon, P. M.: *Medical Malpractice: Theory, Evidence, and Public Policy.* Cambridge, MA, Harvard University Press, 1985.

5. American Medical Association: *Professional Liability in the '80s.* Chicago, AMA, 1984.

6. Slawson, P. F., & Guggenheim, F. G.: Psychiatric malpractice: a review of the national loss experience. *Am. J. Psychiatry* 141:979–981, 1984.

7. Malcolm, J. G.: *Treatment Choices and Informed Consent: Current Controversies in Psychiatric Malpractice Litigation.* Springfield, IL, Charles C Thomas, 1988.

8. Perr, I. N.: Suicide litigation and risk management: a review of 32 cases. *Bull. Am. Acad. Psychiatry Law* 13:209–219, 1985.

9. Gutheil, T. G., Bursztajn, H., Hamm, R. M., et. al.: Subjective data and suicide assessment in the light of recent legal developments. Parts I and II. *Int. J. Law Psychiatry* 6:317–330, 331–350, 1983.

10. Beck, J. C. (ed.): *The Potentially Violent Patient and the Tarasoff Decision in Psychiatric Practice.* Washington, DC, American Psychiatric Press, 1985.

11. Appelbaum, P. S.: *Tarasoff* and the clinician: problems in fulfilling the duty to protect. *Am. J. Psychiatry* 142:425–429, 1985.

12. Felthous, A. R.: *The Psychotherapist's Duty to Warn or Protect.* Springfield, IL, Charles C Thomas, 1989.

13. Kapp, M. B.: Supervising professional trainees: legal implications for mental health institutions and practitioners. *Hosp. Community Psychiatry* 35:143–147, 1984.

14. Appelbaum, P. S.: Civil rights litigation and mental health: section 1983. *Hosp. Community Psychiatry* 32:305–306, 1981.

15. Reynolds, R. A., Rizzo, J. A., & Gonzalez, M. L.: The cost of medical professional liability. *J.A.M.A.* 257:2776–2781, 1987.

16. Nye, D. J., Gifford, D. G., Webb, B. L., et al.: The causes of the medical malpractice crisis: an analysis of claims data and insurance company finances. *Georgetown Law Journal* 76:1495–1561, 1988.

17. Meyers, A. R.: "Lumping it": the hidden denominator of the medical malpractice crisis. *Am. J. Public Health* 77:1544–1548, 1987.

18. Bonnie, R. J.: Professional liability and the quality of mental health care. *Law, Medical Health Care* 16:229–239, 1988.

19. Charles S. C., Wilbert, J. R., & Franke, K. J.: Sued and nonsued physicians' self-reported reactions to malpractice litigation. *Am. J. Psychiatry* 142:437–440, 1985.

20. Gutheil, T. G.: Medicolegal pitfalls in the treatment of borderline patients. *Am. J. Psychiatry* 142:9–14, 1985.

21. Goisman, R. & Gutheil, T. G.: Risk management aspects of behavior therapy. *Behav. Ther.* (In press).

22. American Psychiatric Association: APA guidelines regarding physicians' signatures. *Am. J. Psychiatry* 146:1390, 1989.

23. Wexler, D. B.: Patients, therapists, and third parties: the victimological virtues of Tarasoff. *Int. J. Law Psychiatry* 2:1–28, 1979.

B. INFORMED CONSENT

1. Appelbaum, P. S., Lidz, C. W. & Meisel, A.: *Informed Consent: Legal Theory and Clinical Practice.* New York, Oxford University Press, 1987.

2. Lidz, C. W., Appelbaum, P. S. & Meisel, A.: Two models of implementing informed consent. *Arch. Intern. Med.* 148:1385–1389, 1988.

3. President's Commission for the Study of Ethical Problems in Medicine and Bio-

medical and Behavioral Research: *Making Health Care Decisions: The Ethical and Legal Implications of Informed Consent in the Patient-Practitioner Relationship.* Volume one: Report. Washington, DC, U.S. Government Printing Office, 1982.

4. Faden, R. & Beauchamp, T.: *A History and Theory of Informed Consent.* New York, Oxford University Press, 1986.

5. Lidz, C., Meisel, A., Zerubavel, E., et al.: *Informed Consent: a Study of Decision Making in Psychiatry.* New York, Guilford Press, 1983.

6. Benson, P. R.: Informed consent: drug information disclosed to patients prescribed antipsychotic medication. *J. Nerv. Ment. Dis.* 172:642–653, 1984.

7. Handelsman, M. M. & Galvin, M. D.: Facilitating informed consent for outpatient psychotherapy: a suggested written format. *Prof. Psychol.* 19:223–225, 1988.

8. Wettstein, R. M.: Informed consent and tardive dyskinesia. *J. Clin. Psychopharmacol.* 8 (4):65S–70S, 1988.

9. Munetz, M. R. & Roth, L. H.: Informing patients about tardive dyskinesia. *Arch. Gen. Psychiatry* 42:866–871, 1985.

10. Appelbaum, P. S. & Grisso, T.: Assessing patients' capacities to consent to treatment. *N. Engl. J. Med.* 319:1635–1638, 1988.

11. Gutheil, T. G., Bursztajn, H. & Brodsky, A.: Malpractice prevention through the sharing of uncertainty: informed consent and the therapeutic alliance. *N. Engl. J. Med.* 311:49–51, 1984.

12. Wulsin, L., Bursztajn, H. Gutheil, T. G.: Unexpected clinical features of the *Tarasoff* decision: The therapeutic alliance and the "duty to warn." *Am. J. Psychiatry* 140:601–603, 1983.

C. SEXUAL AND OTHER PROBLEMS IN THE THERAPIST-PATIENT RELATIONSHIP

1. Gabbard, G. O. (ed.): *Sexual Exploitation in Professional Relationships.* Washington, DC, American Psychiatric Press, 1989.

2. Schoener, G., et al.: *Psychotherapists' Sexual Involvement with Clients: Intervention and Prevention.* Minneapolis, Walk-in Counseling Center, 1989.

3. Gartrell, N. Herman, J., Olarte, S., et al.: Psychiatrist-patient sexual contact: results of a national survey, I: prevalence. *Am. J. Psychiatry* 143:1126–1131, 1986.

4. Herman, J. L., Gartrell, N., Olarte, S., et al.: Psychiatrist-patient sexual contact: results of a national survey, II: psychiatrists' attitudes. *Am. J. Psychiatry* 144:164–169, 1987.

5. Gartrell, N. Herman, J. L., Olarte, S., et al.: Reporting practices of psychiatrists who knew of sexual misconduct by colleagues. *Am. J. Orthopsychiatry* 57:287–295, 1987.

6. Pope, K. S., Keith-Speigel, P. & Tabachnick, B. G.: Sexual attraction to clients. *Am. Psychol.* 41:147–158, 1986.

7. Apfel, R. J. & Simon, B.: Patient-therapist sexual contact. I. Psychodynamic perspectives on the causes and results. *Psychother. Psychosom.* 43:47–62, 1985.

8. Apfel, R. J. & Simon, B.: Patient-therapist sexual contact. II. Problems of subsequent psychotherapy. *Psychother. Psychosom.* 43:63–68, 1985.

9. Gutheil, T. G.: Borderline personality disorders, boundary violations and patient-therapist sex: medicolegal pitfalls. *Am. J. Psychiatry* 146:597–602, 1989.

10. Appelbaum, P. S.: Statutes regulating patient-therapist sex. *Hosp. Community Psychiatry* 41:15–16, 1990.

11. Stone, M. H.: Boundary violations between therapist and patient. *Psychiatric Annals* 8:8–21, 1976.

12. Groves, J. E.: Taking care of the hateful patient. *N. Engl. J. Med.* 298:883–887, 1978.

13. Collins, D. T., Mebed, A. A. K. & Mortimer, R. L.: Patient-therapist sex: consequences for subsequent treatment. *McLean Hosp. J.* 3:1, 24–36, 1978.

14. Simon, R. I.: Sexual exploitation of patients: how it begins before it happens. *Psychiatric Annals* 19:104–112, 1989.

15. Stone, A. A.: *Law, Psychiatry and Morality.* Washington, DC: American Psychiatric Press, 1984.

D. CONTRACT AND ALLIANCE

1. Steiner, C.: *Games Alcoholics Play.* New York: Growth Press, 1972.

2. Cooklin, A. I.: Consideration of the contract between staff and patient in relation to current hospital practice. *Br. J. Med. Psychol.* 46:279–285, 1973.

3. Gutheil, T. G. & Havens, L. L.: The therapeutic alliance: contemporary meanings and confusions. *Int. Rev. Psycho-Anal.* 6:467–481, 1979.

E. RECORD KEEPING

1. Gutheil, T. G.: Paranoia and progress notes: a guide to forensically informed psychiatric record keeping. *Hosp. Community Psychiatry* 31:479–482, 1980.

2. Slovenko, R.: On the need for record keeping in the practice of psychiatry. *J. Psychiatry Law* 7:399–440, 1979.

3. Roth, L. H., Wolford, J. & Meisel, A.: Patient access to records: tonic or toxin? *Am. J. Psychiatry* 137:592, 137:592, 1980.

4. Gutheil, T. G.: Clinical and legal aspects of the psychiatric inpatient record, in L. Sederer (ed.), *Inpatient psychiatry: Diagnosis and Treatment,* 2d ed. Baltimore: Williams & Wilkins, 1986.

5

Competence and Substitute Decisionmaking

D. Standards of decision making
    1. Best interests
    2. Substituted judgment
    3. A combined approach

E. Special issues in substitute decision making
    1. Incompetence to consent to admission
    2. Incompetence and hospitalization
    3. Incompetence to consent to research
        a. Incompetence and the risk/benefit ratio
        b. Possible approaches to the problem

III. CLINICAL ISSUES

A. Assessing patients' decision making capacities
    1. Overall strategy
    2. Identifying high-risk groups
    3. Preparing the patient for evaluation
    4. Performing the evaluation
        a. The clinician's tasks
        b. Interviewing the alleged incompetent
        c. Adjunctive sources of information
    5. Assessing the basis for incompetence
        a. Psychodynamic influences on competence
        b. Psychopathological influences on competence
        c. Situational influences on competence
    6. Treating incompetence and repeated evaluation
    7. Evaluating the uncooperative patient

B. Clinical impact of incompetence in fact
    1. Impact on the patient
    2. Impact on the family
    3. Impact on the treatment team

C. Clinical impact of the legal finding of incompetence
    1. Reinfantilization
    2. "Crowding" of the clinician-patient relationship
    3. Impact on self-esteem
    4. Anger at petitioners for guardianship

D. Clinical advantages of guardianship and other substitute consent
    1. Impact on the patient
    2. Impact on the family
    3. Impact on the treatment team

E. Clinical disadvantages of substitute consent
    1. Obstacles to treatment created by the procedure in relation to involuntary treatment
        a. Delay and its consequences
        b. Cost
        c. Lost clinical time
    2. Impact on the patient
    3. Impact on the family

F. Characteristics of the ideal guardian
    1. Availability
    2. Competence
    3. Empathic intuition
    4. Freedom from conflict of interest
    5. Willingness

I. CASE EXAMPLES

A. Case Example 1

A 38-year-old clinical psychologist is voluntarily hospitalized after unexplained and seemingly self-injurious behavior occurring at a religious retreat house where he lives. He was seen striking his head on the ground and deliberately falling down a flight of stairs; when confronted about this, he attempted to plunge through a closed first-floor window.

Extremely bright and articulate, the patient consistently denies after admission that there is anything wrong. Nonetheless, almost daily self-damaging acts continue, and his body begins to accumulate a series of cigarette burns, ecchymoses, and hematomas. A tentative diagnosis of psychotic depression leads the resident psychiatrist to suggest to the patient that he might be benefited by a course of oral tricyclic antidepressants. The patient refuses, claiming that the only medications he needs are natural foods, which will purge his body of impurities, and that he deserves the punishment he is receiving because of unspecified misdeeds earlier in his life. Shortly thereafter, the patient is observed on several occasions eating his own feces, bars of soap, and cigarette butts. He drenches himself in his urine, which he carefully collects in cups in his room.

Throughout this period, he remains pleasant, at times even witty, and delights in philosophical discussions of existential issues. Records of his only previous hospitalization reveal that a similar state resolved after a short course of neuroleptic medication. After months of hospitalization, during which the patient has failed to respond to the milieu or to psychotherapy, the resident is now considering initiating neuroleptics, but the patient refuses, claiming that his previous experience with them did not benefit him and that the side effects were particularly troublesome. State regulations forbid the nonconsensual administration of medication without a judicial declaration of incompetence and the appointment of a guardian.

Because of the peculiar, dichotomous nature of the patient's mental state, the resident believes that this refusal is actually motivated by the patient's delusional desire for continued punishment and is thus not a competent refusal. He confronts the patient with this belief and with the option of initiating a petition to have the patient declared incompetent and a guardian appointed for the purpose of consenting to treatment. The patient's mother, who has been very concerned about his situation, is (as next of kin) the logical choice for guardian; his father is dead and no other friends or relatives are available. Having described a lifelong passive-aggressive mode of struggling against his domineering, success-oriented mother, the patient objects violently to the possibility of her assuming control over this crucial element of his life. The resident wonders how to proceed.

B. Case Example 2

A psychiatrist on a consultation-liaison service in a general medical hospital is asked to see an elderly patient who has been hospitalized for a prostatectomy. The request, though coming from the attending surgeon, actually was initiated by the patient's son, who told the surgeon that he believes his father is no longer able to handle his affairs. He asked that a psychiatrist sign a statement to that effect so that he, the son, could be appointed guardian of his father's property. The son's lawyer has the petition for an incompetence hearing already prepared, save only the physician's statement. Approaching the surgeon before speaking with the patient, the psychiatrist is told that the patient is "a nice old guy," that the surgeon has no idea whether he is competent or not, and that he filed the consult to accommodate the family.

On meeting the patient, the psychiatrist finds that despite the discomfort of an indwelling catheter the man is good-humored, oriented, with an intact memory, and an otherwise normal mental status. He has, in the 20 years since the death of his wife, always lived on his own, handling his own cooking, finances, and housekeeping. The closeknit ethnic neighborhood in which he lives contains his few remaining friends and many acquaintances, and he spends his days walking up and down the streets exchanging pleasantries. He and his son have had increasingly sharp differences over his life-style recently, the son feeling that he was "too old to take care of himself" and urging that he move to a retirement home to which the son had arranged admission. The psychiatrist is perplexed by the inconsistencies before him.

C. Case Example 3

Ms. A. is in her early forties when she is brought by her widowed mother to the hospital and admitted. Her symptoms include hearing voices telling her that she has been chosen for a special, divine mission and having the conviction that her mother is trying to poison her.

The patient has always been extremely tied to her mother, who in effect rules her life. Since her father's death a month earlier—an event ungrieved by the patient in any observable way—she has grown more agitated until, on the day of admission, she threatened her mother with a knife because the mother was "trying to poison me." The mother brings her daughter for help.

On the ward, the patient settles in quietly except for one pervasive difficulty: refusal. She refuses to eat hospital food, to take a bath or shower, to change her clothes, to participate in ward activities, and to take any medication. To all these issues she states, "My divine mission requires purity above all; God's voice tells me not to soil myself with food, bath, medications, etc."

Legal guardianship to permit involuntary medication is the customary approach to treatment refusal in that jurisdiction, and the mother is viewed as a logical candidate to be guardian. When the social worker broaches this plan, the mother's face lights up, her eyes gleam, and she blurts out, "Yes! That's just what I need to solve my problem!"

When the worker points out that the *patient's* problems are the subject under discussion, the mother looks confused and angry. Later, at a meeting of the treatment team, the worker expresses her concerns about the choice of the mother for guardian. A fierce debate ensues.

The social worker points out that the mother seems excessively eager to maintain what is essentially a lifelong symbiotic tie to her daughter. The worker sees her task as helping the mother "let go" of the patient so that the latter can get on with her life; instead, the worker protests, "You're asking me to do the *opposite* of my job for legal reasons. The mother can barely distinguish herself from the patient."

The psychiatric resident argues that the patient is in serious danger and legal action must be undertaken to protect the patient. Bitter experience has taught that judges in this jurisdiction rarely respond to guardianship petitions unless someone is proposed for the role; ergo, the mother appears to be the only choice.

The impasse is referred to a consultation conference.

II. LEGAL ISSUES

In our society, which places such emphasis on individual rights, the right to choose is among the most highly valued of powers. We grant people enormous discretion in deciding with whom to associate, how to dispose of their assets, and in which activities to engage, even when those activities (e.g., mountain climbing) may generate substantial risks of harm. This deference to individual choice is based, in large part, on our view of persons as rational beings, entitled to make decisions for themselves. When that presumption of rationality falls, however, our society steps in to make decisions on behalf of those whom we now deem "incompetent."

Competence can be seen as a threshold requirement for persons to retain the power to make decisions for themselves. An attribution of incompetence is a serious issue, since if substantiated, the person found incompetent can be deprived of many of the rights the rest of us take for granted. In a general sense, there are two kinds of competence: competence to decide (e.g., competence to consent to treatment, competence to contract) and competence to perform an act (e.g., competence to parent). The latter category is the broader one, since it encompasses both decisions and action. But it is the former—decisionmaking competence—with which we will mostly be concerned in this discussion.

Competence is a major issue for psychiatry, given that so many patients with mental illness may have their competence called into question. Although competence is a legal concept and, strictly speaking, can only be determined by a judge, the realities of psychiatric practice require that clinicians often make their own assessments of a patient's likely competence. In a clinical context, for example, a psychiatrist must satisfy herself that the patient has the capacity to make a competent decision about medication before beginning treatment with a neuroleptic. In the forensic setting, a mental health professional may be called upon to assist a court in determining a person's competence to make a contract or execute a will.

In this chapter, we address conceptual and practical issues related to the assessment of competence that will apply regardless of the type of competence being evaluated. Special attention is given in the examples used to competence to consent to medical and psychiatric treatment, because of its relationship to the doctrine of informed consent discussed in Chapter 4 (see Sec. II-B). Chapter 6 (see Secs. II-A and C) addresses issues unique to selected competence assessments in both the civil and criminal areas.

Four issues must be addressed when the question of competence is raised: What standards do we employ to determine whether a person is competent? Who is charged with making that determination? Who assumes decisionmaking authority for the incompetent person? How do they make their decision?

A. Standards for competence

The concept of competence is too broad to consider in an undifferentiated way. It is useful for the purpose of analysis to distinguish between general competence and specific competence. General competence is that state, described in many of the statutes governing guardianship procedures, determined by the ability to handle all one's affairs in an adequate manner. Specific competence is defined only in relation to a particular act: whether one is competent to write a will, make a contract, testify in court, or stand trial for murder.

1. STANDARDS OF GENERAL COMPETENCE

The question of a person's general competence is raised, in the usual case, when an allegation is made that the person no longer has the capacity to make decisions about the entire range of his affairs. A common situation in which this may occur is when the family of an elderly man with dementia fears that he is no longer capable of paying his bills, caring for his residence, or protecting his health. The family may request an evaluation of the person's general competence prior to filing a petition for guardianship, or such an examination may take place after a petition has been filed. In either case, the mental health professional is confronted with the issue of what standards to apply to the determination.

Both statutes and court decisions have done little to move beyond the vaguest descriptions of what constitutes general competence. The Uniform Probate Code, for example, defines incompetence as follows: "A mentally incompetent person is one who is so affected mentally as to be deprived of sane and normal action, or who lacks sufficient capacity to understand in a reasonable manner the nature and effect of the act he is performing." State statutes vary from the nebulous, "Incapable of caring for himself," to the somewhat more specific, "Unable to properly provide for his own personal needs for physical health, food, clothing or shelter." It seems apparent from a review of the law in this area that the tendency has been to give the judiciary maximal flexibilty in determining that an individual is incompetent and is therefore in need of guardianship. This has advantages—individuals in need of assistance are unlikely to fall through any legal cracks—as well as disadvantages—the uncertainty of the standard makes it difficult to prevent abuse in those cases in which the judge is too uncaring or uninformed to conduct a sufficient inquiry before ruling; the frequent failure of the adversary system, leaving the potential ward without adequate representation, exacerbates this problem. In any event, the law provides little guidance for clinicians who are attempting to determine if the patient they are examining is, in fact, incompetent, or who are preparing testimony for a competence hearing.

It may be useful, in beginning to define standards, to note what standards are *not* appropriate to use in such situations. The mere presence of psychosis, dementia, mental retardation, or some other form of mental illness or disability is insufficient in itself to constitute incompetence. General incompetence, as does its counterpart specific incompetence, requires a functional assessment. A reasonable approach to this evaluation follows. It should be utilized in the absence of more specific guidance in most jurisdictions, and is based on an approximation of the standards that most courts apply in these situations.

a. Awareness of situation

An individual should have an adequate sense of the current status of the major elements of her life. Thus, she should be aware of her circumstances of living, sources of support, extent of resources, significant supportive relationships, any limitations on her natural functions, and the presence of any threats to her immediate security (e.g., trust fund running out or major lawsuit pending).

b. Factual understanding of issues

To the extent that the individual suspected of incompetence is required to make decisions about the major elements of her life, those decisions should be grounded in a clear understanding of the facts involved. A patient who is supported by a trust fund may, even given an awareness of the nature of the fund, not be able to comprehend the issues involved in altering the periodicity of the payments.

c. Appreciation of the likely consequences

An understanding of the "dry facts" of a person's situation must be supplemented with a cognitive and emotional appreciation of the implications of those facts. An elderly person may understand at a basic level that once the family homestead is sold, it will no longer belong to him. He may fail, however, to appreciate the consequences of this action, i.e., that he will have to find another place to live that will be unfamiliar and difficult to adjust to. Similarly, the elderly person who fails to pay her utility bills may understand that the bills are requests for money to cover services rendered, but fail to appreciate that her power will be cut off, leaving her without heat or electricity, if she remains delinquent. ("They are always sending me those bills. I don't take them seriously.")

d. Rational manipulation of information

This is the segment of the competence examination that psychiatrists have traditionally been most comfortable performing and sometimes the segment to which they have exclusively directed their efforts. The reason for this single-mindedness of approach is self-evident: psychiatrists have their greatest expertise in the assessment of irrationality. A focus on rational manipulation of information, however important, should not be such as to exclude the other elements of the examination from consideration.

This part of the examination considers the basic components of the patient's mental status: orientation, memory, intellectual functioning, judgment, impairment in rationality (hallucinations and delusions), and alterations of mood. The effect of deficiencies in any of these areas on the patient's actual functioning ought to be tested by means of explicit examples that require the patient to manipulate data and to reach a conclusion. Hypothetical business transactions often meet this need nicely.

e. Functioning in one's own environment

Competence is not a fixed attribute of the individual that remains invariant regardless of environmental factors (see Sec. III-A). A mildly demented patient, for example, might function quite well in the familiar environment of her home, but become confused and disoriented shortly after admission to a hospital. In addition, a person may structure her natural environment in such a way that supports exist there to aid her in her essential tasks. A retarded person, to demonstrate, may have a neighbor or relative available to help with shopping and bill-paying; her inability to perform calculations is thus not crippling in her own environment. The ecology of a person's functioning must be taken into account in a competence evaluation. This may mean examining the person *in situ,* or at the least inquiring about the existence of natural supports.

f. Extent of demands on patient

Patients should not be deemed incompetent because they are unable to perform tasks that they may, in fact, never be called upon to perform. An individual whose primary support is a monthly SSI check, and who turns the entire check over to a halfway house in exchange for the provision of all necessities, should not be considered generally incompetent despite profound difficulties with managing sums of money. On the other hand, a similarly situated individual possessed of a large estate would certainly require the assistance of a conservator for its management and is, in a genuine sense, incompetent.

2. STANDARDS FOR SPECIFIC COMPETENCE

Specific competence is a newer concept than general competence (see Sec. II-C-1-b below). Although the term itself suggests a more focused evaluation, the law, at first glance, appears not to have been terribly helpful here either. Court opinions cite a wide variety of standards to be applied to determinations of a given specific competence (e.g., competence to consent to treatment), sometimes even within the same jurisdiction. There is a tendency for each court to try to derive standards *de novo,* without relying on precedents from other courts. This compounds the confusion.

Careful review of court decisions and statutes in this area, however, suggests that most legal standards are actually composed of one or more of four basic elements. When a clear standard exists in a jurisdiction, the composite elements should be identified and an evaluation structured accordingly. When no clear standard has been formulated by the legal system, evaluators should assess the alleged incompetent on all four of the following standards, allowing the court to select which are relevant in the case at hand.

a. Communication of a choice

It may seem self-evident, but a person cannot be considered competent unless she can communicate the choices that she makes. This capacity refers to more than just being able to say yes or no. A choice should be sufficiently stable that it can be acted upon before the person changes her mind. Although a change in decision is not in itself a sign of incompetence, vacillation of such a degree that it precludes implementation of any choice, especially in the context of mental disorder, may well constitute a basis for a finding of incompetence.

b. Factual understanding of the issues

A competent person ought to have the ability to understand the facts relevant to the proposed decision. For example, if competence to consent to treatment is at issue, the person should understand the information required to be communicated by the doctrine of informed consent: the nature and purpose of the proposed intervention, its risks and benefits, and the possible alternatives, along with their risks and benefits. For competence to make a will, the testator should understand the nature and amount of his property, and the identity and relationship to him of his "natural heirs." Understanding can be tested by asking the evaluee to paraphrase the information provided to him, or to state his understanding of the situation.

c. Appreciation of the situation and its consequences

As in the case of general competence, mere factual understanding may be insufficient. A person can understand what she is being told without grasping the implications of that information for her own situation. For example, a psychotic patient faced with a decision about treatment may understand that the doctors believe she is ill and that medication is needed, but her denial that she is mentally disordered will short-circuit any effort at competent decision making. In the case of someone writing a will, her understanding that she has two sons whom most people would consider the natural objects of her bounty may be distorted by her delusional belief that they have been plotting to kill her so they can inherit her money. She lacks appreciation of the nature of their relationship to her. Appreciation can be assessed by an exploration of the subject's conceptions of the situation at hand, the likely outcomes of alternative courses of action, and the motives of those involved.

d. Rational manipulation of information

Rational manipulation involves the use of logical processes to compare the benefits and risks of various courses of action. When it is employed, the outcomes selected will be logically consistent with the starting premises. It should be emphasized that what is being tested here is a process, not the outcome of that process. If the reasoning process flows logically from its starting premises, though the result might be rejected by most people (e.g., a person refusing potentially life-saving medical treatment), we cannot say that rational manipulation is impaired. Examination of the person's chain of reasoning is required to test this capacity.

3. ISSUES INVOLVED IN THE SELECTION OF STANDARDS FOR COMPETENCE

a. Policy considerations in choosing a standard

Implicit in this discussion has been the idea that there is no single standard of competence. Decisionmaking competence is not a scientifically determinable state, nor a medical condition. It represents a level of functioning at which society is willing to allow a person to continue making her own decisions. As such, both the standards selected and the levels at which cut-offs for incompetence are set should be expected to reflect policy considerations such as: the degree to which individual autonomy in general, and in relation to this particular decision, ought to be encouraged; the extent to which the interests of the decision maker or of third parties ought to be protected, regardless of the wishes of the decision maker; the ability of society to intervene in the name of either of these goals in a manner generally perceived as fair.

Given the differences that are likely to arise when an effort is made to balance these factors, it is not surprising that different jurisdictions have reached varying conclusions concerning standards and cut-offs for a particular competence determination, or that within the same jurisdiction standards and cut-offs may vary for competence to perform different acts. Courts frequently say, for example, that although the standards for competence to write a will are similar to those for competence to contract, the cut-offs for calling the actor incompetent differ. Greater leeway will be given to the allegedly incompetent author of a will (i.e., courts will be more reluctant to call him incompetent) because of the belief that once he is dead there is little point in trying to protect his interests, as distinct from his expressed wishes—and little ability to do so fairly. On the other hand, competence to contract will be judged more rigorously because the interests of a living incompetent may outweigh his wishes as reflected in the contract.

Similar, albeit more controversial, arguments come into play where competence to consent to treatment is concerned. Advocates who believe, for example, that treatment of psychotic persons with neuroleptic medication is undesirable, and that given the choice many psychotic persons will decline treatment, argue for less rigorous standards for competence and/or higher cut-offs for declaring someone incompetent. Those who agree that refusal is likely, but believe that it will usually be deleterious to the patient will urge stricter standards and/or lower cut-offs, so those decisions can be overruled.

There is nothing inherently dishonest about setting standards of competence to achieve policy goals, although mental health professionals accustomed to objectively determined standards (e.g., for the diagnosis of mental disorders) may be uncomfortable with this process. Those involved, however, should recognize the policy-relevant nature of standards of competence and join the debate on those grounds.

b. Sliding scale approaches to competence

Given the relative nature of competence standards, it should not be surprising that suggestions have been offered for varying standards and cut-offs applied in particular cases (not just among different kinds of decisions) according to the values at stake. The argument has been advanced particularly with relation to consent to medical or psychiatric treatment. It has been suggested, for example, that patients consenting to low risk, high benefit treatment should be allowed to do so even if fairly impaired on most measures of competence, because both their autonomy interests and physical well-being will benefit thereby. They might be considered competent if they can merely communicate a choice. In contrast, patients refusing such treatment might be held to higher standards, since they run the risk of serious physical harm. The standards for competence employed in their case might require understanding, appreciation, and rational manipulation.

From a purely abstract perspective, the sliding-scale approach is problematic because of the discretion it appears to allow the evaluator in setting the standard or cut-off employed. Thus, a physician who believed that a patient's decision to reject recommended treatment was wrong could adjust the standard of competence used to insure that the patient was declared incompetent. This is troubling. In practice, however, there is a common-sense feel to the sliding-scale method. It limits the need for formal declarations of incompetence when such procedures would be unlikely to change the outcome (e.g., a marginally competent patient consents to low risk, high benefit treatment). Further, it appears maximally protective of patients' health interests in settings in which it may make sense to give these priority (e.g., a marginally competent patient refuses low risk treatment that will almost certainly save his life). Regardless of the formal standards in place in any jurisdiction, it is likely that a sliding scale approach with regard at least to cut-offs is being employed in practice in health care settings, and probably in courts, as well.

B. Procedural aspects of determining competence

As noted above, a finding of incompetence results in the deprivation of basic individual rights. Such limitations ordinarily occur only after a formal adjudication by a court. Criminal defendants are not deprived of their liberty to choose where to live and how to spend their time unless a court finds them guilty of a crime and imposes a sentence. Even a mentally ill person in need of treatment cannot be held beyond a limited, initial period without court authorization. (See Chap. 2, Sec. II-D-4.) It might be assumed that the deprivation of decision-making power associated with a finding of incompetence similarly requires court action; although that is often true, it is not always the case.

1. PROCEDURES FOR DETERMINING GENERAL COMPETENCE

Consonant with usual models for deprivation of rights, a finding of general incompetence will always involve a judicial proceeding.

Any interested party can initiate a petition to the court of proper jurisdiction (often a probate court) alleging that the individual in question is incompetent and in need of a guardian. The usual standard that has to be met is a finding that the proposed ward is simply "incapable of managing his affairs" or "unable to care for his property or himself." In addition to the mentally ill and retarded, subjects for guardianship proceedings might include alcoholics, drug addicts, the physically disabled, and "spendthrifts." Medical testimony might or might not be required, and notice is not always given to the subject of the petition, though giving notice has become more common.

Whether a physician testifies or not, the petition will be accompanied by an affidavit from a physician attesting to the patient's incompetence, often in global and conclusory terms. Optimally, a framework for assessment such as that laid out above will form the basis for the physician's evaluation. The judge will listen to the testimony, including sometimes the testimony of the alleged incompetent (though in many states that person can be excluded from the hearing), and make a determination as to whether general incompetence has been proven, applying the relevant standards. If so, a guardian will be appointed with power to make all personal and financial decisions for the incompetent ward. This model varies little from jurisdiction to jurisdiction.

A guardian might be selected from among the members of the family or, if the estate warrants more professional supervision and contains sufficient funds, a lawyer or banker might be appointed. The guardian's expenses are defrayed by the ward's estate and, in turn, the guardian is required to file periodic notice with the court of the status of the property entrusted to her care. Guardianship can be terminated by a showing that the ward no longer meets the criteria that warranted initiating the process: that a child has attained majority, a physical infirmity has been ameliorated, or an abnormal mental state has resolved.

2. PROCEDURES FOR DETERMINING SPECIFIC COMPETENCE

Specific competence can also be adjudicated through a judicial proceeding. The proceeding may take place in advance of a decision being made by the alleged incompetent, for example, prior to the person entering into a contract. Or it may occur after the decision has been made, in an effort to void it. With a greater recognition by courts and legislatures that impairment does not have to be global to be worthy of attention, a larger number of adjudications of specific incompetence are taking place.

a. Determining specific competence to consent to medical treatment

In at least one important context, however, specific competence is determined—for all practical purposes—outside of a courtroom. When the capacity to consent to medical treatment is in question, physicians traditionally have conducted their own assessments of patients' abilities to consent. If the patient was thought to lack capacity, her family was asked to consent on her behalf. This model continues to be followed in almost all general health care settings. Only in the absence of family members, or when they are in disagreement among themselves or make a decision that the care-givers believe is not in the patient's best interests, is recourse had to the courts.

To be sure, physicians are not making a determination of "competence" here, although that language is often used. Competence can only be decided by a court, or some other authorized adjudicatory body. But their determinations of functional capacity have the same effect as formal rulings on competence, because the patient loses decisionmaking power.

The desirability of this non-judicial process has been debated widely. On the one hand, it is argued that enormous potential for abuse exists when physicians and family members can collude to deprive patients of decisionmaking rights. The seriousness of the deprivation militates in favor of a judicial proceeding. On the other hand, the evidence for such abuse is all but non-existent, and the health care system would slip into paralysis if it had to delay treatment on the large percentage of severely ill patients who are incompetent until a court hearing could be obtained. Based on these latter arguments, the President's Commission on Ethical Problems in Medicine and Biomedical and Behavioral Research, among others, endorsed continued reliance on informal, physician determinations of decisionmaking capacity.

b. Determining specific competence to consent to "extraordinary" procedures

Competence determinations by physicians, or their functional equivalents, are not accepted for all classes of medical procedures. The courts have identified several categories of treatments that they have termed "extraordinary." Even guardians are not allowed to consent to these procedures without explicit judicial approval. As this doctrine has evolved in the twentieth century, sterilization, psychosurgery, and (in some states) ECT have been included in this category.

More recently, as described in Chap. 3, Sec. II-C-1, courts and legislatures in some states have added treatment with neuroleptic medications to the category of extraordinary treatment. The usual rationale is that, as with the other procedures listed above, they can lead to permanent, adverse effects (tardive dyskinesia and related syndromes); are susceptible to abuse (use to sedate patients solely for the purpose of ease of management); and have the potential to alter mental functioning (though this latter is frequently misinterpreted, since their effects here are usually normalizing). Thus, in many states, physicians cannot, on their own, determine whether patients' consent is acceptable. Especially when patients refuse treatment, some more structured and independent assessment is required. (See Chap. 3, Sec. II-C-2.)

C. Substitute decision makers

Whether a formal or informal mechanism is used to assess patients' competence, a finding of deficient capacities results in someone other than the patient having to make the decision in question. A variety of potential decisionmakers are available and are utilized in different situations.

1. Guardians

Guardians are appointed by the courts after formal judicial hearings at which persons' incompetence is adjudicated. They are given the power to make decisions on behalf of incompetents, with legally binding effect, as if the decisions had been made by the persons themselves.

a. Traditional concepts of guardianship

The role of guardian dates back to Roman times, when it was first recognized that a permanent or temporary disability suffered by an individual left his property subject to dissipation unless an arrangement for its supervision could be provided. Anglo-American law traces the role of the guardian to the traditional power of the lord of the manor to assume responsibility for the property of those who were not able to care for it themselves: minors, the physically infirm, and the mentally retarded. As that prerogative was absorbed by the Crown in medieval times, the mentally ill also came to be seen as worthy of such protection. Yet, historically it was only the *property* of the incompetent individual that was the responsibility of the guardian, not the individual himself. The goal of such intervention was to conserve the property in question for the benefit of potential heirs, dependents, and creditors, and to prevent the ward from becoming a burden on the public purse.

Modern law recognizes a broader potential scope of concern for a guardian—the well-being of the individual himself. This form of guardianship over the person, which might coexist with, or exist independently of, control over the individual's property, grants broad powers of decision making over the personal affairs of the ward, such as living situation, choice of medical treatments, and changes in personal status.

Until the last few decades appointment of a guardian led to major losses of rights for the ward. In general, no distinction was made between guardianship of property and of person; a finding of incompetence usually applied to both. Thus the ward lost the power to make contracts, to allocate and spend his money, to initiate lawsuits, to hire agents (attorneys, doctors, etc.), to marry or divorce, and to decide where to live. All these powers were transferred to the guardian. In many instances, though forfeiting the right to drive a car, the ward retained the power to make a will. When a guardian was appointed for the purposes of managing the estate alone, an exception to the general practice, he was often called a "conservator." In that case, the ward lost only the power to control his economic affairs.

b. Newer concepts of guardianship

The all-or-nothing nature of the traditional guardianship obviously leaves a good deal to be desired. Patients whose illnesses interfere with a closely circumscribed area of functioning, yet who are able to handle many other of their affairs quite well, are faced with the choice of operating without the protection afforded by a guardian or of forfeiting their rights to control every aspect of their lives. Because this situation most frequently arises among the mentally retarded—who, for example, might be incapable of managing their finances, but perfectly able to choose a place to live—the idea of limited guardianship has received the greatest impetus from law in the area of developmental disability.

Under this concept, the needs of each patient are carefully evaluated and a guardian is appointed with powers delimited to the specific incapacities of the individual. The advantages of this approach are that each ward enjoys the maximal possible freedom consistent with his disability; the disadvantages include the expense of the evaluation process and the difficulty of determining, before specific problems arise, the real scope of the patient's incapacity. Some studies have shown that even in the states in which limited guardianship statutes exist, the power to tailor the guardianship to fit the patient is infrequently used, with standard guardians being appointed instead.

There is an obvious congruence between the concept of assessing specific competence and the use of limited guardians. The powers of a guardian can be limited to those functions for which specific incompetence has been found to exist. One of the more promising areas for the application of limited guardianship is consent to medical treatment. Since many patients who incompetently refuse treatment have delusional perceptions specifically related to medication, surgery, or other interventions, while their other areas of functioning remain intact, they are ideal candidates for a guardianship that deprives them only of the right to decide about their treatment course.

c. Advantages and disadvantages of guardians as substitute decision makers

The clear advantage of a judicially appointed guardian lies in the system's ability to hold that person accountable for her decisions. Guardians must make regular reports to the appointing court concerning their actions. These records can be reviewed by interested parties and can be used to challenge a guardian's judgment. The appointing court can be petitioned by an interested party to hold a hearing on the performance of a guardian, and guardians can be removed and even sanctioned if they violate the trust that has been lodged in them. Thus, the system is quite useful when decisions must be made that have low visibility and in which the interests of the guardian and the ward may differ. Management of assets is a good example of a situation for which formal guardianship may be the best available option.

It must be recognized, though, that the use of formal guardianship has certain costs as well. Formal proceedings are expensive and time-consuming, requiring attorneys for all parties, and often testimony from expert witnesses. Privacy of the alleged incompetent is compromised. Subjects of these hearings may feel as though they are "on trial." If a guardian is appointed who is not familiar with the incompetent person, the decisions she makes may not reflect that person's preexisting wishes or interests. When situations exist in which the advantages of a guardianship process are not likely to obtain, there may be good reason to seek some other form of decision making. Decisions concerning medical treatment may be a good example of this. These are usually high-visibility decisions, made in the context of a medical care system that is ostensibly charged with protecting the patient's interests. Although conflicts of interests can exist between decision makers and patients, they tend not to be common. A less formal decisionmaking process than guardianship may be appropriate here.

d. The crisis in the guardianship system

Several factors have combined to increase the demands being placed on the guardianship system. The attention being paid to competence to consent to treatment, the regulations requiring widespread screening of mentally ill and mentally retarded populations for competence (frequently a spin-off of right-to-treatment suits), and the resulting influx of indigent persons into a system that traditionally functioned to preserve wealth—all these have pushed the process for obtaining guardians to the breaking point in many states. In the absence of funds from the patient's estate to pay the guardian, it has become impossible to provide guardians for all who need them. Previously, lawyers or others would serve *pro bono* for those few indigents who required guardianship, but that is no longer an adequate solution when thousands of such cases exist. There is evidence to suggest that these practical difficulties have frustrated the intent of those who support widespread, individualized competence assessments; in many places, despite the law, these are just not being done.

Several possible solutions exist. The state itself could pay guardians directly. Given the amount of time required to perform conscientiously the guardian's role, particularly when such issues as overriding the patient's refusal of treatment must be dealt with, it is unlikely that the states would be willing to provide sufficient funds to entice members of the legal profession—the traditional source of guardians—into that role. The as-yet-undefined liability of guardians who oppose their ward's stated wishes in relation to treatment and other issues is another patent deterrent. In past years, hospital superintendents or other staff were often appointed as their patients' guardians, sometimes serving simultaneously as guardian for thousands of patients, but society appears no longer willing to accept the ostensibly inherent conflicts of interest resulting from combining those two roles.

e. Public guardians and other solutions

Another possible solution is the appointment of state employees to positions as full-time guardians, responsible for the oversight of a number of wards. Ideally, such individuals would have some training in those clinical areas required to understand and to make decisions about their patients' disabilities and would be independent enough of those agencies that deal with their wards to be free of conflicts of interest (see Sec. III-F-4). Social workers might be ideal candidates for such positions. Unfortunately, in some states in which this has been tried it has led either to: (1) a token guardianship, with one person responsible for hundreds of patients, so that no real protective influence is exercised; or (2) a merger of public guardianship into the regular duties of social workers in departments of welfare, leading to conflicts of interest and the interment of a personal relationship under the burdens of a staggering case load. A variation on this approach is to contract out the responsibility for guardianship to nonprofit corporations, a technique that might minimize conflicts of interest but, in the absence of sufficient funding, is prone to the same problems of overburdened workers as the public sector.

What is lacking in all these arrangements, of course, is the sense of intimate concern for the incompetent individual that most people think of when they envision a guardian-ward relationship, and perhaps missing, too, is a sense of trepidation about making decisions for other people that will touch the most fundamental aspects of their lives. To the extent that the protective function becomes bureaucratized, one wonders about the value of interposing a faceless third party between the individual and the professionals with whom he deals, who previously would have taken it upon themselves, acting within the ethical tradition of their profession, to make the decision for the patient.

f. Abuses of the guardianship process

It should be noted that, even today, legal scholars raise a large number of objections to the manner in which the guardianship laws are administered. Despite the widespread trend for reform of state guardianship statutes, many still lack those elements traditionally associated with due process in other settings. The alleged incompetent does not always receive notice of the hearing. When notice is issued, little effort may be made to assure that the person facing the proceedings actually understands what is at stake. Though lawyers may represent the patient, they are frequently not required to do so; if the patient cannot afford a lawyer, often none is available. Even the patient's presence at the hearing may be waived. A number of studies have further shown that the presence of the presumed incompetent and of a lawyer representing her is no guarantee of a rigorous examination of the situation by the court. Lawyers tend to be unfamiliar with the guardianship laws and with possible alternatives, and they are often uninterested in challenging medical or psychiatric testimony. The standards under which incompetence is determined are extremely vague (see Sec. II-A above) and susceptible to almost any interpretation; the distinction between deviance and incompetence is frequently obscure.

From the point of view of the psychiatrist or other mental health clinician who is called to testify in guardianship proceedings, a knowledge of this potential for abuse should signal caution. The careful clinician who is looking toward her patient's best interests will want to investigate who is requesting the competence hearing, what the real basis for the request is, and what the impact is likely to be on the patient of a finding of incompetence. Since no one else of the parties involved may consider possible alternatives short of guardianship, such as the provision of social services that would enable an elderly person to live on her own, the psychiatrist ought to take the initiative in considering such alternatives as a legitimate and appropriate element of her evaluation. The patient should, of course, always be carefully examined, and important or decisive information that is obtained from family members or friends should be corroborated before it is accepted as fact.

2. Judges

As noted above, the courts have reserved for themselves the right to make decisions about "extraordinary" procedures for incompetents. In addition to sterilization, psychosurgery, ECT, and use of neuroleptic medications, this category may include psychiatric hospitalization. The advantages of judicial decision making in these cases are presumed to relate to the more dispassionate attitudes they can take toward these cases, especially in comparison with involved family members. They have the ability to order investigations of relevant matters, as by appointing a guardian ad litem, and to take testimony prior to making a decision. In addition, judges are the quintessential makers of the "tough decisions" in our society. It may seem fitting to relegate these difficult choices to them as well.

On the other side of the ledger, the ability of a judge to learn about a given case is undoubtedly limited by her other responsibilities and the degree of interest she has in the area. Not knowing the incompetent person, the judge starts at a relative disadvantage compared with family members or friends who may be appointed guardian or make decisions informally. The costs of learning what she needs to know may be steep. A judge's ability to monitor the incompetent's state as the situation evolves is also limited, given her usual need to rely on testimony presented in court.

Should judges make substitute decisions? Unless a class of decisions can be identified in which substantial bias is likely to exist amongst other decision makers, it would seem wise not to place these decisions on the judiciary. There may also be some point to using judges for decisions about procedures so controversial that an assurance of absolute independence and incorruptibility is needed. In other cases, though, some other mechanism is preferable.

3. INFORMAL DECISION MAKERS

By informal decision makers, we refer to persons who know the incompetent—family or friends—and who make decisions on his behalf without being formally appointed to that role by a court. Most commonly, this will occur in the medical setting, as discussed above. A number of states, recognizing the advantages of this approach, are beginning to codify it in statutes, at least for particular kinds of medical decisions, such as consent to "do not resuscitate" orders. There will also be many cases in which family members, without formal procedures, will take over responsibility for managing the life and finances of an impaired relative, especially an elderly one. Unless challenged by another disgruntled relative, this procedure usually works fairly well and reduces the cost associated with formal guardianship. The obvious disadvantage is the absence of checks on the good will and disinterested posture of the family member, or less frequently the friend, who assumes this role.

A commonly employed, non-judicial mechanism for allowing someone else to make decisions about an incompetent's finances is the practice of federal and state agencies making disability payments to someone who may be characterized as a "representative payee." Following a physician's determination that a patient is not capable of managing finances, as a result of physical or mental illness, or alcohol and drug abuse, the recipient identifies a person to whom payment will be made. That individual then parcels out the money to the recipient. The system seems to work reasonably well.

a. Durable power of attorney

Mechanisms now exist in most states for a competent person to select a substitute decision maker for a projected time of future incapacity. Documents embodying these choices are called durable powers of attorney. Unlike ordinary powers of attorney, they continue to be in effect, or first come into effect, when the person becomes incompetent. The decision maker selected then has legal sanction, without the necessity of a court proceeding, for making decisions about the issues indicated in the document. Among the advantages of this approach is that it allows a person to discuss his preferences in advance with the substitute decision maker and to select a person whom he believes will act according to his wishes.

b. "Living wills"

In a growing number of states it is also possible to leave instructions regarding particular decisions, especially termination of life-sustaining treatment. These "living wills," as they are often called, provide guidelines for the decision maker, whoever that person turns out to be. How binding these documents are will depend on the particular legislation authorizing them, which can be quite limited in scope. Were they to expand from their current focus on decisions concerning death, living wills (or "decision directives") might prove useful mechanisms for persons with mental illness to specify, during a period of competence, whether they desired hospitalization, medication, ECT, or other procedures when later incompetent. There have been a few efforts to use advance directives in this way, but without legislation their legal status is questionable, especially in the face of subsequent refusal by a now incompetent patient.

4. CLINICAL STAFF

It was once common for clinical staff, especially physicians, to become de facto decision makers for incompetent patients, particularly with regard to medical or psychiatric treatment. If incompetent patients required treatment and no family members were available, the physicians themselves authorized the treatment and administered it. With greater attention to patients' rights, this practice has diminished, but it stills exists in many places. In facilities with a large number of incompetent patients, such as state hospitals, chronic care facilities, or nursing homes, means and resources may simply not be available to seek appointment of a guardian for every treatment decision. When not precluded by state law, physicians may therefore take it on themselves to make these choices.

One could argue that there are certain advantages to this approach, the most salient being its low cost and ready availability. Physicians are also the most familiar, of all possible decision makers, with the medical issues on which many of these decisions are based. And, in many cases, there may simply not be any alternative. As discussed in Chap. 4 (see Sec. II-B), however, the doctrine of informed consent is built on the notion that these decisions are, at their core, personal and not medical. Thus, physicians or other clinical staff who make such decisions on their own run some risk of subsequent liability should something untoward occur.

A better approach when neither formal nor informal options are available may be to formulate a facility-wide policy on how substitute decisions should be made. This could involve the appointment of someone to act as a patient advocate to consult with the physician, representing a reasonable patient's point of view, before a decision is made. Alternatively, a second opinion from another physician or a review panel might be required before proceeding with treatment. Other options are possible, as well, but their common element is to open up the decisionmaking process, soliciting input from others not directly responsible for the patient's care. Experimentation with these models may provide guidance as to which approaches are the most successful.

D. Standards of decision making

To this point, we have focused on the situations in which persons may be deprived of decisionmaking rights, and on the identity of substitute decision makers. But the question of how the decision maker should make her choice has only been alluded to in passing. There are two general ways in which one individual—a guardian, for example—can substitute her judgment for that of another individual: (1) the guardian can attempt to make a decision based on what she perceives as the best interest of the ward, e.g., asking, "Is this investment likely to yield a profit, or is this nursing home going to provide better care than another?" and (2) the guardian can try to conform her choice as closely as possible to the choice that the ward *would* have made, were the ward competent to do so, e.g., asking, "Would my ward, being the person she is, prefer to live in a supervised apartment or in a group home?"

1. BEST INTERESTS

The "best interest" standard, which provides more of an objective approach to the task of decision making, has long been the prevalent one. Ethicists and legal theorists, however, have come of late to recognize that many of the judgments made in the patient's best interest are not as clear-cut as they appear to be, but rather reflect the overt or covert values of the decision maker. Thus, a decision maker who denies a retarded person the possibility of having a sexual relationship, ostensibly because she believes that retarded people have difficulty managing such encounters, may in fact be deciding on the basis of a value system that is resistant to acknowledging the possibility of positive extramarital sexual relationships, for all people and not just for retarded people in particular; the retarded person might feel quite strongly otherwise, as might a large number of competent people.

As long as guardians deal primarily with property, the chance of significant value conflicts arising is diminished. Insofar as a guardianship of the *person* has been established, however, conflicts of values are quite likely to occur. Limited guardianships are one way of mitigating the impact of a clash of values, by excluding areas in which such conflicts are likely to occur from the province of the guardian. A second means of lessening the distortion produced by value-laden decisions is to ask a decision maker to decide based on what he thinks the person would prefer if the latter were competent.

2. SUBSTITUTED JUDGMENT

The substituted judgment standard, which is intended to embody this latter approach, traces its roots back to English common law. Guardians, usually obligated to act in their wards' best interests, were permitted to make gifts from wards' estates (e.g., to an impecunious relative) on the basis that if the ward were competent, he would desire such a gift to be made. The doctrine has been used more recently in this country in several cases permitting transplantation of kidneys from an incompetent person to a close relative.

The best known elaborations of substituted judgment have come in cases dealing with cessation of life-sustaining treatment in incompetent patients. The standard first came to prominence in the *Quinlan* case in New Jersey, in which a father was allowed by a court to authorize the discontinuation of his comatose daughter's respirator on the basis that, given her current condition, she would not have wanted respiratory support continued. From there it was picked up in *Saikewicz v. Superintendent of Belchertown State School,* a Massachusetts Supreme Judicial Court ruling that dealt with a severely retarded patient with acute leukemia. Though his life could have been sustained for several months with chemotherapy, the patient, with an I.Q. of 15, would have had to undergo the agonizing side effects of chemotherapy with no understanding of his condition or of the purpose of the treatment. The court ruled that Saikewicz, if he were competent to decide about receiving treatment under those circumstances, would have declined it, and, therefore, chemotherapy could be withheld (see Suggested Readings—Gutheil and Appelbaum).

Although it attempts to screen out values foreign to the patient, the subjective standard of substituted judgment is highly problematic. In a limited number of instances, it may be possible to determine what the patient would have chosen—as, for example, when a previously competent person has indicated, either informally or in a "living will," what his preferences would be, should he become incompetent to decide. Such a situation is relatively rare. Instead, the decision maker, whether a court, a guardian, or a physician, is left most often to guess at the patient's preferences. From what we know about the influence of the unconscious on people's choices, it seems extremely likely that the guardian's assumptions about the patient's desires will reflect the guardian's own values (what he would want done for himself were he in that situation) or the guardian's prejudices about people similar to the ward (for example, that poor people or the elderly have less of a desire to live when faced with terminal illness than the guardian's own peers do). In sum, it seems unlikely except in rare circumstances that the subjective standard, "deciding as the patient would," offers any real improvement in objectivity or accuracy over the more traditional, "best interest" approach.

3. A COMBINED APPROACH

As the limitations of each of these approaches have been recognized, a consensus has evolved in many jurisdictions as to when each standard should be applied. When it is clear that an incompetent would have selected a particular course of action, most courts will require that the decision maker follow that choice. In the absence of such evidence, however, rather than attempting to intuit—or guess at—what the incompetent would have desired, the decision maker is free to act in the person's best interests, as clearly as she can conceptualize them. This seems a reasonable compromise that is likely to become the dominant approach to this problem.

E. Special issues in substitute decision making

1. INCOMPETENCE TO CONSENT TO ADMISSION

As noted previously (see Chap. 2, Sec. II-C-3), the question of whether patients need to be competent to consent to admission is unclear, but an analogy to the issue of consenting to treatment suggests that they should, indeed, be competent. Most often the question is ignored; but, should the admitting psychiatrist be reluctant to admit the consenting incompetent or desirous of admitting the nonconsenting but noncommittable incompetent, guardianship is not always a solution. A number of state legislatures and state courts have held that a ward cannot be admitted by a guardian without a court hearing, and then only if the ward meets the ordinary standards for involuntary commitment. It should be noted that these holdings are apparently inconsistent with the tone of a 1979 U.S. Supreme Court decision (*Parham v. J. R.*) permitting parents and state agencies to consent to the admission of minors. In general, the guardian, assuming that his powers are not specifically limited by the appointing court, retains the right to admit his ward.

Empirical observations of the way that guardianship is used in practice have turned up some interesting findings. In some areas, patients who cannot be civilly committed under the prevailing standards, usually based on dangerousness, are instead found incompetent, permitting the appointment of a guardian who can then admit them "voluntarily" to a psychiatric facility. While to some this practice may suggest malice on the part of family members or professionals, in reality it is a reflection of the fact that the elimination of *parens patriae* standards from commitment laws has left a large number of persons in need of hospitalization with no way of making it available to them.

The judicial and psychiatric systems, faced with the alternative of abandoning these individuals, have chosen instead to improvise, within the constraints of the current laws, a mechanism for helping those now otherwise excluded from involuntary care. That this has occurred is perhaps the most compelling evidence of the importance of a *parens patriae* approach. A proclamation of the patients' right to be free from confinement unless he is dangerous does nothing to lessen the need for care and treatment of the severely mentally ill. In many ways, both psychiatrists and judges are most comfortable working with a standard designed to care for the helpless, rather than approaching the needs of the mentally ill through a quasi-criminalized dangerousness standard. The lesson must be that if laws are designed so as to ignore realistic needs, in practice the system will find some other way of having those needs met.

2. INCOMPETENCE AND HOSPITALIZATION

Only within the last several decades has the usual route for determining incompetence become a hearing at which those who petition for guardianship and those representing the alleged incompetent can both present evidence before an impartial judge. Prior to that, most persons found to be incompetent attained that status not by virtue of an individualized determination, but rather as a concomitant of psychiatric hospitalization. It was the law in most states that involuntary commitment was the equivalent of a finding of general incompetence with all the deprivations of power that such a finding entailed. Some states modified that approach by creating a rebuttable presumption of incompetence; that is, the patient was assumed to be incompetent and was treated as such unless and until he could convince a court otherwise. Although thousands of patients were held by law to be incompetent, no guardians were appointed to handle their affairs, leaving them in a state of legal limbo.

The laws governing incompetence related to hospitalization were so vague that in some cases they appeared to apply indiscriminately to voluntary as well as involuntary patients, and the means of regaining competent status following discharge were not always clear. In some cases, a proceeding initiated by the former inpatient was required.

Fortunately, it has come to be recognized that mental illness, even illness severe enough to require hospitalization, does not always result in a global loss of the ability to manage one's affairs. The distinction between committability and incompetence has become universal. While this has raised a new set of problems related to inpatient treatment (see Chap. 3, Sec. II-C-1), it has helped to preserve patients' control over their own affairs.

Having moved from presuming incompetence *despite* evidence to the contrary to presuming competence *without* evidence to the contrary, many states are now requiring that newly admitted patients be specifically evaluated for competence by the psychiatric staff and that petitions for guardianship be filed on those who are suspected of incompetence. Recent court rulings on the right of competent patients to refuse treatment have prompted this most individualized of all approaches.

3. INCOMPETENCE TO CONSENT TO RESEARCH

If advances are to be made in the treatment of severely ill psychiatric patients, it will often be necessary to perform research studies with incompetent individuals. The effectiveness of new approaches to the treatment of chronic schizophrenia, for example, whether of a psychosocial or a psychopharmacologic nature, will never be demonstrated unless clinical trials with chronically ill patients, many of whom are incompetent, are performed. While such studies are, therefore, essential, they also raise significant ethical problems.

a. Incompetence and the risk/benefit ratio

If we compare incompetence in the experimental situation with the previously discussed issues of incompetence to consent to admission and to treatment, it is apparent that there are certain analogies. It is generally accepted, and explicitly required in some state statutes and federal regulations, that subjects of human experimentation should provide an informed consent before an experimental procedure takes place. Competence is, of course, a critical element of any informed consent. In the absence of the ability to provide a competent consent, is a substituted consent an acceptable alternative here, as it was in the treatment situation?

In the treatment setting, the object of the substitute decision maker is to serve the patient, either by seeking the patient's best interests or by approximating the patient's own preferences as closely as possible. Since experimentation, unlike treatment, is not always designed to benefit the individual experimental subject, and since there may often be a measure of risk involved, the substitute decision maker here may be in the position of serving other ends: the advancement of knowledge or the well-being of society as a whole. Although it is usually agreed that any individual has the right to act to help others by placing herself at risk, as by participating in research, it is more controversial as to whether someone else can make that decision for the incompetent patient.

The situation is even not always that clear-cut. Experimental procedures by their nature frequently pose an unspecified degree of risk, while holding out the promise of an uncertain amount of gain. Although that is frequently true in the clinical situation as well, there the potential benefits and the probable risks are almost always more well defined. At what point, if any, should we permit one individual to place another at risk?

b. Possible approaches to the problem

An extreme position is that incompetent patients should never be used in research projects. As noted, above, that would stymie many important areas of research, while permanently foreclosing the possibility of eventual amelioration of the condition that is inducing the state of incompetence in the first place. Another approach is to ignore the question of competence and to respect the patient's expressed wishes either to participate or to refuse. This position of "radical autonomy," however, could lead to situations in which very severely disabled patients place themselves at great risk with little hope of gain and little understanding of their choice.

More moderate suggestions consider, in one way or another, the risk/benefit ratio in deciding whether an incompetent patient can be allowed to participate. There is little objection to permitting experimentation, even if no benefits accrue to the subjects, if there is little or no risk. Situations of greater risk require correspondingly greater potential benefits to the subject before a substituted consent is permitted. Various schemes for reviewing risk/benefit ratios and for determining if the participation of incompetents should be permitted have been devised, for example, by the National Commission for the Protection of Human Subjects of Biomedical and Behavioral Research. Some of these schemes include an absolute right of refusal for the incompetent; a substituted consent is permitted to confirm the patient's consent or to take its place in the absence of any indication of the patient's preferences but not to override the patient's overt refusal.

For disorders that are likely to result in predictable periods of incompetence at some point in the future, advance directives offer the possibility of the now-competent person deciding for himself whether to participate in research. This technique has been used in studies of Alzheimer's disease, for example. Mildly demented but still competent patients are asked to consent to research procedures that will continue even when they become more severely disordered. The potential for employing devices of this sort in disorders with cyclical periods of incompetence—such as many of the severe psychoses—is obvious.

III. CLINICAL ISSUES

A. Assessing patients' decision making capacities

1. OVERALL STRATEGY

Whether the question at hand is a patient's general competence or her competence to deal with a specific issue, the competence evaluation should always begin with an assessment of general competence. Given a state of general incompetence, specific deficits of competence are more likely to be found, although it is always possible for a generally incompetent individual to be unusually capable of deciding about a specific task. Conversely, while it is certainly possible for a generally competent person to be specifically incompetent (e.g., a patient with paranoia whose functioning is excellent except in the narrowly circumscribed area of his life that is affected by his delusions), this dichotomy becomes a lesser probability once a good level of general competence has been ascertained.

2. IDENTIFYING HIGH-RISK GROUPS

When a clinician is asked to perform an assessment of a patient's competence-related capacities, as when the patient's competence to contract or make a will is in question, the answer to the question of who should be evaluated is readily apparent. In other contexts, however, as in a psychiatric facility treating a large number of severely ill patients, clinicians must develop a strategy to screen for those patients most likely to have impaired competence to consent to treatment or to perform other relevant tasks (e.g., some states require all inpatients to be evaluated for competence to handle their assets).

Since the resources do not exist in most facilities routinely to screen all patients for competence, the process can be accomplished most efficiently by identifying particular populations whose members are at increased risk of manifesting incompetence. These include acutely psychotic patients, who often suffer from a delirium-like clouding of consciousness; chronically institutionalized patients, who may have lost the capacity critically to evaluate proposed interventions or actions; patients with organic impairment, often elderly, who may slide slowly into an incompetent state; depressed patients, even if nonpsychotic, whose hopeless-helpless thinking may impair reasoning about treatment alternatives and future plans; retarded patients, whose disability may be accentuated by concomitant psychiatric illness; and patients who are being asked to consent to especially risky procedures, or to procedures with little hope of direct benefit to them.

3. Preparing the Patient for Evaluation

Before a meaningful assessment of decisionmaking competence can be performed, the alleged incompetent person must actually have had a chance to learn the relevant information that the examiner will expect her to be able to understand, appreciate and manipulate rationally. As self-evident as this seems, it is not infrequently the case, in the treatment situation, for example, that the patient has not been told about the nature of his condition (e.g., "We believe that you are suffering from a severe depression that will probably respond to medication; the fact that you feel so helpless about your situation now is actually part of your illness") and the issues involved (e.g., the risks and benefits of medication and the possible alternatives). Even if this information has been communicated at some point, it may have been forgotten by the time the competence assessment takes place, or it may not have been explained as clearly as it could have been. Since it is desirable to maximize the number of patients who are capable of making their own decisions, efforts should be made to ensure that the patient has been given every chance to learn about and to understand the issues involved. This means that the clinician who is conducting a competence examination should be present when an explanation or reexplanation of the material takes place in order to assure himself that the problem that the patient appears to be having with the decision does not, in fact, lie elsewhere than in the patient's brain.

4. Performing the Evaluation

a. The clinician's tasks

The job of the evaluating clinician is to collect information relevant to a determination of the patient's competence. When a formal hearing is to take place, the clinician presents that information to the court so that the judge can assess whether or not the patient meets criteria for competence in that jurisdiction. If it is unclear whether a formal hearing is warranted, or when an informal process for assessing competence is to take place (e.g., in most medical treatment settings), the clinician utilizes the information obtained to estimate whether the patient would likely be found incompetent by a court.

The determination of likely incompetence is made by recognizing that no one engages in an ideal decisionmaking process. Were all persons with less than average decisionmaking powers deemed incompetent, we would have the absurd outcome of half the population being deprived of its decisionmaking rights. Rather, if we assume that decisionmaking capacities are normally distributed, those persons whom the courts call incompetent lie at the far lower tail of the curve, beyond two standard deviations. This conceptualization accords with the law's view that deprivation of decisionmaking rights is an extreme intervention to be used only for impairments of considerable magnitude.

Whether a court or an informal evaluator makes the decision about the patient's competence, the information that the clinician must gather is the same, and relates to the patient's functioning on the four commonly used elements of competence (see Sec. II-A above), unless extant law in a given jurisdiction specifies otherwise.

b. Interviewing the alleged incompetent

Appelbaum and Grisso (see Suggested Readings) have suggested a set of model questions to structure this assessment when consent to treatment is at issue. The questions can be modified to apply to other decisionmaking tasks.

Communicating a choice
1. Have you decided whether to go along with your doctor's suggestions for treatment? Can you tell me what your decision is? (Can be repeated to assess stability of choice.)

Factual understanding of the issues
1. Please tell me in your own words what your doctor told you about:
   a) the nature of your condition,
   b) the recommended treatment (or diagnostic test),
   c) the possible benefits from the treatment,
   d) the possible risks (or discomforts) of the treatment,
   e) any other possible treatments that could be used, and their risks and benefits.
   f) the possible risks and benefits of no treatment at all.
2. You mentioned that your doctor told you of a (percentage) chance the (named risk) might occur with treatment. In your own words, how likely do you think the occurrence of (named risk) might be?
3. Why is your doctor giving you all this information? What role does he/she expect you to play in deciding whether you receive treatment? What will happen if you decide not to go along with your doctor's recommendation?

Appreciation of the situation and its consequences
1. Please explain to me what you really believe is wrong with your health now.
2. Do you believe you need some kind of treatment? What is treatment likely to do for you?
3. What do you believe will happen if you are not treated?
4. Why do you think your doctor has recommended (specific treatment) for you?

Rational manipulation of information

1. Tell me how you reached the decision to accept (reject) the recommended treatment.
2. What were the factors that were important to you in reaching the decision?
3. How did you balance those factors?

c. Adjunctive sources of information

Of course, although direct examination of the patient is important, it is not the only source of data about a patient's functioning. Because of the artificiality inherent in the office or hospital situation in which most assessments for competence are performed, an attempt should always be made to secure information from those who know the patient and who have observed her functioning over a period of time. While this can be of invaluable assistance in the examination, a note of caution is warranted: third parties are often far from disinterested and may have selfish interests at stake that turn on whether or not the patient is found to be incompetent. More than one source of information should be employed, and the clinician should always be alert to possible ulterior motives of her informants.

5. ASSESSING THE BASIS FOR INCOMPETENCE

Regardless of the criteria used for the competence determination, it is often too easy to see competence as a legal problem rather than as a clinical issue. This is a mistake, because an individual's status as competent or incompetent is as much a function of his psychological make-up and psychopathology as are any of the more commonly discussed elements of his clinical presentation. As a result, when there is a change in the concerns, feelings, or hopes of a patient, or a change in the severity of his psychiatric illness, there may often be an alteration in his status as competent or incompetent. The clinician who ignores the underlying issues may make a single determination of the patient's status and then erroneously assume that that status is a fixed characteristic.

As paradoxical as it sounds, incompetence itself can be a symptom of a patient's illness and, like any other symptom, can respond to appropriate treatment. A proper assessment for competence does not end when it arrives at the determination that the patient is currently incompetent. The symptom of incompetence requires a differential diagnosis, just as the symptom of dizziness does; an investigation to determine which cause is the most likely precipitant of the symptoms; and the initiation of appropriate treatment. Although the consulting clinician who is performing the competence assessment is often not in the position to perform the investigation or to begin the therapy, he ought at least to call to the attention of the responsible clinician the need for further diagnostic studies and possible modes of treatment. Common causes of incompetence include treatable psychiatric conditions such as depression, use of polypharmacy in a patient with a precarious balance of neurophysiological functioning (especially in the elderly), patient noncompliance with medication, and the presence of undiscovered medical conditions (e.g., tumor). Some of the most common remediable influences on a state of diminished competence include:

a. Psychodynamic influences on competence

Patients who routinely resort to psychotic levels of defense to deal with the stresses they encounter in their lives are susceptible to marked changes in their level of competence as those stresses come and go. Thus, a patient who is faced with the prospect of surgery for breast cancer and is fearful that after the operation her friends will abandon her because she will no longer be a "real woman," may handle the situation by becoming increasingly psychotic, denying or distorting the reality of the situation. A decision to refuse surgery made in that state will be, in all likelihood, an incompetent one. If the patient can be encouraged to talk about her fears, and if their unrealistic nature can be exposed, or if some external disconfirmation of her scenario is provided, as by the sincere expression of concern by her friends, her need for psychotic defenses may be diminished and her level of competence may rise. A reevaluation at that point might yield a result markedly different from the original assessment.

b. Psychopathological influences on competence

This category resembles the situation in which clear-cut psychodynamic influences are present, but differs in that the cause of the fluctuations in the patient's mental status are not always discoverable. Many mildly to moderately demented patients, for example, tend to have marked fluctuations in their level of functioning, dependent on time of day, medications consumed, concurrent physical illnesses, and the like. Although someone whose mental state changes so continuously and so rapidly that there is a steady alternation between competent and incompetent conditions is, for all practical purposes, incompetent, reassessment after the resolution of remediable influences on the patient's mental status can lead to a revised assessment of the patient's competence. This also holds true for many of the functional psychoses, whether acute or chronic.

c. Situational influences on competence

Factors other than the patient's mental state may influence the competence examination. These include the patient's rapport with the examiner; the patient's perception of the purpose of the examination and what is expected from him; and the nature of the setting in which the examination occurs. A patient who is locked in a hostile, withholding struggle with his physician, and who perceives that the doctor's interest lies in obtaining his consent, may deny that "victory" to the doctor by consciously or unconsciously failing to attend to or to understand the discussion or by failing to communicate his responses clearly.

Since patients may simultaneously harbor both rational and irrational reasons for consenting to or refusing a procedure, the reason that is presented may be a function of the setting, as well. Delusional considerations may be presented to the physician in informal discussions, but when the formal examination for competence takes place, perhaps with an outside expert present, the patient may "pull himself together" and justify the same choice with rational explanations. Needless to say, the unequivocal determination of competence in such a situation is extremely complex and may, in point of fact, be impossible.

6. TREATING INCOMPETENCE AND REPEATED EVALUATION

As implied above, remediable causes of incompetence should be treated and a reevaluation conducted. Even in the absence of clearly identified factors contributing to a patient's impaired competence, whenever possible (i.e., in non-emergent situations) evaluation of the patient's competence should be repeated at least once after the initial assessment. This is because multiple factors—not always identifiable—can cause fluctuations in patients' competence. Given the goal of minimizing infringement on decisionmaking rights, a repeated evaluation is highly desirable.

7. EVALUATING THE UNCOOPERATIVE PATIENT

Perhaps the most difficult problem in assessment of competence is when the patient refuses to cooperate with the clinician. This is especially problematic when an emergency exists (e.g., as in the treatment setting), requiring a rapid determination of probable decisionmaking capacity. Neither of the two easy ways out of this dilemma is terribly appealing. Although the law will usually presume a person's competence until incompetence is demonstrated, to adopt such a decision rule in a circumstance like this runs the risk of failing to treat incompetent persons in life-threatening circumstances. Alternatively, to conclude that an uncooperative, even mute, patient is necessarily incompetent will result in overriding the wishes of competent, albeit angry, persons.

The best solution would seem to be to stick with the presumption of competence, but to lower the threshold at which a determination of probable incompetence is made. When, in an emergency, substantial indirect evidence exists of impairment in the patient's capacities (as from relatives, friends, other caregivers, and based on the patient's behavior), it is appropriate to conclude that the person would probably be found incompetent by a court. Informing the patient of this determination gives him the opportunity, if he is in fact competent, to demonstrate his capacities and avoid unwanted interventions.

B. Clinical impact of incompetence in fact

In practice, "competence" in psychiatric terms (as reviewed in Sec. A) is a medical finding that has only the force of an opinion until it is confirmed by a judicial ruling on the evidence. Thus, before a hearing, a patient may be clearly "incompetent in fact," as shown by mentation or behavior, but not yet officially adjudicated incompetent. This clinical (prelegal) status itself poses certain problems for patient, family, and treaters—problems that merit separate consideration before we examine (in Sec. C, below) the consequences of the legal finding.

1. IMPACT ON THE PATIENT

A small but vivid first-person literature reports on the subjective experience of being psychotic (see Suggested Readings) and of being "incompetent in fact" in various areas of decision making and mental functioning (of course, one may be psychotic yet remain competent—see Sec. II-A). Before quoting a few excerpts, we must note that the state of mind that renders a patient incompetent may be extremely euphoric (elating, intoxicating, uplifting, and satisfying); extremely dysphoric (terrifying to the point of panic, crushingly depressing, producing a sensation of being doomed or utterly out of control); as well as encompassing all points of experience in between. One implication of this is that a person may revel in the incompetent state, or may wish passionately to be out of it, depending on the clinical characteristics of the particular disease process.

Example 1: (From *The Inner World of Mental Illness,* see Suggested Readings; a verbatim diary account of his illness by a schizophrenic man):

Doctor help me to slow down a be content whe ever I am at—I wrent to go the thing to fast. Help me to slow down and think mental illness is a emotion the person can not under why he did something he or she did or could not understand. . . . The stillness has to be broken before we feel free to what is the truth and who can you believe . . . Medison (medicine) is from fact for people who don't know God or don't have faith.

While this patient's racing thoughts would clearly benefit from medication, his acceptance *or* refusal of it would probably be incompetent.

Example 2: (Same source, a woman with catatonia describing the illness in retrospect): Shortly after I was taken to the hospital for the first time in a rigid catatonic condition, I was plunged into the horror of a world catastrophe. . . Only a few people—myself and dimly perceived nursing staff—had escaped. . . . All personal matters relating to my family were forgotten. . . . I was also afraid that other people had power to read my mind, and thought I must develop ways of blocking my thoughts from other people. . . . I actually thought very little about my own children.

Here is demonstrated the way a patient may be cut off emotionally from family members by the power of the illness.

Example 3: (Same patient as Example 2): At times during the first episode, certain actions of the nursing staff, such as administration of hypodermics, tightening of the sheets for wet pack treatments, etc., were interpreted as sexual assaults. . . . A different and less terrifying sense of menace was experienced occasionally in relation to men toward whom I was attracted, i.e., doctors and male attendants. A feeling of conscious attraction would be replaced suddenly by a feeling that the other person possessed special and vaguely threatening power.

This excerpt demonstrates how the illness can lead to distortion of the roles, actions, and intentions of hospital staff, including their performance of medication-related procedures.

Example 4: (Same source, excerpt from Clifford Beers's *A Mind That Found Itself*): The very instant I caught sight of my letter in the hands of my brother, all was changed. The thousands of false impressions recorded during the seven hundred and ninety-eight days of my depression seemed at once to correct themselves. . . . To me, at least, my mind seemed to have found itself, for the gigantic web of false beliefs in which it had been all but hopelessly enmeshed I now immediately recognized as a snare of delusions. . . . Though insight regained seemingly in an instant is a most encouraging symptom, power to reason normally on all subjects cannot, of course, be so promptly recovered. My new power to reason correctly on some subject simply marked the transition from depression, one phase of my disorder, to elation, another phase of it. Medically speaking, I was as mentally disordered as before—yet I was happy!

As Beers articulates so clearly, the manic side of manic-depressive illness is characterized by an absolute self-confidence and sense of great understanding that bears no relationship to the patient's actual capacities and, hence, competence. The reader is referred to the Suggested Readings for further examples. In addition, it should be noted that certain organic disorders (e.g., Alzheimer's dementia) leave some areas of functioning intact so that the patient may remain aware of the deficit—an extremely painful experience for the individual, evoking rage, blame, grief, terror, and despair, as well as attempts to deny any problem.

2. IMPACT ON THE FAMILY

Beyond the effect on the patient herself, serious mental illness that results in incompetence can disrupt a family to the point of devastation of their resources—personal, emotional, financial, and spiritual. The effects on families of patients who are violent, destructive, suicidal, raving, or wasteful are readily comprehensible and visible; more subtle are the effects on the family of the patient's psychotic withdrawal, chronic grinding depression, pervasive but quiet thought disorder that garbles all attempts at communication, or progressive senility with memory loss that encroaches on all areas of functioning and communication. Families may react, as do the patients themselves, with anger, blaming, and despair; denial of the illness or attempts to "cover up" to protect their image in the neighborhood; misinterpretations of the illness (e.g., seeing the psychotic symptomatology as willful malingering); or bafflement, confusion, uncertainty, and paralysis.

Added to these burdens are the human conflicts around the problem posed by the illness. Children forced to "take over" for a senile or otherwise incompetent parent, for example, may readily reexperience earlier conflicts (e.g., even from infancy) about control, domination, and rivalry, as well as about aggression and coercion.

3. IMPACT ON THE TREATMENT TEAM

The patient who is incompetent in fact poses a challenge to the treaters who are attempting to enlist his participation in the treatment process. The search for problems and approaches to them that would ordinarily lead to forging a treatment contract tends to be impaired by incompetence in fact, which vitiates informed and responsible collaboration in the treatment effort; the patient can be acted only on or for, not acted with. Ironically, the fact that staff in many jurisdictions now have to seek substitute consent before proceeding with treatment places the entire matter on an even less collaborative, more adversary footing.

C. Clinical impact of the legal finding of incompetence

The clinical effects of the formal legal finding of incompetence on the patient, the family, and the clinical setting will be considered here. When family members are chosen as substitute decision makers, as is often the case, the impact may differ from cases in which others are so appointed.

1. REINFANTILIZATION

For many of the seriously ill, especially younger patients, the struggle to separate autonomously from their families is central to their difficulties in growth and development, to their falling ill, and, consequently, to the therapeutic work. Regardless of the patient's age, the formal finding of incompetence in effect reverses the separation-individuation process; the patient becomes like a minor child. Thus, for the individual patient, the legal finding may deal a regressive blow to her strivings for independence and adulthood.

It should be noted, similarly, that in some cases pathologic *family* functioning is reinforced by the finding of incompetence in the patient; that is, families that habitually tend to infantilize the subject patient or that, for reasons of pathologic family psychology, need to see her as "incompetent," receive from the legal finding an "official authorization" for this antitherapeutic encouragement of dependency rather than autonomy.

2. "CROWDING" OF THE CLINICIAN-PATIENT RELATIONSHIP

A second effect might be termed the "crowding" of the clinician-patient relationship; judges, lawyers, and guardians swell the treatment dyad. Ordinarily, the treatment contract is "signed" only with the patient. With a finding of incompetence the contract exists essentially between the clinician who proposes the contested treatment and the substitute decision maker who may consent to it. The incompetent patient, *past* whom the contract is negotiated, becomes a passive bystander to his own treatment. While this is, from the legal viewpoint, the very purpose of appointing a substitute, the clinician and patient may be discomfited by the absence of the experience of direct dealing with each other.

The situation with regard to the therapist-patient alliance is also complex. Ideally, the alliance is formed between the therapist and the healthy side of the patient; when the patient is found incompetent, it is unclear with whom the therapist is collaborating: is it the patient or the substitute decision maker? In the special case of treatment refusal, the therapist is in a complicated alliance with the consenting substitute, but remains in opposition to the treatment-refusing side of the patient (it could perhaps be argued that by proceeding responsibly to effect treatment the clinician is still allied with the submerged healthy side of the patient that "would consent," were that side in dominance). Psychiatric treatment, complex enough to begin with, becomes more so under this ambiguous arrangement.

3. IMPACT ON SELF-ESTEEM

The patient whose illness is severe enough to raise questions of competence is likely to suffer a blow to self-esteem from being so impaired from the illness itself; the actual legal (and hence public) finding of incompetence further assaults self-esteem, the more so in those areas of life-functioning where the patient took pride in skill or ability. The formerly skilled financier who prided himself on his deft handling of money, and whose present organic dementia compels conservatorship, experiences significant impairment of his self-image.

4. ANGER AT PETITIONERS FOR GUARDIANSHIP

While resentment at the family or the treatment team for initiating guardianship or similar proceedings is not universal, it is neither an uncommon nor an incomprehensible reaction on the part of the patient. As a study of families involved in guardianship revealed (see Suggested Readings—Isenberg and Gutheil), the families' fear of just this response acted as a deterrent to their willingness to participate in the process. For the treatment team as well, this matter represents a problem of delicate and diplomatic negotiation in the service of being as supportive as possible to patient *and* family in what is essentially a shared crisis. The professionals involved must maintain a clear perspective on the goals of the procedure as being ultimately in the patient's interests; they must reject the patient's accusations that they are merely attempting to coerce and control her for self-serving motives such as the exercise of personal power.

D. Clinical advantages of guardianship and other substitute consent

From the *clinical* viewpoint, the advantages of substitute consent constitute a considerably briefer list than the disadvantages; however, we can outline certain clinically positive effects.

1. IMPACT ON THE PATIENT

While most patients have considerable concerns about substitute consent, as noted in Sec. E-2 below, an occasional patient describes some feeling of security or reassurance—feelings deriving from two sources. On the one hand, in the case of refusal of treatment the patient sees that a distressing disagreement with treatment staff is being taken seriously via a "referee," as the guardian or judge may be considered. The exertion of these efforts may convey the dedication of the staff and of the "system" as a whole to protecting the patient's interests. Similarly, a patient concerned about his own ability to handle financial affairs may be reassured when a trusted guardian or conservator is designated to take care of him.

Along the same lines, some treatment-refusing paranoid patients experience successfully obstructing their treatment as being "out of control," a threatening state; such patients, told they must take their medication because it has been authorized by the guardian or judge, often willingly cooperate. The substitute's decision has relieved them of the need to make the conflicted acknowledgment that they are ill and need treatment—an acknowledgment that would be implicit in their accepting treatment voluntarily. The experienced clinician recognizes here the familiar parallel to a patient's feeling safer when he understands that limits and controls are available from the "outside," as in this example:

> *Example 5:* (also from Suggested Readings, *The Inner World of Mental Illness;* a violent, psychotic woman):
>   So the monster was out and the ghost of some old berserker ancestor rose up within me... and I knew that no power on earth but a strait-jacket could hold her.
>   So I went to the nurse and said, "Tie me." ... But the nurse was so stupid she mistook the whole meaning and because I displayed no

agitation she sent me back to bed. . . . They were going to make me control that which there is no holding. . . . All my energy was being expended to hold the thing down till I could be tied. (Finally, she is given a strait-jacket). When I was tied down securely and could relax my hold upon myself, all my shame flowed out in a wild flood of tears . . . that I had not had the courage to do the thing I had such an urge to do—but more, they were tears of relief that I had not done them. . . .

Finally, some realistic benefits accrue to the extent that substitute consent actually protects the patient's best interest. In matters of treatment refusal in jurisdictions where guardianship is required to permit involuntary treatment, the advantage is clearly that the patient receives the needed treatment. When a patient's personal affairs are jeopardized by his incompetent handling of his property, the substitute decision maker can secure the patient's financial interests to the patient's clear benefit.

2. IMPACT ON THE FAMILY

Though rife with conflicts in their own right (as noted in Sec. E-3, following), substitute decisions may serve to diminish uncertainty and ambiguity in the crisis facing the family. In consequence, fears, tensions, anger, and guilt concerning what should be done about the patient may diminish, particularly if the process is uncomplicated and uncontested; if the decision maker is a respected person outside the family, and thus, from the family's point of view, more objective, the decrease in tensions may be even greater, to the potential benefit of the patient.

3. IMPACT ON THE TREATMENT TEAM

The major effect of substitute consent on the treaters is also reassurance, but here the system of due process communicates a sense of decreased risk of liability in the issue at hand. Treatment attempted or carried out with an oppositional patient under the shadow of threat of suit is almost invariably poorer treatment, since the approach is inherently more defensive and oppositional than in the ordinary situation; hence, in this narrow sense, substitute consent may lead to more confident and therefore better treatment.

E. Clinical disadvantages of substitute consent

1. OBSTACLES TO TREATMENT CREATED BY THE PROCEDURE IN RELATION TO INVOLUNTARY TREATMENT

Some of the obstacles to treatment created by the process of obtaining substitute consent have been alluded to earlier; in addition, the arrangement itself may create difficulties once it is in force.

a. Delay and its consequences

The first and most critical problem is *delay*—a problem from which other problems stem. Even at its most highly lubricated, the mill of the law grinds slowly; with some emergency exceptions (such as immediate hearings on some matters), due process simply does not have the inherent urgency so frequently encountered in the clinical situation. In the usual clinical setting, for example, the absence of the doctor is managed by coverage from colleagues or superiors; however, the absence, illness, or vacation of any of the parties to the legal proceeding may lead to postponement of the hearing.

The net result is delay in the initiation of treatment and the often consequent extension of the duration of the hospital course, as in the case examples for Chapter 3. This can lead to the promotion of chronicity; increased narcissistic injury deriving from the experience of being utterly out of control for long periods of time; increased likelihood of social labeling as a "chronic" patient; and loss of contact with current developments in school, job, or community.

Delay is one of the most common manifestations of so-called "critogenic" harms, a term meaning "judge caused" and intending to parallel the concept of iatrogenic harm, or doctor-caused harm. Critogenic harms refer to usually unrecognized costs of the operation of the legal system, even when the system is working as well as possible. Besides the factors listed below, other critogenic harms most commonly include adversarialization of the relationship, such as inevitably occurs when conflicts are resolved or decisions made by means of the legal system.

b. Cost

Closely related to delay is cost, another critogenic harm. A prolonged stay in hospital naturally costs more, and this cost must somehow be borne, if not by the patient or family, then by some third-party source or by the citizenry through taxation. In addition, the legal proceedings and personnel also consume money as well as time; the guardian, if not a family member or volunteer, *should* be paid for the time, responsibility, and liability involved. The cost of legal proceedings can be significant and may represent a formidable obstacle for impoverished patients, thrown on overcrowded legal aid resources.

c. Lost clinical time

Related to delay and cost is the concept of clinical time out. Treatment personnel must be irreplaceably on the scene in any court proceedings to present the clinical facts and arguments; to do so, even if the judicial procedure occurs in the hospital (as in some jurisdictions), mental health professionals must take time out from care of patients. In complex cases extending over long periods with many depositions, this time out may have to be taken repeatedly. The detriment to care is evident.

2. IMPACT ON THE PATIENT

One effect on the patient is the experience of *coercion*. While we may readily distinguish judicially sanctioned coercion from that not so sanctioned, the patient *feels* the loss of autonomy almost regardless of the process that sanctions it. Because of the nature of certain illnesses, this fact has two distinct implications: (1) For patients in whom narcissistic issues predominate, lasting grudges, resentments, and hatreds may arise around being forced to take medication or surrender their savings to another's care. These feelings may operate to the detriment of future collaboration. (2) Because of the selective effects on competence of major mental illness, the patient found incompetent in a certain area is not necessarily "out of it," uncomprehending, or, in fact, incompetent in other areas. As a result, the patient may have a number of personal reactions to being the ward of someone who is empowered by a court to rule over certain of his affairs, including finances, residence, and the like. A seventy-two-year-old man, for example, albeit found incompetent with regard to his finances because of dementia, may yet resent receiving an allowance from a guardian or conservator as though he were a seven-year-old. A rebellious 20-year-old woman may resent being placed "voluntarily" (i.e., by substituted judgment) in a residential setting that she detests.

In regard to this last point, a caution is in order. Guardianship is onerous; demands on a guardian's time decrease when a ward is institutionalized. This fact of life may lower the threshold, as it were, for institutional placement as a solution to difficulties experienced by the ward. The ethical guardian remains alert to this temptation to a "fast solution."

3. IMPACT ON THE FAMILY

Another effect of substitute consent may be the reinforcement or reenactment of family pathology (see Suggested Readings—Isenberg and Gutheil), in addition to the reinfantilization earlier noted (Sec. III-C-1). Family members may be forced to deal with guilt over opposing the patient's stated wishes and compelling her to accept treatment involuntarily or to surrender control of choices about finances or residence. In addition, since hospitalization of the patient is itself a burdensome crisis for the family, the family may resent the onus of bearing this additional responsibility for the patient; the acute crisis may resonate with situations in the past where the patient or her anger has burdened the family. Families may actively fear the patient's retaliatory anger at their opposition; and related conflicts about aggressive, punitive, or sadistic feelings may be generated by the implicit coercion. These feelings, some of which can be extremely powerful, may touch off preexisting strains in the family's dynamic equilibrium.

In addition, because of these preexisting and/or exacerbated familial difficulties, the family member as guardian may not act in the *patient's* best interests (as in Case Example 3) in the vicarious and empathic way envisioned by the theory of guardianship. The critogenic harm of adversarialization of the relationship may exert its influence in seeming to pit family against patient, even when the ultimate goals of both are quite comparable.

When a guardian is not a family member, closely bound or paranoid families may attempt to vie with, extrude, or thwart this perceived "invader" of the family circle.

F. Characteristics of the ideal guardian

In discussing the procedure of guardianship, it is important to identify the characteristics of the ideal person to fill the role. This is no idle exercise, since the use of professional guardians is becoming the answer increasingly sought to the thorny problem presented by incompetence in the mentally ill person (especially since the judicial system persists in seeing formal guardianship as a panacea, despite the frequent deleterious clinical results).

1. Availability

Since decisions in the clinical sphere often must be made rapidly on short notice and at unpredictable times, ideally the guardian must be geographically and temporally available. One implication of this desideratum is that if a guardian ever wishes to take a vacation, some sort of coverage must be arranged, in advance of need, by another party empowered in the same manner, since there is no guarantee that the ward's clinical state will remain stable during the interim. The same, of course, is true for the patient's financial and social status. Unfortunately, this potentially critical detail is rarely addressed at the time of the appointment.

2. Competence

The requirement of competence for the guardian of an incompetent ward might seem tautological, were it not for the empirical finding that disturbed patients not infrequently come from disturbed families in which *no* family member possesses sufficient capacity to grasp the complexities of major decisions. Attainment of sufficient background knowledge, even in a stable family member, might require formal training in the issues of concern to the patient's life. For a patient who requires a decision about psychiatric treatment, this might include attainment of an educated layman's knowledge of rudimentary psychopharmacology; the course of treated versus untreated major mental illness; the benefits, risks, and consequences of treatment with medications, ECT, psychotherapy, and milieu; and advantages and disadvantages of inpatient and outpatient treatment, group home, and halfway house residence. Guardians appointed to aid in managing financial affairs might require similarly explicit training.

3. Empathic intuition

This term refers to the often desirable quality in a guardian of being able to make a difficult determination according to what the patient *would* want were she sane, competent, and possessed of sound judgment. At issue here is the guardian's ability to make truly *vicarious* decisions (see Sec. II-D-2).

4. Freedom from conflict of interest

The guardian should be free from contamination of purpose by any conflicting interest. Such interests might include psychological, psychosocial, or socioeconomic concerns that would or might interfere with objective substituted judgment. When family members serve as guardians, as noted earlier, these matters wax complex. There is a trade-off in appointing family members: one may obtain the empathy desired of guardians, but one is burdened with their inevitably ambiguous psychological and practical involvement with the patient.

5. Willingness

Guardianship can at times be a sinecure, but occasionally it can be a burdensome, even overwhelmingly demanding role. It may require not only expenditure of time and energy but tolerance of disruption of one's schedule and private life, tolerance of the emotional conflict deriving from the role, and tolerance of the ingratitude, vituperation, and sometimes the litigation of one's ward.

It is not surprising that even adequate remuneration often has been insufficient to persuade potential guardians, including attorneys, to take the job.

6. ADEQUATE REMUNERATION AND PROTECTION FROM LIABILITY

Although these are not virtual characteristics of the guardian but of the surrounding legal system, they should be articulated since they represent the practical pillars on which must rest the creation of a cadre of professional guardians. It cannot be overemphasized that for the population of patients without families and friends—a sizable percentage of chronically mentally ill persons— these provisions may represent the only hope for ethical treatment under current legal guidelines. This is especially true in those jurisdictions that require the petitioning party to propose a person to be appointed. The onus of arranging for both remuneration and protection from liability lies on the legislatures, prodded by professional societies and lay groups interested in mental health.

We might also note a clinical dimension of the idea of remuneration for the professional guardian, somewhat analogous to the therapist-patient contract around the fee. A guardianship fee has several effects:

a. Formalization of the relationship

The role of guardian is a job, governed by contractual considerations; it is not a vocation, a charity, a favor, or other ambiguous and potentially conflicted function.

b. Inculcation of responsibility

Like other employees in other jobs, the guardian is expected to discharge his task in a responsible and accountable manner.

c. Decrease in emotional conflict

Treating guardianship as a "serious business" avoids clouding of the issues by the patient's feeling of obligation to the guardian, the physician's feeling about an "intruder" in the dyad, and other complicating views.

It should be noted, however, that the "job" aspects of guardianship should not dominate over the guardian's sensitive concern to the ward's interests, as indicated in Sec. F-3 above.

IV. PITFALLS

A. Inappropriate finding of incompetence

In this instance the clinician mistakes illness, psychosis, maladaptive functioning, and obstreporousness as equivalent to incompetence. Formal testing in the specific area under question is frequently ignored in favor of these more global impressions. Specificity is central to the issue here, since some clinicians (and a surprising number of judges) fail to grasp how the specificity of mental illness and its remarkably selective effects may operate to preserve competence in one area while clouding it in another. Witness one judge's attempt at irony that demonstrates how easily this point may be missed:

. . . . . defendants took the position that, although a committed mental patient would be presumed competent to deed his home to his doctor, he would not be presumed competent to decide whether to follow that doctor's advice concerning taking of medication. Such an argument would make a doubter of the most credulous. (*Rogers v. Okin*)

Credulousness is not the issue here; the fact is that, as both clinical data and common sense suggest, people have feelings about their houses that differ from their feelings about their bodies. Mental illness may affect competence in regard to one and not the other.

All these essential distinctions can be blurred by the countertransference. For example, the overinvested clinician resists finding the patient incompetent for fear that this would be seen as deprecatory; the clinician angry at the patient or in·a struggle with the patient finds the latter incompetent on affective grounds, as it were, rather than by assessment in terms of formal criteria.

B. Inappropriate finding of competence

Certain forms of mental illness may present disturbance of the mental mechanism involved in decision making in ways that are subtle and difficult to detect. Most often these mental disorders affect the patient's interpretation of risks and probabilities but leave cognition or speech largely intact, permitting the patient to express herself in a logical, fluent, or even glib manner. Examples of these disorders include the "glib" paranoid patient, whose basic suspicion of the doctor's intention may co-exist with a clear sensorium and fluent speech; the depressed patient, whose profound pessimism may distort any realistic appreciation of the probabilities of the success of treatment but may leave the patient able to express these pessimistic views in coherent and logical-sounding sentences; the manic or hypomanic patient whose disorder may lead to total denial of any illness, while not impairing the patient's ability to make apparently logical explanations for his decision; and the patient with anorexia nervosa whose incompetence is limited to the narrow area of food, nutrition, and body image and who may be able to express very clear and logical sounding reasons for avoidance of certain foods or treatments.

In all these cases, the clinician may be discouraged from petitioning for an evaluation of competence because of the patient's apparent lucidity; many attorneys will also misperceive the patient's underlying incompetence. The clinician must make efforts through careful assessment and consultation to define and document even subtle forms of incompetence in order to present these data effectively in court and thus to keep the patient from being deprived of needed treatment.

C. Inappropriate petitioning for substitute decision making

Inappropriate reasons for such petitioning include excesses of therapeutic zeal leading to the wish to take over and control the patient by these legal means; and wishes to coerce, take advantage of, or bypass the patient as a participant in decision making. This last point may be a result of the treater's quite understandable wish to deal with a rational person, since the patient's irrationality is so frustrating.

D. Inappropriate failure to seek substitute decision making

As earlier noted, seeking a substitute decision, as an experience for the clinician (due process aside), may evoke conflicts around coercion, sadism, and the like. Anxiety in this area, conflicts over opposing the patient's stated wishes, laziness, fear of courtroom procedures or yielding to the family's wish to evade the role of decision maker—all these elements may deter or inhibit the clinician from seeking substitute decisions.

E. Approaches

The confusion around competence noted in Sec. II-A above is best remedied by education of the clinician in the use of clearly specified criteria, applied in a strict manner, in the clinical setting.

The countertransference difficulties noted above are managed in the customary manner through consciousness raising, introspection, supervision, consultation, and peer review.

V. CASE EXAMPLE EPILOGUES

A. Case Example 1

The resident contacts the mother, who agrees to serve as guardian and to hire a lawyer who would initiate proceedings. Based on the psychiatric testimony, the patient is found to be incompetent for the purpose of consenting to or refusing treatment, and his mother is appointed temporary guardian with power limited to approving or disapproving a treatment plan.

Furious at his mother for again intervening in his affairs, the patient refuses to meet with her and further regresses, again eating his own feces. When confronted, however, with the possibility of forced injections of neuroleptics—a treatment consented to by his mother after a discussion of risks and benefits with the doctor—he agrees to take oral medication. His response to relatively low doses of neuroleptic is dramatic: within five days his self-abusive behavior disappears and he becomes willing to discuss previously hidden areas of concern. Plans are made for discharge to a halfway house.

B. Case Example 2

The psychiatrist, puzzled by the discrepancy between his findings on examination and the reported opinion of the patient's son, is uncertain whether his examination has overlooked some crucial datum or whether the request represents an attempt to "railroad" the patient. He decides to contact the patient's son directly, explaining that he has examined the patient and, having found him of apparent sound mind, is wondering what the son was concerned about.

Somewhat sheepishly, the patient's son indicates that he, too, knows that the patient is able to manage his own affairs, but that he is concerned about his father living alone in an area distant from him, should something unfortunate occur. On the advice of his lawyer, he had hoped to use the hospitalization as an opportunity to have the patient declared incompetent, either mentally or physically, to handle his financial affairs, hoping that once he was in control of his father's meager finances, he could coerce him into a retirement home.

While empathizing with the son's concern for his father, the psychiatrist suggests that perhaps social service agencies could provide services, such as a homemaker or a daily hot lunch program, that would ease his worries and improve his father's everyday situation. The son thanks the psychiatrist for his suggestions, but, in saying goodbye, mutters something about contacting the father's personal physician to see if *he* will sign the certificate of incompetence.

C. Case Example 3

Before the consultation conference on Ms. A., additional data emerge. Her mother, developing a better relationship with the social worker, confesses that she has been putting some of her own sedative capsules in her daughter's tea, "to calm her down after her father died." It was, in fact, the discovery of a partially dissolved capsule in her tea that prompted Ms. A. to express fear of being poisoned.

This evidence, of both the mother's pathology and her difficulty in distinguishing the patient's distress from her own, proves decisive for the consultation. Efforts are made to reach other family members and, after many false starts, an uncle in a distant city is found willing to serve. The judge, though reluctant to appoint a nonresident of the locale as guardian, finally appoints the uncle, who consents to treatment, which then proceeds. The psychosis largely remits under treatment; however, the patient now incorporates the uncle into her residual delusional system.

VI. ACTION GUIDE

A. Evaluation of Competence

1. *Work* with low threshold of suspicion of incompetence, especially with:
   a. Acutely psychotic patients who often suffer from delirium-like clouding of consciousness;
   b. Chronically institutionalized patients who may have lost the capacity to evaluate critically the proposed interventions or actions;
   c. Patients with organic impairment, often elderly, who may slide slowly into an incompetent state;
   d. Depresed patients, even if nonpsychotic, whose hopeless-helpless thinking may impair reasoning about treatment alternatives and future plans;
   e. Retarded patients whose disability may be accentuated by concomitant psychiatric illness;
   f. Patients who are being asked to consent to especially risky procedures, or those with little hope of direct benefit to them.
2. *Screen* for general competence.
   a. *Use* this as indicator of probability that more specific impairments exist.
   b. *Assess* awareness of nature of situation.
   c. *Evaluate* factual understanding of issues.
   d. *Determine* appreciation of basic consequences.

  e. *Assess* basic elements of mental status:

   i. Orientation,

   ii. Memory,

   iii. Intellectual functioning,

   iv. Judgment,

   v. Impairments in rationality—delusional thinking, hallucinations, etc.,

   vi. Mood alterations.

  f. *Relate* performance to patient's functioning *in his/her own environment;* for example:

   i. Mildly demented patient may be disoriented in hospital, but function quite well at home.

   ii. Moderately retarded person with difficulty performing calculations may have neighbor or family member who accompanies him on shopping trips.

  g. *Consider* the level at which the individual must function—e.g., someone with a large estate may require assistance, while a similarly impaired patient who gives his monthly SSI check to a halfway house may not.

  h. *Solicit* information from those who know the patient and who have observed her functioning over a period of time—but be aware of hidden motives.

  i. If at all possible *observe* and *interview* the patient on more than one occasion, to minimize the effect of chance flucutations in mental state.

3. If the patient appears to be generally incompetent, *assess* the therapeutic measures that might restore competence.

  a. *Have* medical status evaluated.

  b. *Pay* particular attention to medications that might be impairing mental functioning, e.g., tranquilizers in the elderly.

  c. *Look for* treatable psychiatric conditions and *recommend* indicated course of therapy, e.g., depression in elderly patients presenting as dementia and amenable to treatment with tricyclic antidepressants.

4. *Consider* possibility that apparent general incompetence may actually be limited to specific areas.

5. *Screen* for specific competence (e.g., competence to consent to psychiatric treatment).

  a. *Examine* patient's capacity to communicate a choice.

  b. *Assess* patient's factual understanding of issues: illness, proposed interventions, including their risks, benefits, and the possible alternatives (e.g., use of medication: risks—possibility of tardive dyskinesia; benefits—probable resolution of psychotic episode; alternatives—ECT, psychotherapy if feasible given patient's condition).

  c. *Test* patient's appreciation of the situation and its consequences.

  d. *Examine* patient's use of rational processes for manipulating information to arrive at decision (e.g., absence of delusional basis for deciding to accept or to refuse treatment).

  e. *Remember* that patient must be adequately informed before assessment can be meaningful—examiner should always be present when patient is informed to judge adequacy of presentation.

  f. *Rule out* spurious indicators of specific incompetence:

       i. Psychodynamic (e.g., patient's fears evoke nonrational defenses);

      ii. Psychopathological (e.g., poor medication compliance, unknown to primary clinician, leading to impaired thought processes);

     iii. Situational (e.g., enmity between patient and primary clinician leads patient to "act crazy" to frustrate clinician).

6. *Remember* that in presence of general incompetence specific deficits should always be suspected, but specific incompetence can also coexist with general competence (e.g., paranoid schizophrenic may be incompetent to make a will, because of delusions about family, but may easily handle everyday affairs).

B. Identification of Potential Decision Makers if Indicated/Required

1. *Assess* clinical impact on patient if that nominee were chosen as proxy: regressive elements, perpetuation of family's pathologic interaction, ability to see patient's wishes/needs with reasonable objectivity and protect patient's actual interests.

2. If immediate family unable, unwilling, or inappropriate, *extend* search to more distant relatives, or, if needed, neighbors, friends, clergy, attorneys, or other professionals associated with patient or family.

3. *Assess* wilingness of local Legal Aid agencies and similar groups to serve.

4. *Evaluate* guardian, if one is required, for suitability according to standards in Sec. III-F; in sum:

    a. Availability,

    b. Competence,

    c. Empathic intuition,

    d. Freedom from conflict of interests,

    e. Willingness,

    f. Availability of remuneration and protection from liability *or* proxy's willingness to serve without compensation.

C. Contact with Potential Proxies

1. Directly, as part of clinical outreach to family;

2. Indirectly, as in urging family to petition with their own attorney;

3. *Support* efforts as needed, including therapeutic interventions directed at coping with conflicts aroused by procedure itself, as well as exacerbations of previous conflicts.

D. Attempts to Maintain Bases for Treatment

1. *Agency:* clarify with patient (if possible) that efforts are directed to his interests, albeit involving other persons or facilities (e.g., court).

2. *Alliance:* despite potential oppositionality of procedure, attempt collaboration with most adult side of patient; elucidate procedure as part of treatment effort in patient's interests or as achievement of needed safeguards for impaired patient.

3. *Ongoing working relationship:* after proxy is appointed, explore with

patient what experience is like (may include mourning of previous competence, autonomy, self-sufficiency, self-esteem).

E. Observation of patient with reversible illness for signs of returning competence; as soon as feasible, *retest* for competence and—if competence has returned—*initiate* procedures to withdraw substitute decision mechanism (this section would ordinarily not apply to fixed, chronic, functional illness or to fixed or progressive organic illness like dementia).

F. Awareness of pitfalls, including inappropriate findings of competence *or* incompetence; inappropriate seeking *or* failing to seek substitute decision, and failure to detect subtle incompetence.

VII. SUGGESTED READINGS

A. COMPETENCE

1. Appelbaum, P. S., Lidz, C. W. & Meisel, A.: *Informed Consent: Legal Theory and Clinical Practice.* New York, Oxford University Press, 1987, chap. 5.

2. Faden, R. & Beauchamp, T.: *A History and Theory of Informed Consent.* New York, Oxford University Press, 1986, chap. 8.

3. Feinberg, J.: *Harm to Self.* New York, Oxford University Press, 1986, chap. 20 and passim.

4. Freedman, B.: Competence, marginal and otherwise. *Int. J. Law Psychiatry* 4:53–72, 1981.

5. Grisso, T.: *Evaluating Competencies: Forensic Assessments and Instruments.* New York, Plenum Press, 1986.

6. Appelbaum, P. S., and Grisso, T.: Assessing patients' capacities to consent to treatment. *N. Engl. J. Med.* 319:1635–1638, 1988.

7. Appelbaum, P. S., and Roth, L. H.: Clinical issues in the assessment of competency. *Am. J. Psychiatry* 138:1462–1467, 1981.

8. Drane, J. F.: Competency to give an informed consent: a model for making clinical assessments. *J.A.M.A.* 252:925–927, 1984.

9. Kaplan, K. H.: Assessing judgment. *Gen. Hosp. Psychiatry* 9:202–208, 1988.

10. Murphy, J. G.: Therapy and the problem of autonomous consent. *Int. J. Law Psychiatry* 2:415–430, 1979.

11. Culver, C. M., Ferrell, R. B. & Green, R. M.: ECT and special problems of informed consent. *Am. J. Psychiatry* 137:586–591, 1980.

12. Pavlo, A. M., Bursztajn, H., Gutheil, T. G., et al.: Weighing religious beliefs in determining competence. *Hosp. Community Psychiatry* 38:350–352, 1987.

13. Gutheil, T. G. & Bursztajn, H.: Clinicians' guidelines for assessing and presenting subtle forms of patient incompetence in legal settings. *Am. J. Psychiatry* 143:1020–1023, 1986.

14. Miller, B. L.: Autonomy and the refusal of lifesaving treatment. *Hastings Cent. Rep.* 11(4):22–28, 1981.

15. Winograd, C. H.: Mental status tests and the capacity for self-care. *J. Am. Geriatr. Soc.* 32:49–55, 1984.

16. Searight, H. R., Oliver, J. M. & Grisso, T.: The community competence scale in the placement of the deinstitutionalized mentally ill. *Am. J. Community Psychol.* 14:291–301, 1986.

17. Nolan, B. S.: Functional evaluation of the elderly in guardianship proceedings. *Law, Medicine and Health Care* 12:210–218, 1984.

18. Saunders, A. G. & Simon, M. M.: Individual functional assessment: an instruction manual. *Mental and Physical Disability Law Reporter* 11:60–70, 1987.

19. Goldstein, J.: On the right of the "institutionalized mentally infirm" to consent to or refuse to participate as subjects in biomedical and behavioral research, in National Commission for the Protection of Human Subjects of Biomedical and Behavioral Research: *Research Involving Those Institutionalized as Mentally Infirm*, Appendix. Washington, DC, DHEW Publication No. (05)78–0007, 1978.

B. SUBSTITUTE DECISION MAKING

1. President's Commision for the Study of Ethical Problems in Medicine and Biomedical and Behavioral Research: *Making Health Care Decisions: the Ethical and Legal Implications of Informed Consent in the Patient-Practitioner Relationship.* Vol. 1. Washington, DC, USGPO, 1982.

2. Buchanan, A. & Brock, D. W.: Deciding for others. *Milbank Q.* 64 (suppl. 2):17–94, 1986.

3. Areen, J.: The legal status of consent obtained from families of adult patients to withhold or withdraw treatment. *J.A.M.A.* 258:229–235, 1987.

4. Solnick, P. B.: Proxy consent for incompetent non-terminally ill adult patients. *J. Leg. Med.* 6:1–49, 1985.

5. Developmental disability model legislation series: Guardianship and conservatorship act. Introduction and short-form model statute. *Mental Disability Law Reporter* 3:264–290, 1979.

6. American Bar Association: *Exercising Judgment for the Disabled: Report of an Inquiry into Limited Guardianship, Public Guardianship, and Adult Protective Services in Six States.* Washington, DC, ABA, 1979.

7. American Bar Association: Guardianship: an agenda for reform. *Mental and Physical Disability Law Reporter* 13:271–313, 1989.

8. National Conference of the Judiciary on Guardianship Proceedings for the Elderly: *Statement of Recommended Judicial Practices.* Washington, DC, American Bar Association, 1986.

9. Wettstein, R. M., & Roth, L. H.: The psychiatrist as legal guardian. *Am. J. Psychiatry* 145:600–604, 1988.

10. Pleak, R. R. & Appelbaum, P. S.: The clinician's role in protecting patients' rights in guardianship proceedings. *Hosp. Community Psychiatry* 36:77–79, 1985.

11. Isenberg, E. F. & Gutheil, T. G.: Family process and legal guardianship for the psychiatric patient: a clinical study. *Bull. Am. Acad. Psychiatry Law* 9:40–51, 1981.

12. Iris, M. A.: Guardianship and the elderly: a multi-perspective view of the decisionmaking process. *Gerontologist* 28(suppl.):39–45, 1988.

13. Parry, J: Life services planning for vulnerable persons. *Mental and Physical Disability Law Reporter* 10:517–522, 1986.

14. Parry, J.: A unified theory of substitute consent: incompetent patients' right to individualized health care decision-making. *Mental and Physical Disability Law Reporter* 11:378–385, 1987.

15. Gutheil, T. G. & Appelbaum, P. S.: Substituted judgment: best interests in disguise. *Hastings Cent. Rep.* 13(3):8–11, 1983.

C. PATIENTS' DESCRIPTIONS OF THE INCOMPETENT STATE

1. Kaplan, B.: *The Inner World of Mental Illness.* New York, Harper & Row, 1964.

2. Beers, C. W.: *A Mind That Found Itself (1923).* Quoted in ibid.

3. Vonnegut, M.: *The Eden Express.* New York, Praeger, 1975.

4. Green, H.: *I Never Promised You a Rose Garden.* New York, Signet Books, 1964.

5. Hatfield, A. B.: Patients' accounts of stress and coping in schizophrenia. *Hosp. Community Psychiatry* 40:1141–1145, 1989.

6

Forensic Evaluations

2. COMPETENCE TO CONTRACT
   a. Legal criteria
   b. Ethical issues in the assessment of capacity to contract
3. EMOTIONAL HARMS
4. MENTAL DISABILITY
   a. Workers' compensation
   b. Social Security Disability Insurance

III. CLINICAL ISSUES

A. Problems of agency in the forensic evaluation

1. AGENCY IN THE "PURE" EVALUATION MODEL
   a. General considerations
   b. Factors contributing to confusion over agency
      i. Regression
      ii. Transference
      iii. Countertransference
2. AGENCY IN THE MIXED EVALUATION/TREATMENT MODEL
   a. Inpatient criminal forensic evaluations
      i. Dealing with conflicts in agency
      ii. Effects on treatment
   b. Outpatient forensic evluations
      i. Dealing with the conflicts in agency
      ii. Effects on treatment

B. Performing the forensic evaluation

1. APPROACHES TO THE EVALUATION OF COMPETENCE TO STAND TRIAL
   a. Informed consent
   b. General level of function; establishment of rapport
   c. Appreciation of the charges
   d. Appreciation of range and nature of possible penalties
   e. Ability to appraise likely outcomes
   f. Capacity to disclose to attorney available pertinent facts
   g. Ability to appraise legal defenses available
   h. Level of unmanageable behavior
   i. Quality of relating to attorney
   j. Planning of legal strategy
   k. Ability to appraise the roles of various participants in court
   l. Understanding of court procedure
   m. Capacity to challenge witnesses
   n. Capacity to testify relevantly
   o. Manifestation of self-serving vs. self-defeating motivation
   p. Interviewer responses
   q. Assessment
2. APPROACHES TO THE EVALUATION OF CRIMINAL RESPONSIBILITY
   a. M'Naghten Test
   b. Irresistible impulse test
   c. ALI standard
   d. Federal insanity standard
   e. Role of "outside observers" of the crime
3. APPROACHES TO THE EVALUATION OF TESTAMENTARY CAPACITY
4. APPROACHES TO THE EVALUATION OF COMPETENCE TO CONTRACT
5. APPROACHES TO THE EVALUATION OF EMOTIONAL HARMS
6. APPROACHES TO THE EVALUATION OF MENTAL DISABILITY
   a. Workers' compensation
   b. Social security disability insurance

I. CASE EXAMPLES

A. Case Example 1

A 25-year-old man appears at the admitting office of a community mental health center escorted by two police officers. The patient is known to the center by virtue of 4 previous hospitalizations for psychotic episodes dating back 7 years. He carries a diagnosis of chronic schizophrenia, generally responds well to medication, but invariably discontinues his medication after discharge from the hospital. Now he again appears to be psychotic.

The police officers present an order from the court stating that the patient has been committed to the center's inpatient unit for 20 days of observation to assess his competence to stand trial and his criminal responsibility on charges of car theft. The only information given about the alleged crime is that it occurred more than one year ago. In addition, they deliver a letter from the psychiatrist in the court clinic, who examined the patient earlier that day. While providing a review of the patient's clinical history, the letter gives no indication of the patient's current legal status or why the questions of competence or responsibility were raised. In fact, the only justification for the hospitalization that is offered appears to be that the patient is psychotic.

Following admission, the resident assigned to the case requests forensic consultation. She is confused about why the patient was referred, what her obligations are to the court, and whether the patient should be treated during his hospitalization.

B. Case Example 2

A 54-year-old man is sent to the state hospital for evaluation of competence to stand trial for assaulting his wife, with the additional question of criminal responsibility.

The resident on the case, just beginning her psychiatric training and feeling pressured and uncomfortable about her role in relation to the court, begins by interviewing the patient in the customary way. The patient takes to her immediately and shares the following history:

The patient, originally a Jewish tailor in Poland, spent his early twenties in hiding from the Nazis. For five years he slept in barns, haystacks, woods, and ditches, eating stolen food or cattle feed, befriended by farmers but constantly plagued by the fear that the friendliest host might secretly be planning to betray him to the Gestapo.

He claims in relation to the alleged crime that his wife, a younger American-born woman, "makes him crazy" with her nagging; in his broken English he explains that he reached his limit and hit her.

The resident seeks out the service chief. "Listen," she says, "my parents were concentration camp survivors; I know what the situation over there was like. This man is somewhat paranoid but, my God, who wouldn't be with a story like that?"

The service chief interviews the patient in front of the resident, and presses him hard to understand what it means that "his wife makes him crazy"; could this mean the benign marital complaint, "You're driving me crazy," or the more ominously psychotic, "You're influencing my mind"? The patient becomes extremely upset during the interview but—to her own surprise—so does the resident.

When the patient returns to the ward, the resident turns in fury on the chief. Berating him for sadism, insensitivity, and anti-Semitic prejudice, she voices her intent to see the hospital legal consultant and storms out of the room.

C. Case Example 3

A young forensic psychiatrist just beginning private practice eagerly opens a case that he has received for examination from a plaintiff's attorney. An employee had apparently been held up at gun point while working in a fast food restaurant and during the robbery had felt paralyzed, helpless, and in danger of death, the more so because his paralysis made the gunman increasingly impatient. Though the robbery occurred without any injury or bullets being fired, the young man left work early and has claimed subsequent inability to work. The place of employment is being sued for negligently failing to take adequate security measures, resulting in emotional harms to the complainant that have destroyed his social life, family relations, work capacity, and peace of mind. Feeling that the subject is the best source of clinical information, the psychiatrist arranges for an interview with the victim as the first step.

On interview the subject presents as a mildly disheveled young man with poor eye contact and a tendency to stare fixedly over the psychiatrist's left shoulder. He also displays a tendency on occasion to use almost the correct word instead of the correct one. Although rambling and far ranging, his speech does not appear to meet strict criteria for either loose associations or flight of ideas, and no other significant stigmata of mental illness are present.

Though the examinee denies any pre-existing psychiatric difficulties, the psychiatrist's uncertainty about the clinical presentation leads him now to call the law firm and contact the paralegal who works for the litigating attorney. He confronts her with suspicions of an underlying, pre-existing disorder. The paralegal acknowledges that, indeed, the patient has a significant psychiatric history and agrees somewhat indifferently to send the records to the psychiatrist.

Review of these materials reveals a significant psychiatric history dating to childhood, with recurring hospitalizations and ongoing diagnosis of chronic paranoid schizophrenia. More specifically, the examinee, on several occasions during his frequent hospitalizations, even subsequent to the robbery, has dated the origin of all his difficulties to a sexual scene that he may have either witnessed or participated in when he was nine years old, almost ten years before the time of the robbery. The forensic psychiatrist considers how to proceed.

II. LEGAL ISSUES

Mental health professionals are called on by the legal system to provide testimony in a wide variety of cases, both criminal and civil. In the criminal area, forensic clinicians may be asked to comment on the competence of a person to make decisions throughout all the phases of criminal investigation, trial, and punishment. These include: competence to waive one's rights (e.g., the right not to be searched without a warrant, the right not to answer investigators' questions or make a confession), to stand trial, to plead guilty, to be sentenced, to waive appeal (especially in capital cases), and to be executed. The first section of this chapter focuses on the most common of the criminal competence assessments, competence to stand trial. We then consider the most well-known and controversial role that mental health professionals play in the trial process, evaluating defendants' criminal responsibility.

On the civil side, clinicians perform a similarly broad range of functions. They may assess a number of civil competences, including competence to make a will, contract, make decisions about one's person and property, and marry. Clinical experts will also be called upon to testify about a person's mental impairments insofar as they relate to ability to work or as they have been caused by an allegedly negligent act ("emotional harms"). These evaluations are considered below.

Clinicians who work with children are frequently involved in evaluations and testimony concerning juvenile delinquency, child custody, termination of parental rights, and newer issues such as competence of children to testify and how they may be protected in the courtroom. Since child-related evaluations are the basis of a newly-emergent and rapidly growing subspecialty of child forensic practice which cannot be addressed in adequate detail here, readers are referred to texts dealing specifically with these issues. (See Suggested Readings—Schetky & Benedek).

A. Competence to stand trial

Probably the most common request by the judicial system of the psychiatric system is for the assessment of the competence of a defendant to stand trial. It is estimated that roughly 25,000 competence to stand trial evaluations are performed in the United States each year. About one-quarter of these result in a finding that the defendant is incompetent to stand trial. The best available data suggest that, at any point in time, approximately 3,400 incompetent defendants are hospitalized for treatment.

Until quite recently psychiatrists performed almost all competence to stand trial evaluations, but that has changed dramatically in the last decade. Psychologists have assumed this role as rapidly as states have changed their statutes to permit them to perform evaluations. Some jurisdictions also permit social workers to evaluate competence to stand trial, a trend which is likely to grow. (See Sec. III-B-1 for a discussion of practical approaches to performing the assessment of competence to stand trial.) This section will review the historical evolution of the legal standards concerning competence to stand trial and will then discuss the forensic evaluator's approach to the issue.

1. HISTORICAL BACKGROUND

The determination of competence to stand trial has a rather inglorious history. Under English common law, in the medieval period, the proceedings of a trial were stopped cold by the failure of a defendant to plead to the charges. Officials therefore had to resort to means of convincing the defendant to enter a plea. The procedure commonly used was referred to as *peine forte et dure*; it consisted of placing increasingly heavy rocks on the body of the defendant until either he voiced a plea or the necessity for the trial disappeared. While many of those who refused to plead were undoubtedly criminals seeking to avoid capital punishment, some of those who succumbed to the weight of the court's persuasion were probably mentally ill and mentally retarded individuals who did not have sufficient capacity to understand what was required of them.

As the law worked its way into more enlightened times, the rocks were dispensed with in favor of the recognition that there might be some categories of individuals who were incapable of pleading and who, in addition, might not be able to participate adequately in the subsequent proceedings. These individuals were arraigned before a 12-man jury and evidence of their mental state was presented. If the jury determined that the defendant was not able to plead, the defendant was sent to prison, there to remain until he became competent again. For many, that meant a lifetime of incarceration. Those who were thought to be malingering were tried despite their failure to plead.

The grounds on which the jury was to make its determination of competence were at first not spelled out at all. Beginning in the late 1700s, a series of cases led, by virtue of somewhat more explicit judicial decisions, to a consensus on the legal standard to be applied: the defendant needed to be possessed of sufficient reason to understand the charges against him and to participate in the trial in his own defense. The heavy cognitive component of this standard, insofar as it stressed understanding to the exclusion of impairments of rationality or affect, was characteristic of the time and is also reflected in the nearly contemporaneous M'Naghten rule for criminal responsibility determinations (see Sec. B below).

2. MODERN-DAY STANDARDS

Modern standards for competence to stand trial differ little, in most jurisdictions, from the nineteenth-century common law rule. Each state determines the standards that govern most criminal trials in the state, except those under federal jurisdiction. There the standard enunciated in the federal case of *Dusky v. United States* applies: "The test must be whether he has sufficient present ability to consult with his lawyer with a reasonable degree of rational understanding, and whether he has a rational as well as a factual understanding of the proceedings against him."

A tripartite definition of competence can be formulated that will apply in most jurisdictions: the defendant must have an understanding of the nature of the charges against him and of the nature and purpose of court proceedings; and he must be able to cooperate with an attorney in his own defense.

The rationale that underlies this standard has also undergone considerable evolution since the days of *peine forte et dure*. No longer is the law strictly concerned with the ritualistic aspects of lodging a plea. Rather, the requirement that a defendant be competent in order for a trial to take place is seen as protecting the fundamental fairness of the proceedings, guaranteed by our constitution, and as ensuring that all relevant information that the defendant can provide is made available to the court. It can be argued that some aspects of the trial as ritual persist: to the extent that public faith in the criminal justice system requires a perception of inherent fairness in the process, the exclusion of those whose competence is impaired makes the entire system more legitimate. Thus, judges are constitutionally required to order competence evaluations whenever the defendant's behavior or the representations of any party raise "a bona fide doubt" about the defendant's competence to stand trial.

3. ROLE OF THE MENTAL HEALTH PROFESSIONAL IN DETERMINING COMPETENCE

Unlike the English courts of several centuries ago, contemporary American courts do not rely on the unassisted lay judgment of a jury to decide a defendant's competence to stand trial. Although a few jurisdictions still employ juries, the defendant will usually first be examined by a clinician appointed by the court, and the clinician's report will then provide an important basis for the jury's decision. In most jurisdictions, the trial judge will determine the defendant's competence, again almost always with clinical assistance. Some states make use of panels of experts to assess competence.

Regardless of who is the ultimate decision maker, empirical studies of courtroom procedure have shown that the opinion of the forensic evaluator is highly influential in the final determination. Unfortunately, it is not always clear what standards are being used by the clinician in making her assessment.

a. Standards for assessment

Until quite recently, little attention has been given to how mental health professionals should operationalize the standards to be used in assessing defendants referred because of a question of incompetence. The impression of researchers who have conducted field studies of hearings on this issue is that clinicians, as well as attorneys and judges, frequently confuse the question of competence with the questions of the presence of psychosis, suitability for civil commitment, and responsibility for criminal acts—determinations that should be clearly distinguished from each other. Evaluators' opinions have tended to be stated in a conclusory manner with little or no justification given for the opinion that the defendant is not capable of standing trial.

In order to focus clinicians' attention to those areas of functioning that are most relevant to a determination of competence to stand trial—and to fill the void left by the absence of clear guidelines from the courts—a number of checklists have been devised. The most carefully constructed of these is the work of McGarry et al. (see Suggested Readings), which was empirically validated by cross-reference to the ultimate judicial disposition of the defendants on whom it was tested. The McGarry scale attempts to operationalize the competence assessment questions by looking at 13 areas of functioning, including the defendant's:

1. Ability to appraise the legal defenses available,
2. Level of unmanageable behavior,
3. Quality of relating to attorney,
4. Ability to plan legal strategy,
5. Ability to appraise the roles of various participants in the courtroom proceedings,
6. Understanding of court procedure,
7. Appreciation of the charges,
8. Appreciation of the range and nature of possible penalties,
9. Ability to appraise the likely outcomes,
10. Capacity to disclose to attorney available pertinent facts surrounding the offense,
11. Capacity to challenge prosecution witnesses realistically,
12. Capacity to testify relevantly, and
13. Manifestation of self-serving versus self-defeating motivation.

Although the McGarry scale comes with an elaborate scoring system for each of these factors, the average clinician outside of a research setting will probably find that the use of the checklist to structure his own interview is sufficient to ensure thoroughness (see Sec. III-B-1). It appears that responses to several of the criteria depend upon previous experience with the legal system (i.e., factors 1, 4, 5, 6, and 9). Clinicians should not regard poor showings on these factors as determinative of incapacity, unless the defendant demonstrates an inability to be educated about these issues.

In addition to ensuring a thorough and systematized evaluation, the use of a scale, whether the McGarry checklist or one of the other published works, enables the clinician to organize his report to the court in such a way that the basis for her decision about the patient's competence or incompetence is immediately clear. This avoids the problem of offering blanket statements that judges and attorneys have either to reject or to accept on their face.

b. Answering the ultimate question

Because competence to stand trial is, in the end, a legal determination, many experts feel that a clinician should not offer an opinion as to the ultimate legal question. That is, they maintain that while all the relevant data that a judge might need in order to decide if a defendant is competent (for example, those factors in the McGarry scale) should be presented clearly, the evaluator should *not* offer an opinion as to whether, based on this information, she considers the defendant competent or incompetent. These experts feel that the question of whether a defendant should stand trial is not a clinical decision, but one based on a balancing of values concerning fairness to the defendant and the public's interest in resolving the criminal charges. Clinical evaluators have no special expertise in resolving these questions and are thus likely to rely on their own sociopolitical biases in reaching a decision, an outcome that is unfair to the defendant. In addition, it is argued that the clinical professions lose credibility with the public when they attempt to usurp the role of society's appointed fact-finders in this fashion.

On the other side of the argument some forensic clinicians advocate that evaluators who work in court settings should, in fact, view themselves as an arm of the court and should attempt to be as useful to the court as they possibly can. If answering the ultimate question would be helpful for the court, then that is a function mental health professionals should perform. These forensic clinicians would probably aver that objectivity in assessment is illusory anyway, and that to the extent that bias exists, openly recognizing it is more likely to mute its effect than ignoring it altogether.

There is something to be said for both sides of the issue, but, in the end, the clinician is an expert in human behavior and not in law. Regardless of professional considerations, it is unfair to the defendant for his legal status to be decided by clinical, rather than by judicial, fiat. Unfortunately, because the presentation of the bare clinical facts, even utilizing a scale such as McGarry's, leaves the judge or jury with the task of making the conceptual leap from the clinical formulation to the legal desiderata—an extremely difficult chore that they prefer to avoid—attorneys and judges frequently press evaluators for a more direct response to the legal issues. Clinicians in this situation are faced with two options: (1) caving in to the pressures exerted by the judge; or (2) protesting to the judge that their expertise lies in assessment of the patient and does not extend to legal matters, and stating that therefore they would prefer not to answer the question.

c. Ethical issues in competence evaluations

Whether the examiner intends to restrict his report to the court to descriptions of the defendant's mental state or to respond to the ultimate question of whether the defendant is competent to stand trial, he is performing a role different from the one usually assumed by a clinician; rather than collecting data that might be of aid in the treatment of the individual, his intent is to collect data that will be useful to a third party—the court—and that may or may not be used in the best interests of the individual.

There are two schools of thought about participating in evaluations that are undertaken primarily at the request of third parties.

The case for abstinence.   Two arguments are generally posed in favor of clinicians abstaining from all participation in forensic evaluations. The first centers on the distortion of the clinician-patient relationship inherent in court evaluations and on the consequent effects on clinical practice as a whole. The position is advanced that the mental health professional in such cases is exploiting the defendant by using her clinical skills to obtain information for the court, often in the face of the defendant's reluctance to provide that information, and often to the person's detriment. Despite the fact that a true clinician-patient relationship does not exist—the defendant has usually not requested the evaluation, and no treatment is planned as a result of it—evaluees may sometimes be seduced into providing information as though the clinician with whom they are talking were, in fact, concerned only with their well-being. Similar issues arise in every setting in which a clinician is employed by someone other than the subject and renders reports to that third party, who may then act to the person's detriment: this includes evaluative aspects of mental health work in prisons, the military, some university health services (although many try to approximate the private practice model), and industry.

There is additional concern about the generalization of this redefinition of the clinician-patient relationship. Some fear that having been tainted with the label of an "agent of social control" in the court setting, clinicians will be unable to shake that appellation in other settings as well. To the extent that the public begins to perceive mental health professionals as working for the state or other social institutions, rather than for the individual patient, the trust that lies at the core of every therapeutic relationship will be significantly impaired.

The second line of argumentation against participation focuses more directly on the courtroom proceedings themselves and asks whether clinicians can make any unique contribution to the competence evaluation. Since the sine qua non of competence is the ability to defend oneself in court, it is reasoned that the judge and the defense attorney are in a better position to determine whether a person is competent for that narrow task than is the clinician who may be only vaguely familiar with actual courtroom procedure. Why, then, are mental health professionals dragged into the picture? Some believe it is because judges dislike making difficult or controversial decisions and would rather merely ratify a clinician's assessment. Others point to the extralegal use by judges of the competence assessment statutes to detain, treat, or evaluate defendants; clinical participation is always helpful and occasionally essential for those controversial functions (see Sec. 4 below).

The case for participation.   Those who advocate clinicians' involvement in competence (and other forensic) evaluations urge both that forensic assessment of defendants can be invaluable in protecting the fairness function of the courts and that clinicians have an obligation to render whatever help they can to the courts. Assuming the utility of the evaluations, with which the majority of clinicians would probably agree, the avoidance of participation because of discomfort with the model or fears of some nebulous impact on the profession implies that mental health professionals are willing to shrug off their obligation to society— the obligation of every citizen to aid the smooth functioning of the justice system—in order to avoid grappling with the apparent ethical dilemmas that these evaluations raise.

A synthesis.   There is an alternative to total abstinence from participation in competence evaluations that at the same time tries to protect the rights of the defendant and to preserve the ethical standards of the professions. Its basis is the utilization of the model of informed consent to guide the practitioner through the ethical shoals. (See Chap. 4, Sec. II-B.) This requires that the defendant:

- Be informed in advance of the interview as to its purpose and as to the likelihood that the information revealed will be disclosed to the court. The defendant's lawyer should also be informed, since she is responsible for guarding her client's rights. The ethical reason for desiring such a warning are clear: to counter the natural assumption of most people that an individual who introduces herself as a physician and begins to ask questions is doing so for reasons that will be of direct benefit to them. Moreover, the courts in many jurisdictions have required that this information be revealed to the defendant so that he can exercise his privilege against self-incrimination in choosing whether to respond. Many state laws provide that information obtained in competence examinations pertaining to questions of innocence and guilt cannot be admitted in court in any event—a valuable safeguard.
- Be competent to understand the information presented to him about the nature of the interview. If it appears that the defendant is so psychotic or retarded that he cannot understand that the purpose of the interview is not therapeutic but evaluative, the interview should be deferred. The evaluator may, depending on the situation, want to obtain the substituted consent of a judge, the defendant's attorney, or someone else acting on behalf of the defendant.
- Be consenting voluntarily. Any intimation that this might not be the case should be grounds for the clinician's terminating the interview.
- Be continually aware of the nature of the interview. Evaluees who begin talking about personal matters often become so caught up in the events and feelings they are describing that they lose track of the social conventions controlling the situation. Subjects who seem to be slipping into the "therapeutic" frame of mind, revealing material that they would probably not reveal if they were aware of the actual nature of the interview, ought to be stopped and reminded again of the purpose of the discussion.

Such procedures should diminish the qualms many clinicians feel about entering situations in which their real masters are third parties and not the patients by making clear to the subjects of the interviews exactly what the situations entail.

4. MISUSE OF COMPETENCE EVALUATIONS BY THE COURTS

Several empirical studies have demonstrated that a large number, in some cases a majority, of the defendants ostensibly referred by the courts for competence examinations are, in fact, being referred for other reasons. This usually occurs when the prosecutor or the court is interested in finding an alternative to holding a defendant in jail until the time of the trial or releasing him on bail. When the competence assessment is done on an outpatient basis, or in the courthouse, the judge may use it as a way of finding a reason for denying bail (e.g., as a consequence of a finding that the defendant is mentally ill and dangerous) or for committing the defendant to a state hospital or other psychiatric facility (e.g., as a consequence of a finding that the defendant needs further evaluation for competence).

Even more subject to abuse are referrals to inpatient facilities for competence assessments. Most states permit involuntary commitments of defendants for periods of up to several weeks, with renewals for periods of up to several months. Judges are most likely to use such alternatives when defendants have a history of treatment for mental illness or have been behaving oddly, even if there is no good evidence that they are incompetent to be tried. Commitment for evaluation allows judges to avoid criticism for returning likely recidivists to the streets on bail. It also serves a judge's wish to sequester people whose behavior is so deviant, without actually being violative of the law, that they are a perpetual discomfort to society. These individuals can be arrested on a petty charge such as disorderly conduct and then, without a trial or a chance at obtaining bail, be committed by the judge to a hospital for a substantial period of time.

This use of the system by the judiciary obviously deprives defendants of their constitutional rights to bail and to a speedy trial and often results in unnecessary detention. On the other hand, the competence referral is frequently used for a more benevolent, though still extralegal, purpose, namely, the treatment of mentally ill individuals who will not accept voluntary hospitalization but who are in need of treatment. Restriction of civil commitment statutes in many states to criteria emphasizing dangerousness has left a large number of severely ill, but nondangerous people roaming the streets with no means for the state to provide the care that they need. Benevolent judges often seek to thwart the intent of such statutes by committing these people after arrests on minor charges; formally, a competence evaluation is requested, but in actuality, the reason for commitment is the judge's wish that these individuals receive psychiatric care, even if only for a short period of time. This misuse of the competence assessment laws is a result of the pressures exerted on society by civil commitment statutes that are entirely governed by dangerousness criteria (see Chap. 2, Sec. II-D-2). It is another confirmation of the need for involuntary treatment laws that permit treatment for the patient's own welfare, not merely because someone else is being threatened by the patient's behavior.

It should be noted that abuse of the competence referral sometimes emanates from the defendant's attorney, too. In addition to failing to protest extralegal referrals made by the courts, defense lawyers sometimes *request* competence evaluations when the real issue is their desire to delay the court hearing— whether for their own convenience or for strategic purposes—or to obtain a sounding on the level of the defendant's psychopathology as it relates to the possibility of later offering an insanity defense. Lawyers have also been known— without consultation with the client—to waive their client's rights to be released from the hospital after the statutorily permitted period of evaluation has expired.

Unfortunately, there is little that clinicians can do to thwart such abuse of the system. Court clinic personnel can try in their evaluations to be as scrupulous as possible about relating their evaluations to the specific criteria for competence to stand trial (see Sec. II-A-3-a above). In addition, they can avoid labeling defendants as incompetent simply because they are mentally ill. Inpatient services have no option but to accept court commitments, but they can try to accomplish the evaluations as expeditiously as possible with an eye toward returning the patient promptly to court. The most effective move to prevent abuses—and to make the system function more efficiently—is probably to require that competence to stand trial evaluations be performed on an outpatient basis, unless the defendant otherwise meets commitment criteria or close observation is required as part of the competence assessment. Some states have successfully implemented such outpatient-oriented assessment systems.

5. THE PROBLEM OF DISPOSITION

As noted above, medieval English courts had a ready solution for the problem of what to do with the defendant who was charged with a crime for which he could not be tried. The defendant was simply sent to jail until his condition improved enough to allow his trial to take place. If his condition did not improve, the trial did not take place, and the defendant remained incarcerated indefinitely. Surprisingly, this solution to the problem remained the common one in this country until the U.S. Supreme Court decision in *Jackson v. Indiana* in 1972. The court held that Jackson, who was severely retarded, and therefore unlikely ever to reach a state of competence for trial on charges of stealing nine dollars worth of property, could not be given the virtual life sentence to which indefinite detention would amount. The state was ordered to release Jackson when it became clear that it was unlikely that he would ever become competent.

Most states were forced by *Jackson* to amend their statutes concerning competence assessments. The usual post-*Jackson* statute provides for a period of evaluation, followed by a period of treatment, at the end of which, if no improvement has occurred and the patient is not otherwise committable under state law, the patient must be released and the charges dismissed. These changes have had the effect of preventing the criminal justice system from using incompetence to stand trial as a means of indefinitely hospitalizing those chronically ill, nondangerous patients whom the civil commitment laws also no longer permit to be detained against their will.

On the whole, this result represents a substantial contribution to the fairness with which the system operates. Chronic but harmless patients, many of whom are probably not likely to benefit from treatment, can no longer be picked up on minor charges and hospitalized for life by the court. It is unfortunate, though, that potentially treatable patients in this group cannot be guaranteed care through the more appropriate channel of the civil system. There are, in addition, a small number of patients who are chronically ill, who repeatedly violate the law in significant ways, but who are incompetent and quite unlikely ever to regain competence. Assuming that their crimes do not render them a danger to themselves or to others, in most states there is no way to deal with the problem that they present. If arrested, they cannot be tried and, after an evaluation period and a brief attempt at treatment, must be released. When released, they invariably become involved in illegal activities again, resulting in their arrest and a repetition of the cycle. Since they are not dangerous, they cannot, in most places, be committed.

Our society's devotion to individual rights leaves us with no means of dealing with the majority of this admittedly small, but troublesome, class of offenders. It may be the price that we as a society have to pay to prevent worse abuses.

6. Treating incompetence

It is suggested elsewhere in this book (see Chap. 5, Sec. III-A-6) that insofar as incompetence is the result of a psychopathologic process, it ought to evoke a search for the underlying illness and an effort at treatment. Some facilities have begun innovative attempts at "treating" incompetence to stand trial through an active program of education concerning the role and function of the court, including opportunities to rehearse actual participation in a trial. While these efforts at education are commendable and perhaps should be made routine for all defendants, not just the mentally ill, they do not constitute genuine treatment of the underlying disorder that has led to the incompetent state, since simple ignorance of courtroom procedure should never, in itself, be the basis for a finding of incompetence. A genuine treatment for incompetence involves intervention directed at the defendant's psychopathological state.

The treatment of defendants who are incompetent to stand trial has become a topic of unnecessary controversy, generally stemming from a misunderstanding on the part of many lawyers and judges of the nature of action of psychotropic medications. Their objections affect both voluntary and involuntary treatment.

a. Voluntary treatment

Although one would expect that a defendant who wanted to take psychotropic medication that would ameliorate his psychosis and simultaneously restore him to competence would be permitted, indeed, even encouraged, to do so, there have in the past been a number of objections to the practice. Some members of the legal profession have felt that the state induced by the medications represented "artificial competence," which differed in some way from the "true competence" that the patient would attain if only he were allowed to improve without medications. People who offer such arguments generally fail to recognize the normative effect of psychotropic medications: these medicines do not create an artificial state of functioning, but return the patient in the direction of his nonpsychotic baseline. In addition, to ask that many chronic patients attain competence without medication is to require the impossible; if these patients are to be tried at all, it can only be while under treatment. Since the *Jackson* rule has precluded the indefinite detention of incompetents, objections to voluntary treatment have fallen off. The criminal justice system is usually eager for a trial to take place before the defendant must be released to the streets.

b. Involuntary treatment

Involuntary treatment remains a controversial area. The objections to treating incompetent defendants against their will include those that are applied to involuntary treatment in general (see Chap. 3, Sec. II-C). Additional arguments that are offered include (1) the "artificial competence" argument; (2) the feeling that it is unethical to infringe the patient's autonomy, not for his "best interests," but merely to serve society by readying him for trial; (3) the fear (on the part of the defendant's attorney) that an insanity defense will be undermined by the defendant's nonpsychotic appearance.

The ethical argument is a complicated one, but seems to come out on the side of treatment. Not only does society's interest in trying the defendant outweigh his desire to maintain autonomy, but since his exercise of autonomy has already been massively impeded by his arrest and incarceration, it comes down to a choice of *means* of societal coercion, not to a question of whether coercion will take place at all. Adding to this the interest of society in maintaining the integrity of the criminal justice system by preventing those who would avoid its grasp (in this case, by refusing medications) from doing so, the balance seems to tip in favor of treatment.

As far as the objection that treatment will undermine the insanity defense is concerned, a careful explanation to the jury of the effect of the medications should counter that. While one can never be certain that the jury will be able to discount the effect of seeing an apparently normal defendant before them, our system entrusts the jury with many more complicated assessments; to take the effect of medications into account does not seem an unreasonable thing to ask of them.

Attempts to resolve this issue in the courts are ongoing. Some states have allowed defendants to refuse treatment that would restore competence; others have not. At this writing, the U.S. Supreme Court has yet to rule on the constitutional aspects of the issue.

7. PROPOSALS FOR ALTERING THE CURRENT PROCESS

The abuses of the competence to stand trial evaluation process referred to above, plus the enormous expense of evaluating several tens of thousands of defendants each year, have led to a number of proposals for altering the system. The most imaginative of these have in common the removal of an outright bar to trying defendants who may lack competence. Two versions of these proposals have been offered.

It has been suggested, and actually implemented in some jurisdictions, that incompetent defendants be permitted to stand trial, with their attorneys making the best defense they can. If the defendant in such a trial is acquitted, she is permitted to go free. If she is convicted, the trial is vacated and she is committed for restoration of competence, and ultimate retrial. This approach has the virtue of maintaining adherence to a core value underlying the rules on competence to stand trial—fairness to the defendant. It also diminishes the need to evaluate and treat those defendants who would be found innocent anyway, thus reducing costs and making abuse of the competence assessment system more difficult. On the negative side, it runs the risk of permitting some trials in which the defendant's inability to assist in her defense or behave properly in the courtroom mock the adjudication process. If very many second trials were required, they might also eat up whatever monies are saved as a result of reducing evaluations and hospitalizations.

A second, related suggestion would go even further in mitigating the effect of a finding of incompetence. An incompetent defendant would be permitted to waive his right not to be tried in that state, as long as his attorney—acting, in effect, as a limited guardian—concurred in the decision. The defendant would then take his chances at trial or in a plea bargain. Arguments in favor of this approach (see Suggested Readings—Winick) emphasize reduced costs and the fact that many defendants play little role in preparing or presenting their defense, with their lawyers making the decisions for them, including the decision to keep them off the stand. Not much would be lost in such a case were the trial to proceed even with the defendant still incompetent. This would allow defendants and their attorneys, as a matter of strategy, to risk a finite, often short, sentence rather than accept long-term hospitalization for restoration of competence. Substantial constitutional, ethical, and practical objections to trying incompetent defendants, however, stand in the way of adoption of such proposals.

B. Criminal responsibility

The purpose of the insanity defense is to permit the exoneration of those individuals whom society does not feel should be held morally responsible for their acts. This lack of responsibility could stem from an absence of free will in their behavior, or the ineffectiveness of punishment in deterring their behavior. Because it is in the interest of society to excuse as few people as possible from the dictates of the criminal law, the defense of moral nonculpability historically has been limited to young children (below the age of seven) and to the mentally disturbed. From the days of the "wild beast test"—under which the defendant was exonerated if he "doth not know what he is doing, no more than . . . a wild beast"—the defense evolved considerable sophistication; yet its use traditionally was limited to the psychotic defendant. Recent studies of those acquitted by reason of insanity reveal that this is no longer the case. Between 10% and 30% of not guilty by reason of insanity (NGRI) acquittees carry diagnoses of personality disorders. The tests that have evolved over the centuries share a common requirement—that the defendant be considered mentally impaired—but differ from each other in substantial ways, as will be considered below.

It is safe to say that the insanity defense is the single most controversial legal doctrine relating to the mentally ill. The idea that someone who has committed a crime should escape punishment—regardless of his degree of mental impairment—strikes many people as intuitively wrong. A number of misconceptions about the insanity defense contribute to popular discontent. Research has shown that lay people and legislators tend to overestimate greatly the number of NGRI acquittals that occur. The best available data, which predate the most recent period of reform, indicate that about 1500 defendants per year are found NGRI. Successful insanity defenses occur in fewer than 1 in every 2000 felony cases. Most determinations of NGRI result from negotiated pleas between the prosecutor and defense, rather than from a trial. Nor does a finding of NGRI typically lead to immediate release to the streets. The duration of hospitalization after an NGRI acquital varies across jurisdictions and according to the seriousness of the charges, but the average acquittee spends several years in a state hospital. Recidivism by NGRIs appears to be no greater than rearrests for convicted criminals, when the initial charges are the same.

Thus, the salience of the issue of criminal responsibility is due less to the large number of cases or its purported role as a way to beat the system than to the pointed manner in which it raises basic questions about how we apportion responsibility for one's actions. (See Sec. III-B-2 for a discussion of practical approaches to assessment of criminal responsibility.)

1. THE THRESHOLD QUESTION OF MENTAL ILLNESS

All the formulations of the insanity defense require that the impairment claimed in mental functioning be a result of mental disease or defect. "Defect" is usually taken to refer to mental retardation. Defining disease is problematic. Few of those in either the legal or the mental health professions would disagree that any psychotic illness, as long as it is not deliberately induced by the defendant's use of mind-altering agents, legitimately may be considered a disease for the purpose of criminal responsibility determinations. On the other hand, the personality disorders, especially antisocial personality disorder, and other disorders present problems a good deal more controversial.

With the exception of the American Law Institute test for legal insanity described below, the law has undertaken no definitive clarification of what it means by disease. It is clear that, in theory, disease is not limited to psychosis (though the actual practice may be quite different). A prominent court offered the following definition: "A mental disease or defect includes any abnormal condition of the mind which substantially affects mental or emotional processes and substantially impairs behavior controls." It should be evident that such a definition sets virtually no limits on what is classified as a disease.

An embarrassing example of the consequences of failing to address this conceptual void arose in the well-known *Blocker* case. The defendant was originally convicted of murder despite his claim of insanity because, although his psychiatrists diagnosed him as having a "sociopathic personality disturbance," they asserted that he was not suffering from a mental illness. Shortly after his trial, the doctors at St. Elizabeths Hospital in Washington, where Blocker had been examined, decided that henceforth they would testify that sociopaths were indeed victims of a mental disease. Blocker's conviction was overturned on appeal on the basis that he deserved "a verdict based upon the most mature expert opinion available"—in other words, the latest swing of the pendulum.

The issue is clearly not academic. Every clinician who testifies in court in a case in which the insanity defense is employed will be required to state her opinion as to whether the defendant suffers from a mental disease. As of now, the answers of any set of examiners who concur in the diagnosis of a personality disorder or an adjustment reaction, for example, will not necessarily agree with each other. The resulting confusion discredits the professions and perplexes the courts.

The inherent circularity of the definition of disease in this context should not be ignored. Mental disease is a prerequisite for exculpation presumably because society recognizes something in the popular understanding of disease that reduces moral culpability. The law could, in fact, define disease in just that way: a state of reduced moral culpability. One noted judge has made a suggestion along these lines (Bazelon, concurring in *U.S. v. Brawner*).

To the extent that any psychiatric definition of disease deviates from the tacit moral principles that underly the insanity defense, therefore, it is likely to be rejected by the court. For example, if organized psychiatry declared that every disorder in the current *Diagnostic and Statistical Manual* were actually a "disease," courts would still properly refuse to accept "tobacco dependence disorder" as a disease for the purposes of the law. As new disorders are defined, the courts must determine whether they more nearly resemble schizophrenia or tobacco dependence disorder in their potential effects on moral culpability. This process is now occurring for such entities as pathologic gambling, post-traumatic stress disorder, and premenstrual syndrome.

Despite this circularity—the law asks for a definition of disease to aid in determining moral responsibility but will accept only definitions limited to those conditions that appear to impair moral responsibility—there is some point to the exercise of attempting to formulate a psychiatric definition of disease. First, clinical testimony, for whatever use the courts wish to make of it, will then be consistent and reproducible. Second, in that consistency the law will find a starting point from which to begin the process of clarifying its own approach to mental disease. As things now stand, any individual evaluator remains free to decide for herself whether or not the defendant she is evaluating is mentally ill, as long as she can defend that definition in court.

2. THE TESTS OF CRIMINAL RESPONSIBILITY

Mental disease in itself does not exculpate a defendant from responsibility for his criminal acts. There must be something more. The mental disease whose presence has been established by the threshold test must bear such a relation to the criminal behavior that the perpetrator appears to be morally nonculpable. Exactly what that relation should be has been the subject of voluminous discussion in the legal and psychiatric literature, the result of which has been the formulation of a number of tests of criminal responsibility. Those tests will now be examined.

a. The M'Naghten test

The most durable of the tests of criminal insanity (it should be apparent by now that "insanity" in the law is a term of art describing a state of nonresponsibility and is not related to the presence or absence of psychosis) is the *M'Naghten* rule, first formulated in Great Britain in 1843. It states that ". . . to establish a defense on the ground of insanity, it must be clearly proved that, at the time of the committing of the act, the party accused was labouring under such a defect of reason, from disease of the mind, as not to know the nature and quality of the act he was doing; or if he did know it, that he did not know he was doing what was wrong."

A literal reading of M'Naghten would seem to leave little room for applying it to most mentally ill individuals. Few defendants manifest a "defect of reason" such that they "know" neither the nature and quality of their act nor that it was wrong. But some courts have been more generous in their interpretations, removing "know" from a strict cognitive context and allowing it to connote an affectively infused appreciation of one's acts. A schizophrenic, in this more generous reading, convinced that her landlord was an agent of the devil bent on turning her mind to thoughts of sex, and who therefore had to be killed, could be held not to "know" the wrongness of her act of murder, though she might respond in the abstract that to murder was wrong.

"Wrong" is the other key word in the M'Naghten test. Courts are split on whether the knowledge that an act is wrong refers to a recognition that the behavior is forbidden by the law or an awareness of its moral wrongfulness. The latter is more consistent with the usual legal holding that ignorance of the law is no excuse, but it allows a significant degree of subjectivity to enter into the assessment by focusing on the offender's capacity for distinguishing varying shades of moral error. Assuming an impairment in moral awareness is discovered, the forensic examiner has the added burden of determining whether it is a result of the mental illness.

M'Naghten has been the subject of criticism for two reasons: first, by focusing on "knowing" that an act is "wrong," it is said to limit the scope of expert testimony to cognitive assessments alone; second, in so doing it is alleged to adopt the outdated "faculty" psychology of the nineteenth century, which divided the mind into several discrete, nonoverlapping compartments, thereby ignoring modern understanding of the interrelationship between a variety of mental functions. Nonetheless, the M'Naghten rule in some form is still the law in the majority of American jurisdictions.

b. The irresistible impulse test

The second standard test of criminal responsibility is the "irresistible impulse" test: the defendant is not liable if, by reason of mental illness, she is unable to exert control over her acts. Once again, this test of volitional control can be construed narrowly, as its eponym suggests, to be applicable only to suddenly arising impulses acted upon without reflection, or it can be given a broader interpretation, to encompass all acts that result from defective control regardless of the length of time between the initial thought and the act. This test is usually used in conjunction with the M'Naghten test.

The problems for forensic evaluators should be evident immediately. There is first the difficulty in differentiating between an uncontrolled act and an uncontrollable act; the *post hoc* temptation is to assume that every act that has occurred was inevitable. But even more difficult is the acceptance of the test's underlying premise: that there are disorders of the mind that so impair the will as to leave the individual a prisoner of her impulses. Much of the approach of modern inpatient psychiatry is built on a negation of that assumption. Even psychotic patients are encouraged to bear full responsibility for their acts and are discouraged from attributing their behavior to impulses over which they have no control. Behavior modification programs, often used with the most regressed or retarded patients, work from similar premises.

Since the defense is frequently employed, however, there must be forensic evaluators who disagree and who believe that patients *do* lose control over their behavior. One suspects that in many of these cases the irresistible impulse test is superfluous because such individuals would fail the "knowing" test of M'Naghten. An example might be an individual in a toxic delirium. But for those instances in which this test is relied upon exclusively—and recent data suggest that there are a significant number of defendants who are reported to qualify for a volitional, but not a cognitive, standard of non-responsibility—the question remains open whether any mental illness so impairs behavioral controls as to render the defendant helpless to exert *any* domination over her impulses.

c. The American Law Institute (ALI) standard

The third major test of criminal insanity, the standard devised by the American Law Institute (ALI) and published as part of its Model Penal Code, gained in popularity through the early 1980s. It was adopted in the majority of federal jurisdictions and a significant number of states. It reads, in full: "(1) A person is not responsible for criminal conduct if at the time of such conduct as a result of mental disease or defect he lacks substantial capacity either to appreciate the wrongfulness of his conduct or to conform his conduct to the requirements of the law. (2) As used in this Article, the terms 'mental disease or defect' do not include an abnormality manifested only by repeated criminal or otherwise anti-social conduct."

In drafting the Model Penal Code, an effort was made to incorporate both of the two older standards in their broadest forms. Thus the "know" requirement of M'Naghten was replaced by the "appreciate" test, an alternative designed to suggest the affective as well as the cognitive awareness of the nature of one's acts that the law requires. Similarly, the capacity "to conform one's conduct to the requirements of the law" allows the broadest possible reading of the irresistible impulse standard.

Unique to the ALI test is the requirement that the defendant have only a lack of "substantial capacity" either to appreciate the wrongfulness of her conduct or to control her behavior—this in place of the total deficits that the older tests seemingly required. Psychiatrists, reluctant to attribute a complete absence of behavioral controls to the defendant, might feel more comfortable testifying to a partial impairment, subject, of course, to the inevitable quibbling over what constitutes "substantial capacity." In a similar vein, a partial lack of appreciation of wrongful conduct might be more plausibly asserted than a complete one.

The full ALI test pointedly excludes any mental disease or defect "manifested only by repeated anti-social or otherwise abnormal behavior." While not all jurisdictions that have adopted the ALI standard have accepted this qualification, in those that have it is clear that the intent is to exclude the antisocial personality disorder from the advantages of the insanity defense. The potential impact of changes in psychiatric diagnosis on the law is nowhere more evident than here. At the time that the Model Penal Code was published, many psychiatrists argued and many judges accepted that, "as the majority of experts use the term, a psychopath is very distinguishable from one who merely demonstrates recurrent criminal behavior." The subsequent *DSM-II* definition of antisocial personality confirmed this, stressing such elements as selfishness, impulsiveness, absence of loyalty, inability to experience guilt, and a low frustration tolerance, and stating expressly, "A mere history of repeated legal or social offenses is not sufficient to justify this diagnosis." The *DSM-III-R* diagnostic criteria, on the other hand, allow the diagnosis to be made on the basis of a history of legal and social infractions alone; plainly, in any jurisdiction that recognizes the second half of the ALI test, most defendants with *DSM-III-R* antisocial personality disorder will need to look elsewhere to establish a workable defense. Despite the many protestations of the judiciary that the law, and not the psychiatric profession, will determine who is eligible for the insanity defense, this is clearly one example where the interaction between the two is decisive.

d. Other approaches

Modified ALI standard.   In the wake of the trial of John Hinckley, Jr., who attempted to assassinate President Reagan and was found not guilty by reason of insanity, a great deal of discussion took place about narrowing defendants' opportunities to employ an insanity defense. One of the most widely endorsed approaches, which received the approval of both the American Bar Association and the American Psychiatric Association, involves removing the so-called "volitional prong" (or modified irresistible impulse standard) from the ALI test, leaving the "cognitive" or appreciation test standing on its own. The rationale for this change was the belief that volitional impairments are particularly difficult to ascertain, and account for much of the conflicting testimony by experts that so distresses legislators and the public.

Persuaded by this argument, although without empirical data to support it, a Congress intent on restricting the use of the insanity defense altered the federal test for criminal responsibility in 1984 to include only a defendant who, "as a result of a severe mental disease or defect, was unable to appreciate the nature and quality or the wrongfulness of his acts." The use of the term "severe mental disease or defect" was designed to limit the use of the defense by persons with all personality disorders, not just antisocial personality disorder. Dropping the volitional test was thought to eliminate the most dubious cases in which the defense would be used. Whether either of these results have been achieved in the federal courts is unclear.

Abolition of the insanity defense. The furor following the Hinckley trial led some states to experiment with an attempt to abolish the insanity defense. The defendant's mental state could not be removed from consideration entirely, because the law has always required that the criminal act (in legal terminology, the "actus reus") be accompanied by an evil intent (the "mens rea"). The nature of the intent required differs from one crime to another. Several states, however, abolished an independent defense of not guilty by reason of insanity, allowing expert testimony on mental state only when, in the words of the Montana statute, "it is relevant to prove that the defendant did or did not have the state of mind which is an element of the offense." Since the states involved are among the less populated in the U.S., and thus insanity defense trials were rare to begin with, it is unclear at this point whether there has been a real reduction in the number of successful mental state defenses offered. As the Hinckley trial recedes into the background, the momentum for abolition appears to have faded.

The Durham standard. The *Durham* test, which prevailed in the District of Columbia from 1954 until 1972, allowed a finding of NGRI if the accused's unlawful act "was the product of mental disease or defect." This "product" test was designed to allow psychiatrists maximal leeway in introducing evidence relevant to the accused's mental state. A similar test has long been used in New Hampshire. As it was clarified in a later case, it represented a "but for" approach to causation: "but for" the existence of mental disease the act in question would not have occurred. This standard is perhaps most compatible of all with the exculpation of many of the personality disorders, for almost everyone would acknowledge that the "inflexible and maladaptive traits" (*DSM-III*) that are their characteristic elements contribute substantially to the resultant behavior. *Durham* died, however, not because of the breadth of its potential scope, but because the court believed that the psychiatrists who testified under it were defining "product" in conclusory terms that eroded the fact-finding function of the jury.

Diminished capacity. "Diminished capacity" is a defense based on impairment of the mind that has evolved in several states, beginning in California (which has now abandoned it). It supplements, rather than replaces, the insanity defense, allowing evidence of any interference with the normal functioning of the mind (though in some incarnations of the defense such interference must once more be the result of mental disease or defect) to be introduced to prove that the defendant did not have the ability to formulate one of the specific mental elements required for the crime charged. Thus, an intoxicated individual accused of assault with intent to murder might reasonably claim that he was too drunk to formulate an intent to murder the victim of his assault; the result would be a guilty finding on the reduced charge of assault and battery. The defense has somewhat arbitrarily been limited to crimes that are said to require a higher-level "specific intent" rather than the "general intent" common to all criminal acts.

Guilty but mentally ill. "Guilty but mentally ill" is another variation on the usual techniques for dealing with the mentally disordered offender. Juries can find a defendant pleading insanity "guilty but mentally ill" if they believe that his illness existed at the time of the crime, but did not contribute to the act to such an extent that a finding of not guilty by reason of insanity is warranted. The mental health professions' role is not much different here from that in an insanity defense; the contribution of the individual's illness (again the definition-of-illness problem arises) to his act must be assessed. Persons found GBMI are then referred for evaluation and are supposed to receive psychiatric treatment, if that is warranted.

The guilty but mentally ill verdict caught on in popularity after Hinckley's trial, in large part because it was seen as a way of persuading juries that they could recognize a defendant's mental illness without finding her NGRI. In this light, it is something of a fraud. Those found GBMI are treated the same as those who are convicted in an ordinary manner; any prisoner can be evaluated for treatment and should receive it if needed. To the extent that jurors are led to find a defendant GBMI in the belief that such a verdict differs materially from a finding of guilty and is akin to a verdict of NGRI, they have been tricked. Nonetheless, about one-quarter of the states adopted a GBMI option, largely in the hope that just such misunderstandings would occur.

3. Mechanics of the Insanity Defense

a. Raising the defense

The procedural details of implementing an insanity defense vary from jurisdiction to jurisdiction, but in general any party in a criminal proceeding can raise the issue of a defendant's criminal responsibility at any point in the process. Prosecutors will often use the request for an examination of responsibility as a technique for detaining without bail those defendants whom they would prefer not to see released prior to trial; judges often go along with these requests for similar reasons. Examinations of this sort are usually conducted in inpatient facilities whose security varies with the seriousness of the alleged offense. It has been noted that allowing the prosecutor and the judge to request responsibility examinations provides an interesting potential for them to redefine "political" crimes as the act of a madman; how often that opportunity is exploited in this country is unknown. Defense attorneys who intend to raise an insanity defense are required in many states to notify the prosecution in advance of the trial or forfeit the option.

b. Obtaining an examination

Any defendant is entitled to employ his own expert witness, and since the U.S. Supreme Court's decision in *Ake v. Oklahoma*, states have been obligated to provide forensic mental health professionals to defendants facing major charges who cannot afford to hire their own. Which cases this applies to and what level of funding the states must offer are among the issues that are still being hammered out by the lower courts. If the defense attorney elects not to use the testimony of a forensic expert who has examined her client, presumably because it does not support an insanity defense, there is some difference among jurisdictions as to whether the prosecutor can later call the expert at trial. Clinicians should be aware of the rules in their own jurisdictions, at least in part so that they can provide accurate information to the defendant they evaluate concerning the level of confidentiality that attends the examination.

c. The burden of proof

The states have a variety of rules concerning who bears the burden of proof in insanity defense cases. Following the Hinckley trial, many states and the federal government placed the burden on the defendant to prove legal insanity by a preponderance of the evidence. This is now the majority rule. Some states still retain the requirement that the prosecution prove the absence of legal insanity beyond a reasonable doubt, reasoning that since a *mens rea* is an essential element in any crime, the prosecution should bear the burden of proving that the defendant was actually criminally responsible. In order to trigger this burden for the prosecution, the defendant need only present evidence to the contrary. In such cases the job of the expert witness for the prosecution, who must convince a jury beyond a reasonable doubt that a given mental state did not exist, is considerably more arduous than the task of the defense's expert, whose testimony must only raise some measure of doubt.

4. DISPOSITION

Historically, defendants were loath to raise an insanity defense because a finding of not guilty by reason of insanity led almost invariably to an indefinite, potentially lifetime commitment to a psychiatric hospital, usually one for the "criminally insane." Since all but major crimes like murder held out the hope of eventual release from prison, and since there was in addition a chance that even the most seemingly guilty defendant could convince a jury of his innocence, it was almost always in the noncapital defendant's interest to eschew the insanity defense.

This situation changed with a number of court decisions that declared it to be a violation of a defendant's right to due process to be incarcerated indefinitely regardless of his current mental status or the severity of his crime. Current rules in most states allow a period of hospitalization for evaluation, often up to several months, following a verdict of not guilty by reason of insanity. Persons who are deemed to be mentally ill and dangerous can be hospitalized for an extended period with periodic reviews of their status. If they remain ill and dangerous despite treatment, recommitment must take place on a regular basis. In some states, this process will operate with rules identical to those used for civil committees. In others, there will be differences designed to make it more difficult to release acquittees, for example placing on them the burden of proving non-dangerousness.

The revolution in disposition procedures has heightened the desirability of employing the insanity defense and has probably been responsible for an increase in the frequency of its use. Also contributing to the increased utilization of the insanity defense is the shift of responsibility for the care of some categories of mentally ill minor offenders from the penal to the psychiatric systems. With a greater sensitivity to the presence of mental illness, the criminal justice system now frequently channels such offenders to the state hospitals. Once labeled as psychiatric cases, these offenders are more likely to want to employ and to be successful in employing an insanity defense in response to future charges. Obviously the more rapid turnover of not guilty by reason of insanity acquittees— mandated by the court decisions requiring a finding of dangerousness for continued incarceration—may also contribute to the increased subsequent utilization of the defense.

The most important innovation in post-acquittal procedures has been the Psychiatric Security Review Board model initiated in Oregon and since adopted in a number of other states. Insanity acquittees in Oregon are committed to the PSRB for the maximum time that they might otherwise have been incarcerated, if they had been found guilty. The PSRB can place them in inpatient or outpatient treatment, and can follow them after discharge from an inpatient facility. If the acquittee begins to deteriorate, or fails to comply with discharge conditions, she can be rehospitalized expeditiously, followed by a hearing before the Board. This approach, endorsed by the American Psychiatric Association as a model for the rest of the country, gets around the problem that exists now in most states: once an acquittee no longer qualifies for inpatient hospitalization, often according to civil standards, the state loses all control over her. It allows long-term monitoring of a class of people about whom society has every reason to be concerned. The PSRB approach appears to be successful, based on recidivism rates, and warrants careful consideration in every state.

5. THE MENTAL HEALTH PROFESSIONAL'S ROLE IN DETERMINING RESPONSIBILITY

Many of the issues here are analogous to those discussed above with reference to competence to stand trial (see Sec. II-A). Despite the proliferation of legal standards for determining responsibility, little attention has been devoted to translating those standards into clinically meaningful terms. Law and psychiatry have yet to find a common basis for discourse.

The basic legal doctrine can be stated simply: "Our criminal laws are premised on the view that human beings are normally capable of free and rational choice between alternative modes of behavior, that an individual who chooses to harm another is morally blameworthy or guilty, and that he is liable to punishment if his behavior and the resulting harm have been proscribed by the law" (Brakel & Rock, *The Mentally Disabled and the Law*). From these basic presumptions the law formulates its expectations of the mental health professions.

Clinicians, accustomed to speaking their own private language, are forced to speak a foreign tongue. They are asked whether individuals have acted with appreciation of the nature of their acts or with the free will to avoid violations of the law if they so choose. They are sometimes asked to evaluate the effect of a complex disease process on a given act, remote in time, which they did not witness, and which the alleged actor may be maintaining has never occurred. They are asked to define mental disease and to apply the definition to the defendant. All the while, they must keep in mind that the system for which they are working denies a fundamental theoretical premise of much of psychiatry: that all behavior is influenced by unconscious forces beyond the control of the actor and is thus to some extent *both* involuntary and predetermined.

It should not be surprising that in this situation a number of studies have cast doubt on the objectivity of forensic evaluators. Their judgments concerning the presence or absence of criminal responsibility have been shown to relate to their political and social views, in addition to taking into account the characteristics of the defendant. Part of the public discomfort with the insanity defense undoubtedly relates to the perception that mental health professionals are allowing their own opinions to influence the outcome of major trials in ways that confuse, rather than clarify, the issues to be decided by the finder of fact.

A strong argument therefore can be made that forensic clinicians should avoid offering testimony on those aspects of the insanity defense that require more political or moral, than clinical, judgments. This means avoiding testimony on the ultimate issue of the defendant's responsibility. Just such a limitation was adopted by Congress for the federal courts as part of the post-Hinckley reforms. Clinicians may also benefit, even in this more limited role, from the development of structured assessment instruments to guide their evaluations. Several instruments exist to date, but they suffer from deficiencies that will, it is hoped, be rectified in subsequent research.

C. Civil forensic evaluations

Legal interest in the opinions of mental health professionals is by no means limited to the criminal realm. As is frequently the case in criminal proceedings, however, civil forensic evaluations often focus on the competence of a person to perform a given act. In general, this concern reflects a societal consensus that it is improper to allow an individual with particular impairments of mental functioning to engage in acts that will have significant consequences for himself or for others. The criteria for determining competence in these situations vary according to the particular societal concern that is being protected. Clinicians are asked by the courts, as experts in the evaluation of mental impairment, to ascertain the presence or absence of the indicia that are of interest to the law. The ambiguities of psychiatric evaluation and of the translation of clinical findings into legally relevant data make these assessments extremely challenging. (See Secs. III-B-3 through 6 for discussions of practical aspects of performing these evaluations.)

1. COMPETENCE TO AUTHOR A WILL

a. Legal criteria

The basic legal requirements for competence to write a will, also known as testamentary capacity, vary somewhat across jurisdictions. A common formulation is that those who would write a will "retain the power to understand the nature and extent of their property, their relationship to those persons who are usually the objects of a person's bounty, and the nature and operative effect of will making." In this brief definition itself, the societal interest in competent will making is quickly evident. It is an interest primarily of the heirs, or—more accurately—the presumptive heirs, in assuring, first, that the estate is not carelessly dissipated (hence the requirement for an understanding of the extent of the property and of the fact that one is executing a document that controls its disposition) and, second, that they are, in fact, the beneficiaries (thus the phrasing "those persons who are usually the objects of a person's bounty").

Challenge to the competence of a will is usually undertaken by expectant heirs whose hopes have been disappointed. In some cases they seek to prove that the deceased lacked understanding of the extent of his property or of the nature of his acts, but that is obviously a difficult task except when there is reason to believe that an individual was suffering from dementia. The more common challenges is on the basis that the author of the will was subject to "insane delusions" (a legal term of art) that affected his perception of the usual objects of his bounty. Practically, this means that the deceased held the delusional belief that his wife had been unfaithful to him or that his son had been plotting to steal his money.

b. Ethical issues in the assessment of testamentary capacity

The entire process of evaluating testamentary capacity in court and of declaring the will of a deceased individual invalid on the basis of incompetence has been the subject of considerable attack on ethical grounds. What the process accomplishes, the critics charge, is to rob the defenseless deceased of her last wishes for the disposition of her property on the grounds that her desires do not conform to the usual expectations of society as to how an individual should distribute her wealth. Clinicians' roles in the process are also the target of invective, particularly because they testify about the condition of persons whom they usually have never examined. Some mental health professionals would agree with this criticism and would maintain that clinicians should never testify about anyone whom they have not examined personally. Certainly the violation of this rule should occur only when the evaluator is faced with incontrovertible evidence of a given mental state. The clinician must decide for herself, as well, whether the case represents an attempt to thwart the competent wishes of the deceased or is truly an instance in which an injustice would be done to the natural heirs as a result of real mental impairment in the testator.

2. COMPETENCE TO CONTRACT

a. Legal criteria

Many of the issues discussed in Section 1 above apply to contracts as well. The traditional standards for competence to contract were oriented along cognitive lines: that the party to the contract had "such mental capacity . . . that he could collect in his mind without prompting, all the elements of the transaction and retain them for a sufficient length of time to perceive their obvious relations to each other, and to form a rational judgment in regard to them." As with wills, the presence of "insane delusions" might be one bar to forming rational judgments. More recently, these standards have broadened somewhat in an effort to include among the incompetents grandiose manics whose acts are performed with good cognitive understanding and in the absence (often) of overt delusions, but whose distorted overassessment of their own abilities leads them to make contracts that are ultimately deleterious to them. Recognition of this problem leads to the formulation of standards that add an "appreciation" test (see Chap. 5, Sec. II) to the usual "understanding" test employed in these cases. Alternatively, some of the more recent formulations have approached a "but for" test of incompetence: if "but for" the mental illness the individual would not have signed the contract, it should be voided.

Courts will generally be willing to void contracts on the appeal of one of the parties that she was incompetent at the time the contract was signed, as long as several conditions are met: the party's incompetence is proven in court, the status quo prior to the signing of the contract can be restored (i.e., money or real property can be returned), or, if the status quo cannot be restored, then the contract was an unfair one. Whether the second party to the contract had knowledge of the incompetent status of the first party, and was thus presumptively taking advantage of her, may also play a role in determining if the contract should be voided. Scholars of contract law maintain that courts commonly conflate the questions of incompetence, undue influence, and fraud in deciding whether contracts should be enforced. Thus, it has been said that the fairness of the contract is a more important factor than any objective data that might be presented concerning the condition of the alleged incompetent party (see Suggested Readings—Green).

It should be noted that incompetence to contract may preclude a person from deeding a gift of real property or chattels, or entering into marriage, both actions with contractual qualities. Courts frequently say that the standards they use to determine competence to contract are higher than those applied to testamentary capacity (i.e., a person may be incompetent to make every other kind of contract, but will be given the benefit of the doubt when it comes to making a will); careful review of both classes of cases reveals little support for this proposition.

b. Ethical issues in the assessment of capacity to contract

There are those who charge that any attempt to void a contract retroactively on the grounds of mental incompetence robs the alleged incompetent of the autonomy to make decisions for herself and is unfair to the other party to the contract, assuming that he acted in good faith. This argument is supported by the suggestion that many efforts to void contracts are made, not by the incompetent party, but by guardians—often family members—or heirs, who are concerned that the incompetent's actions have damaged their own interests. While this may occasionally be the case, it is certainly too broad a remedy to propose abolishing all efforts to void contracts of incompetents. Even more than in the case of an invalid will, the incompetent herself may stand to suffer substantial harm as a result of acts performed while mentally ill, and it would appear to be consonant with society's general interest in equity to void such acts.

3. EMOTIONAL HARMS

Persons injured by another's negligence ordinarily have a remedy in suits brought under the law of torts. This principle underlies such familiar causes of litigation as medical malpractice. (See Chap. 4, Sec. II-A.) Traditionally, however, persons alleging that the harms they suffered affected their mental, rather than physical, well-being have faced strict limitations on their ability to recover damages. Limitations of this sort have been based on the belief that plaintiffs will fabricate claims of emotional distress and that mental health professionals will not be able to distinguish between real and malingered distress.

The earliest exceptions to the common law rule excluding claims of negligent infliction of emotional distress developed in the mid-nineteenth century under what came to be known as the "impact rule." Under this standard, as long as a negligent act had led to a physical touching, resulting emotional distress could be compensable. The rationale seemed to be based on the assumption that emotional distress is more likely to occur after physical impact (but not necessarily physical *injury*), and thus such claims are more probably legitimate. An undercurrent of sentiment may also have existed in favor of saddling a defendant who demonstrably caused negligent physical impact with all the consequences of his actions. Nearly 20% of the states still follow this approach.

Many jurisdictions found the physical impact rule too confining, however, excluding what appeared to be legitimate cases of emotional harm. Efforts at liberalization led in several directions. The "ensuing physical injury rule" allowed claims when the emotional distress led to physical symptoms (e.g., neck or back pain, headaches, ulcers). Proponents of this modification seemed to believe that subsequent physical symptomatology increased the probability that the emotional distress was not faked—a dubious proposition, given that many of the physical symptoms identified in these cases are diagnosed solely on the basis of self-reports. The "zone of danger rule" permitted recovery if the plaintiff had been threatened with physical harm, but escaped (e.g., a driver who left a car stalled on railroad tracks seconds before an oncoming train reached it). Persons whose distress resulted from their observation of loved ones being injured were allowed, in some jurisdictions, to recover under a "bystander rule." As exceptions to the underlying restrictive doctrine proliferated, the rationale for the system as a whole became less coherent.

The ultimate step taken by some courts has been the abolition of all distinctions between recovery for physical and emotional injuries. This is accomplished by the adoption of a "foreseeability rule": liability can be imposed if the emotional distress was a foreseeable result of the defendant's behavior. Only a small number of states have gone this far, although courts in all jurisdictions are likely to allow recovery when the emotional distress was intentionally inflicted (e.g., a landlord's harassment of a tenant).

From a psychiatric perspective, rules distinguishing between physical and emotional harms appear to be based on a number of untested empirical assumptions. These relate to the probability of emotional distress occurring in particular circumstances, such as following physical impact. Yet it is clear that severe emotional distress can occur without any of the limiting conditions being present. Restrictions on recovery seem unfair and arbitrary in these cases. Adoption of a uniform foreseeability approach would be highly desirable.

4. MENTAL DISABILITY

Assessments of mental disability are probably the most common civil evaluations that mental health professionals are called upon to perform. Work-related disability can result in eligibility for insurance or entitlement programs including: workers' compensation, Social Security Disability Insurance (SSDI), Supplemental Security Income (SSI), private disability insurance, and veterans' benefits. Each source of compensation for disability has a distinctive history and unique rules that shape the nature of the required evaluation. Two of the largest programs are considered here.

a. Workers' compensation

Workers' compensation plans in the United States developed in the early twentieth century as a mechanism for dealing with claims of workers injured on the job. Throughout most of the nineteenth century, workers were generally precluded from recovering damages for job-related injuries in the courts by such legal doctrines as assumption of risk, contributory negligence, and the fellow-servant rule. As these barriers began to break down in the Progressive Era, industrialists and social reformers alike agreed on the desirability of a non-fault based compensation system that operated outside of the courts. The result was the establishment by the states of mandatory insurance schemes that preempted recourse to the courts, providing some (often fixed-amount) compensation for work-related injuries.

Early workers' compensation schemes focused exclusively on physical injuries. In the last few decades, however, a growing number of states have broadened their plans to cover some categories of mental disabilities induced on the job. Because there is still considerable concern that liberal rules regarding coverage of mental disorders will lead to difficult-to-detect malingered claims, most states still limit mental disability claims in some way. These parallel the restrictions discussed above on recovery for negligent infliction of emotional distress. They may, for example, require that a physical injury precede the alleged mental disability (the so-called "physical-mental" case), thus excluding claims based solely on mental stress. Alternatively, mental stress on the job alone may constitute an accepted causal basis for a claim, but only if it results in physical effects as well as mental disability (known as "mental-physical" cases). Finally, some states will permit claims alleging that mental stress caused a purely mental disability, but usually with limitations such as the requirement that the causative factor be perceived as stressful by a reasonable person ("mental-mental" cases).

Workers' compensation claims are adjudicated by disability determination commissions set up by the states. Disability need not be total to be compensable. Although fault need not be shown (i.e., the question of whether negligence caused the injury is irrelevant), evidence must be introduced to establish the fact of disability and its causal link to the work place. Both issues usually require testimony by mental health professionals.

b. Social Security Disability Insurance

SSDI is a federal disability program to which all workers contribute as part of their social security taxes. It is available only to workers who have paid into the insurance fund, and benefits are partially linked to prior payments. It differs in this way from SSI, which is available to all disabled persons, regardless of past work history. The program is administered by the Social Security Administration (SSA), which has created an elaborate set of requirements governing SSDI eligibility.

To be compensable under SSDI, a disability must result in an inability to work that lasts for at least 12 months. The disability must be total. If the claimant is capable of performing any work (not necessarily her former job) available to a substantial extent in the national economy, she is not disabled for purposes of this program. The evaluation process for claims follows a fixed sequence. First, one of the classes of psychiatric disorders that are generally agreed to result in disability must be diagnosed. Then, the degree of restriction of function is addressed, focusing specifically on four categories: activities of daily living; social functioning; concentration, persistence and pace in job-related activities; and history of deterioration or decompensation in work or work-like settings. If impairment is not sufficient in these four areas to warrant a finding of disability, the claimant's "residual functional capacity" can be considered.

SSDI claims are reviewed by state disability agencies, acting under contract to the federal government. Adverse findings can be appealed to the agency, then to an administrative law judge, to a national appeals board, and under certain circumstances to the federal courts. During the 1980s, substantial evidence accumulated to indicate that SSA was not following its own regulations in processing mental disability claims and performing periodic reviews. The agency's aim appeared to be to reduce costs by eliminating hundreds of thousands of claimants from the rolls. Action by the federal courts and Congress resulted in revision of SSA procedures and restoration of benefits to many chronic mentally ill people who were unfairly denied them.

III. CLINICAL ISSUES

A. Problems of agency in the forensic evaluation

The role of a forensic evaluator is most clearly distinguished from the role of a treating clinician by a dramatic change in agency, i.e., the entity for whom the mental health professional works. In the clinical setting, the mental health professional is primarily the agent of the patient, although the demands of the law— for example, the duty to protect potential victims of a patient's violence—may sometimes induce situations in which conflicting obligations arise (see Chap. 4, Sec. II-A-3-e). Many of the most challenging aspects of dealing with mental health law for the clinician revolve around the need to remain primarily the agent of the patient.

In marked contrast, the forensic evaluator is most definitely *not* the agent of the subject of the evaluation, even when the subject is paying her bill (see Sec. 2-b-i below and Chap. 8, Sec. II-C-1). The purpose of the evaluator's involvement is not primarily to benefit the subject, although that may be an incidental outcome of her work, but to produce an objective report that is responsive to the question motivating the examination. That the evaluator's conclusions may be to the detriment of the subject is (or ought to be) taken for granted by all parties. Without this possibility, the evaluation would be of no use to either side in the case.

This alteration in agency results as well in a shift in terminology. As far as the subject of a forensic evaluation is concerned, he can no longer properly be termed a "patient"—at least in relation to the evaluator. We will thus be using the terms "subject," "examinee," or "evaluee" to describe this person's role. Although there may be circumstances in which the subject-patient boundary becomes blurred (see Sec. 2 below), these situations are problematic at best, and are most successfully dealt with by attempting to reestablish the distinction.

1. AGENCY IN THE "PURE" EVALUATION MODEL

a. General considerations

Under this model, evaluator and examinee are strangers to each other who meet only for the specific occasion of the examination, evaluation, or consultation. The clinician's agency is quite explicit and should be made clear to the examinee at the very outset of the conversation. Explicitness is also required about which side of the case has retained the examiner, as in this example.

> *Example 1:* The clinician invites the examinee into the office and shows him in which chair to sit. He then says: "Mr. Smith, I want to make two points clear before we start. First, since this is an evaluation related to the lawsuit you have filed, what we say to each other is not confidential, in the same way it would be with a psychiatrist who was actually treating you. In other words, what we talk about might appear in writing and might come up in open court, if it's relevant to the case. Second, you need to know that since I've been retained by the attorneys for the defendant physician, I might be considered to be working on the 'opposite side of the case' from you. We need to have that clear before we start. If you have any questions, please ask them now."

Alternatively, if the clinician were working for the evaluee/plaintiff's side, that would also be conveyed. Experience dictates that clarity should be achieved at the outset that this does not necessarily mean that the clinician's opinion will mirror the subject's.

b. Factors contributing to confusion over agency

Even with a conscientious effort made to apprise the subject that the evaluation does not have therapeutic ends and that the evaluator will not necessarily arrive at favorable findings, subjects often slip back into a therapeutic mindset. There are a number of reasons for this.

Regression. Except for persons with antisocial personality disorder and those overly familiar with the court system, the stress of being involved with the courts, whether one is mentally ill or not, may promote a regressive eagerness to find someone to be of help or to confide in; this attitude, of course, contributes to formation of a sound working alliance in customary treatment but may pose a problem where the subject's openness may yield evidence damaging (in the sense of self-incriminating) in court.

Transference. In concert with regression, transference operates ubiquitously, whatever the official parameters of the relationship. The mentally ill person sent for evaluation may turn to the evaluator as parent, lawyer, savior, advocate, ally, or simply "my clinician"; in doing so, the subject may draw upon the images of figures from the past and consciously or unconsciously transfer feelings associated with them onto the present evaluator. Insofar as the evaluator does not in fact serve any of those roles, these images are unrealistic.

While such a process is both inevitable and not really preventable, its operation should be taken into account by the conscientious clinician in formulating her true posture in relation to the subject. How challenging the matter can be is illustrated in this example:

> *Example 2:* A psychiatrist employed by an organization always told his interviewees that what they told him would *not* be kept confidential from the organization; he noticed, however, that interviewees seemed to reveal more when told this. He realized that his frankness, though ethically required, was acting as a "seduction" to candor by conveying openness and honesty.

Countertransference.   As in the second case example at the beginning of this chapter, the evaluator may become personally involved—positively or negatively—with the patient, the alleged crime, or some aspect of the system or question at hand. The homosexual defendant evaluated by a clinician who is also a gay rights activist, the rapist evaluated by a clinician who has been raped, or the defendant assessed for criminal responsibility by an evaluator who doesn't believe in the insanity defense—all represent areas of possible contamination of objectivity that may be sensed by the subject, who may then respond as if the evaluator is or is not "on my side."

2. AGENCY IN THE MIXED EVALUATION/TREATMENT MODEL

Notwithstanding the desirability of distinguishing between treatment and evaluation roles, situations may arise in which these roles become blurred together or merged.

a. Inpatient criminal forensic evaluations

Dealing with conflicts in agency.   Criminal forensic evaluations are often performed on an inpatient basis in state mental facilities. When this occurs, the facility is charged with the responsibility of both conducting the evaluation and treating a psychotic, depressed, or otherwise disordered patient. When staff time is at a premium, as is commonly the case, there is a temptation to ask the treating clinician to serve also as evaluator, the assumption being that time will thereby be conserved.

This is a problematic situation. The newly admitted defendant is being asked to confide, for treatment purposes, in the same person from whom she may have a right to withhold information, lest it be used to her detriment. (E.g., information gathered during this inpatient evaluation may later be introduced in court at the time of sentencing, affecting the nature and severity of the punishment inflicted on the defendant.) Even if the evaluee/patient is able to distinguish between the two roles filled by the clinician, there may be no way for her to resolve the conflicting messages the clinician conveys concerning the desirability of disclosure.

The optimal means of dealing with this situation is to split the clinical and evaluative roles, assigning one person to treat the patient and another to examine the evaluee. Information communicated to the treating clinician ideally should not be shared with the evaluating clinician, although that degree of separation may be difficult to accomplish in an inpatient facility in which patients become well known to all members of the staff.

What if this solution is not feasible, e.g., the only clinician qualified to treat the patient is also the only one available to perform the evaluation? The Code of Ethics of the American Psychological Association proscribes such approaches, while the comparable document of the American Psychiatric Association is silent on the issue. It is likely that these situations will occur in practice, regardless of the positions taken by professional organizations. Should they come about, the clinician embedded in them should attempt as clearly as possible to explain his dual role to the defendant—not a satisfactory solution, but perhaps the only one available. The clinician might say, "What you tell me will not necessarily be kept confidential from the court, since I am working for them in doing this evaluation. With that reservation, however, I will try to be as helpful as I can."

Effects on treatment.   The confusion of agency inherent in this situation may also affect the treatment the patient/evaluee receives. Because patients sent from the court must be admitted regardless of actual clinical indications, treatment staff may resent their helplessness to influence the process. The glib psychopath who has convinced a judge he is "mental"; the alleged murderer, rapist, or child molester; and the moderately mentally ill defendant who would not be sick enough to be admitted on purely clinical grounds—the presence of all these on the ward may evoke in staff feelings of resentment and the sense of being inappropriately "used" by the court.

This attitude may be intensified by the feeling that the patient is "not like our usual type of patient." This latter view may be appropriate (e.g., for the malingering psychopath) or inappropriate (e.g., for the sizable number of truly mentally ill persons who arrive on a court paper) but seems to derive in part from the sense of the patient's "belonging" to the court. Inexperienced staff members may employ this altered agency to justify a "hands off" policy toward the patient, preventing them from engaging him in treatment and leading essentially to rejection of the patient. The burden falls on supervisory staff to redirect attention to the patient's needs and to the requirements of the task at hand.

When a patient is accused of a dramatic, violent, perverse, or unusual crime, clinical staff may react to or recoil from the patient (sent on a court paper) as if she were already guilty, i.e., convicted, even though that adjudication remains in the future. The patient, of course, may turn out not to be the criminal in question; even if caught "red-handed," the patient may not be clinically any different from other patients whose illnesses are uncomplicated by criminal involvements. Thus, "preconviction" may deprive the patients of careful attention and objective assessment of their actual state. Again, the remedies are supervisory and consultative in nature.

b. Outpatient forensic evaluations

Dealing with the conflicts in agency.   Even more common than the dilemmas created by inpatient forensic evaluations are the problems that arise in the outpatient setting. Clinicians who are treating patients will frequently be asked to evaluate them for a variety of forensic purposes. Patients in treatment may request assessments of their ability to care for their children, their ability to work, the emotional harm they suffered from an accident, or even their competence to stand trial. The common assumption is that the treating clinician is privy to the information required to respond to all of these questions by virtue of previous therapeutic contact.

The problems of mixed agency are as troubling here as in the inpatient setting. In addition, the necessity for the clinician to reveal her opinions concerning the patient's diagnosis, functional state, and the like, as well as the possibility that the clinician's opinion will not be favorable to the patient/subject, are likely to interfere with subsequent therapy. Furthermore, given the specialized nature of the data that are required to answer forensic evaluation questions, the underlying assumption that the clinician will, as a matter of course, already possess the needed information may well be false.

Again, the best solution is to refer the patient for evaluation by another mental health professional. And again, this will not always be possible, particularly when administrative agencies require evaluation by the treating clinician.

Practitioners in this situation will do best to discuss the problem thoroughly with their patients, preparing them especially for unexpected or negative opinions.

The nature of the subject's claim on the clinician's loyalty is complicated by the previous relationship in which the subject has purchased the clinician's services and, presumably, allegiance. In this new situation, the evaluee may confuse this with being purchaser of the clinician's viewpoint; in consequence a subject may expect, in effect, to dictate the result of the evaluation by "my" therapist-evaluator.

> *Example 3:* Asked to evaluate a patient's fitness as custodian for a child, a therapist declined to take either a pro or con position, explaining that he had never directly observed the patient in a childcare situation nor had he any access to sources of data on this point other than the patient's own (subjective) report. The patient became enraged, shouting, "I'm the one that's paying you, you're supposed to be on *my* side."

As the above example hints, the patient is not alone in experiencing the private practice version of the tensions inherent in altered agency. For the clinician deriving her livelihood from the patient's fees, the economic pressure to "give the patients what they want" can be considerable.

Although the matter becomes focused with greater intensity in the forensic situation, the issues are no different in substance from other kinds of pressures—personal, social, political, or economic—tending to corrupt the therapeutic position. The ethically concerned clinician calls the situation as she sees it on clinical grounds, selling only her skills in evaluation, not her conclusions (see Chapter 8, Sec. II-C).

Effects on treatment.   A variety of consequences may ensue for an ongoing relationship that has experienced this alteration but then reverts to a treatment contract after the evaluation has been completed and the court satisfied. It is not infrequently the case that patient and therapist find it difficult to return to their former footing.

If, for example, the clinician has merely "cleared" the patient to drive a car, little strain on the alliance should result. The strain would increase if the findings resulted in loss of license, loss of child custody, and the like; Case Example 2 in Chapter 1 gives such an illustration.

The clinician has little tactical alternative but to treat the phase of altered agency as yet another event in therapy, with both objective and subjective elements suitable for therapeutic exploration, and as a shared experience that had an impact on both members of the dyad. The therapist's subsequent consistency in maintaining neutrality as the agent of the patient may make it possible for the treatment process to resume its customary evolution.

B. Performing the forensic evaluation

The following brief descriptions of approaches to specific forensic evaluations are designed to provide an overview for clinicians unfamiliar with them. More detailed guides to performing many of these evaluations can be found in the Suggested Readings, including attempts to devise structured assessment instruments. The Action Guide to this chapter contains suggested outlines for reporting the results of criminal and civil evaluations.

1. APPROACHES TO THE EVALUATION OF COMPETENCE TO STAND TRIAL

The McGarry Competence Assessment Instrument, described earlier in section II-A-3-a and cited in the Suggested Readings, represents an outline of critical issues in competence assessment. The following guidelines may help to convert this set of variables into a clinically efficient interview that has a logical flow and maximizes the examinee's performance on the evaluation. For each of the criteria given in the headings, a set of sample questions is offered that might be asked of the interviewee. The wording should, of course, be adapted to the personal style of the examiner and the examinee's linguistic, cultural, or intellectual idiosyncrasies.

a. Informed consent

"We are talking today because I've been asked by the court to write a letter evaluating your ability to stand trial. You should be aware, therefore, that the purpose of our discussion is for me to be able to give my opinion to the court, not particularly to decide how you will be treated. You don't have to talk with me if you don't want to and you don't have to answer any particular questions, but if you do, it will make it easier for me to give the court an accurate picture of your ability to stand trial. You can talk with your lawyer first if you like. Keep in mind that anything you tell me will not necessarily be confidential, so you shouldn't tell me anything that you would not want the court to find out. Do you have any questions? Can I go ahead and ask *you* some questions?"

b. General level of function; establishment of rapport

"Can you tell me how you happened to come here?"

c. Appreciation of the charges

If the examinee in response to question b above does not indicate admission was related to court proceedings, but indicates that he is being evaluated for treatment, or is present to take care of the other examinees, to do research, to learn how to be a doctor, or to save the world, the examiner at this point should correct these impressions in some manner like the following.

"I understand that you were sent here by the court or brought here by the police. Can you tell me what it is they are accusing you of having done?"

Examinees occasionally will completely deny having done anything. Needless to say, it is fruitless to attempt to discuss an event that, allegedly, has not occurred. Thus, some time may be required to clarify that the examiner's job is neither to indict nor to exonerate, and that he is, at this time, not actually concerned with what was done, but merely with the examinee's understanding of the charges, whether true or false. Efforts should be made to see if the examinee can make this distinction.

d. Appreciation of range and nature of possible penalties

"I don't know what the court or the law is going to do in this situation, but if, for example, the court finds you guilty of having done [specify charges], do you know what they could do to you? What are some of the sentences you could get? What could the judge make you do?"

If the response to this line of inquiry is inadequate, it is acceptable to ask specifically about the possibility of prison, fine, probation, and the like or—as in other competence assessments—to perform some educational efforts in clarifying sentencing procedure and then asking for the examinee's predictions. This will also convey a sense of whether the examinee grasps the relative seriousness of the crime.

e. Ability to appraise likely outcomes

"What do you think is the most likely thing to happen when you get to court? What do you think will actually happen if you are found guilty? Do you think they might find you not guilty?"

f. Capacity to disclose to attorney available pertinent facts

"Could you describe for me exactly the things that happened just before you were arrested? What was going on that led to the police getting involved?"

It is understandable that the interviewee may refuse to respond to this phase of the questioning, since this portion of the story could readily be incriminating; indeed, the examinee may have been explicitly instructed by his attorney not to discuss the offense. The examiner might respond:

"I can understand your not wanting to talk with me about what happened (I can understand your attorney telling you not to discuss what happened), but do you think you'll be able to discuss these things with your attorney? Have you been able to do that so far?"

g. Ability to appraise legal defenses available

"How do you intend to plead when they ask you if you plead guilty or not? Has your attorney given you any suggestions about this?"

If the response to this is inadequate, ask specifically about guilty, not guilty, NGRI, and other possible pleas.

h. Level of unmanageable behavior

This assessment is usually made on the basis of clinical observation of the examinee in the office or, for inpatient evaluations, on the ward. Some determination of the examinee's ability to control impulses or to remain silent when urged to do so would be most relevant here. In some circumstances, however, direct questions may be useful in this regard.

"Do you think you'll be able to control your behavior in court? I noticed in the group therapy meeting your tendency to shout out when you didn't like what people were saying. Since that could get you into difficulty, do you think you'll be able not to do that in court?"

i. Quality of relating to attorney

"Have you met your lawyer yet? (if so) Do you think you'll be able to work with him/her? Does he/she seem like the kind of person you could cooperate with in this work? (if not) Do you think in general you would be able to work with an attorney? Have you done so in the past?"

j. Planning of legal strategy

"I don't know what's really going to happen, but let's just say that your lawyer told you that he didn't think you stood a chance of being found innocent, but that if you pled guilty he could make a deal with the D.A. to get you off with only a suspended sentence. Could you go along with that? Why? What do you have to gain, what do you have to lose?"

Both affirmative and negative responses may be reasonable here, depending on the circumstances. Attorneys regrettably occasionally fall far short of their duties to inform their clients of the full spectrum of possibilities here and some probing for the examinee's awareness of these issues may be extremely useful, as may some explicit teaching to remedy deficiencies in this area.

k. Ability to appraise the roles of various participants in court

"Have you ever been in court before? (this provides the background necessary for interpreting subsequent responses). Can you tell me what the job of each of these people is in court? The defense attorney, the prosecuting attorney, the judge, the jury, the witness? Do you know the meaning of the oath?"

l. Understanding of court procedure

"Do you know which side presents its case first in court? What happens next? What does it mean when people call witnesses?"

m. Capacity to challenge witnesses

"Let's just say that one of the policemen who arrested you is testifying on the stand and says that you did something that you knew you didn't do; what would you do about it? What else might you do?"

n. Capacity to testify relevantly

This criterion is usually ascertainable from the interview as a whole and, in the case of inpatient evaluation, from more longitudinal observations by clinical staff. Sometimes, however, it will be useful to ask the interviewee directly about the possibilities.

"Do you think you'll be able to tell your side of the story in a crowded courtroom, with the judge staring at you and the prosecutor asking sharp questions? Do you feel that if the attorneys pressure you a bit, that you'll be able to keep your cool?"

o. Manifestation of self-serving vs. self-defeating motivation

Again, this will often be evident from either the statements the interviewee has made in response to earlier questions or from contemporary observations on the inpatient unit. Most commonly depressive guilt is the significant pitfall here, since individuals charged with crimes or incarcerated would experience normal depression even without preexisting illness.

"If you could pick the result you wanted, how would you like to see this all end up? What do you think would be the best outcome?"

p. Interviewer responses

In the face of inadequate responses to sections c,d,e,g,k,l, and m, the interviewer should make an attempt to educate the interviewee in all relevant areas. Follow-up questions should then assess the examinee's educability. At times, the teaching and reassessment should occur on repeat evaluations over time, since some examinees will be in the process of gradual recovery from psychotic states.

q. Assessment

Significant impairments due to mental disease or defect on more than one question (or the interviewee's inability to be educated concerning more than one question) should raise substantial doubt about the defendant's competence to stand trial. Moderate impairments on several questions should have a similar effect. The interviewer should keep in mind that the attorney's role is often pivotal in this situation and that various legal strategic decisions (such as not having the examinee testify at all) may compensate fully and appropriately for minor defects in the sophistication of the examinee's grasp of courtroom issues.

2. APPROACHES TO THE EVALUATION OF CRIMINAL RESPONSIBILITY

In performing this evaluation, it is important to recall the intrinsic difference from the examination for competence to stand trial. The latter examination is like a snapshot; the clinician need only know what the actual charges are and something about the subject's clinical history to perform a reasonable assessment of her competence to stand trial. Criminal responsibility, on the other hand, is like a movie, which may begin as early as childhood and should capture a longitudinal view of the examinee, embracing the totality of the examinee's clinical history (with continuing focus, of course, on the period immediately surrounding the alleged crime).

The initial steps of attaining informed consent are similar to those for competence to stand trial. The examinee's capacity to understand the warning about non-confidentiality becomes critical here, since in describing material related to the alleged crime, the examinee confronts directly material likely to lead to self-incrimination, and which in some jurisdictions may be susceptible to subpoena by the prosecution, even if elicited by an examiner for the defense. Any question about the examinee's competence to understand this aspect of the warning requires immediate termination of the interview and consultation with the defense attorney.

Once acceptable consent has been obtained, the examinee should be interviewed in great detail concerning her behavior on the day of the alleged crime and all relevant mental states, as well as matters impinging on mental state (intoxication, medications, fatigue, sleep disturbance, etc.). Detailed descriptions from contemporaneous observers, including statements of victims, bystanders, arresting officers, and family members must be obtained for external corroboration, since the heart of this forensic evaluation is its transcendence of the examinee's unsupported self-report (see Sec. e below). The examiner should review this material, whenever possible, prior to assessing the defendant.

Particular attention obviously should be paid to assessment of conditions that are most likely to impair the understanding or appreciation of the nature and/or wrongfulness of one's acts and to impair the ability to control one's behavior. Typical examples of these conditions include: dementia; delirium; grandiose, persecutory or other paranoid delusions; command hallucinations; moderate to severe mental retardation; psychomotor epilepsy; and dissociative states, as well as intoxications of various kinds (though the latter are usually not considered exonerating if voluntarily attained).

In addition to these determinations, the examiner should elicit a full clinical history from the defendant, as is usually done in the treatment context. This should include personal, social, psychiatric, and medical histories, as well as a current mental status examination. The examiner should compare the defendant's responses to questions concerning mental status at the time of the alleged crime with expected responses based on his total evaluation of the examinee. Allowance must be made for significant time lapse between examination and crime.

Clinicians should investigate specifically the areas of mental functioning at the time of the crime that are relevant to the standard of criminal responsibility used in that jurisdiction. (See Sec. II-B-2 above.)

a. M'Naghten test

The examinee should be interviewed to determine his understanding of the nature and wrongfulness of the criminal act. Issues of wrongfulness are usually focused on the legalistic sense of the concept (i.e., wrong means illegal), but some jurisdictions focus on the broader concept (i.e., wrong means morally wrong). The defendant who says, "Murder is wrong, but killing an agent of the devil is right," poses special problems for the fact finder when the narrower test is applied.

b. Irresistible impulse test

Assessment focuses on ability to control behavior. This is a sensitive and complex evaluation since, as the APA position statement on the insanity defense noted, "The line between an irresistible impulse and an impulse unresisted is probably no sharper than the line between twilight and dusk." To be considered irresistible in many jurisdictions, an impulse need not be sudden. A person who ruminates for months about a delusional perception of malevolence by a colleague at work, until he can no longer control the impulse to retaliate, may still qualify for this plea. When successful pleas are made under this test, they usually involve mental disorders that induce a subjective sense of loss of volitional control, including psychotic disorders with command hallucinations and delusions, dissociative disorders, and anxiety disorders.

c. ALI standard

This standard differs from the M'Naghten test, in part, in that it seeks not mere understanding or knowledge but appreciation of the wrongfulness of the criminal act. Here, affective components that may cloud a persons' judgment may be highly relevant. Note that only substantial incapacity, not a total lack of appreciation, is required. The same is true for the examinee's ability to control her behavior. But a defendant choosing not to control behavior or seeing no reason to control behavior does not manifest the requisite "substantial incapacity" to control behavior.

d. Federal insanity standard

For this hybrid standard, applicable in federal jurisdictions, the examiner must assess the ability to appreciate the nature and quality or the wrongfulness of the act.

e. Role of "outside observers" of the crime

Whenever possible, the clinician should make every effort to contact and interview others who have witnessed the events in question. Particular attention should be paid to the elements of corroboration and disconfirmation supplied by these other sources; efforts should be made to correlate witnesses' accounts of the examinee's behavior with the examinee's self-report. Whenever possible, as well, family members or significant others should be interviewed to ascertain their observations of the examinee's behavior shortly before, during, or after the events in question. The clinician's diligent search for such data may assist to some degree in minimizing the effect of the major inherent problem in this assessment, namely, the fact that it is performed retrospectively, often considerably later in time, by an evaluator who was not an eyewitness to the events in question.

3. APPROACHES TO THE EVALUATION OF TESTAMENTARY CAPACITY

Foremost among the difficulties in performing an assessment of an individual's testamentary capacity is the fact that in the usual case he is already dead. (Some testators, however, anticipating a challenge to the validity of their will, may request a competence evaluation at the time they endorse their will to make later attempts to overturn their disposition of their property more difficult.) The evaluator is forced to speculate on the basis of such information as may be available from written materials and the testimony of friends and relatives (who may be far from disinterested) as to the deceased's mental state. (See Sec. II-C-1 for a discussion of the relevant legal standards.) In many cases it simply will be impossible to draw a reasoned clinical forensic opinion from the available data. Even when reports exist of flagrant symptomatology, the conclusion that the symptoms directly influenced the action of the deceased in writing the will as she did can never be reported in anything but probabilistic terms. Any attempt to draw firmer conclusions leaves the clinician open to devastating cross-examination.

As with other forensic determinations (see Sec. II-A-3-b), the question of whether the examiner should attempt to answer the ultimate question rather than merely to report the clinical findings will arise here and in the evaluations considered subsequently in this section. The pressures will be great, but again they should be resisted in favor of leaving the drawing of legal conclusions to the court.

4. APPROACHES TO THE EVALUATION OF COMPETENCE TO CONTRACT

Since the signing of the contract generally occurred at a time far removed from the challenge, the examining clinician is once again faced with the problem of determining an individual's mental status retrospectively. However, unlike the case of evaluation of testamentary capacity, the alleged incompetent is still alive and available for examination. In this respect, the evaluation is not much different from that for criminal responsibility (see Sec. 2 above), with its attendant problems, except that this evaluation might be called an assessment of civil responsibility. A good lawyer for the party requesting the examination will guide the evaluator through the legal requirements that are specific to that jurisdiction, enabling him to focus his examination on the most relevant aspects of the individual's mental state. (See Sec. II-C-2 for a discussion of the relevant legal issues.)

5. APPROACHES TO THE EVALUATION OF EMOTIONAL HARMS

Assessment of emotional harm requires attention to several issues related to the legal standards (see Sec. II-C-3). A thorough psychiatric evaluation is in order, similar to the kind of work-up that would be undertaken for a patient entering treatment. In addition, particular attention should be paid to the evaluee's mental state as it existed prior to the alleged tortious act and since that time. The plaintiff need not meet diagnostic criteria for a particular mental disorder to recover for emotional distress, although the existence of a clear-cut diagnosis probably enhances the chances of a favorable verdict.

Some conclusions must be drawn in these cases about the causal relationship between the alleged tortious act and the plaintiff's subsequent mental condition. Post-traumatic stress disorder (PTSD) has become a popular and controversial diagnosis in these cases, since it (along with adjustment disorders) is one of the few diagnostic categories that carries with it the implication that symptoms are related to a particular event.

Preexisting mental disorder can lead to especially difficult evaluative problems. Since compensation is available only for disability caused or precipitated by the tortious act, the question of what caused the ultimate emergence or worsening of psychiatric symptoms is important to the evaluation. Yet the connection between environmental stresses and subsequent mental disorder is a controversial one and, in the individual case, may be impossible to ascertain. Clinicians must be wary of going beyond their expertise in this area.

Given the financial rewards available to the successful plaintiff, malingering must always be considered. Careful attention must be paid to the consistency of the subject's report, both internally and with known psychiatric syndromes. As in the criminal realm, corroboration of reports by third parties, including family, friends, neighbors, co-workers, and supervisors (though each of these may have interests of their own in the outcome) can be crucial, as can review of documentary evidence such as evaluations of work performance.

Evaluators whose findings are favorable to the side employing them can expect to be asked to write detailed reports of their findings, to be deposed by the opposing side, and to testify at trial.

6. APPROACHES TO THE EVALUATION OF MENTAL DISABILITY

a. Workers' compensation

As with all disability evaluations, the workers' compensation assessment differs from the ordinary clinical evaluation in requiring focal attention to functional, not merely symptomatic, issues. (See Sec. II-C-4 above for a discussion of the relevant legal standards.) A full assessment requires a description of the onset of the mental disorder and its connection to the work environment, documentation of the subject's current mental state, some prognostic judgment, and evaluation of the impact of the subject's symptoms on his functional capacity. The importance of this last element cannot be overemphasized, since it is the key to the disability determination process. Given the well-known lack of correlation between diagnosis and functional state, the existence of a psychiatric disorder, even of some severity, does not by itself establish disability. Only a consideration of the evaluee's actual abilities can address that issue.

Functional capacity can be estimated by careful history-taking regarding the subject's daily activities, including those related to meeting basic needs, handling money, managing interpersonal relationships, and recreation. Recent attempts to work, or efforts at performing in work-like situations, are especially relevant.

The workers' compensation evaluation also raises issues of the veracity of the evaluee's reports that are much more salient than in the ordinary clinical situation, in which rewards for exaggerating symptomatology are usually less prominent. Precautions similar to those suggested for emotional distress evaluations should be observed. (See Sec. 5 above.) As compensation is dependent on demonstrating a causal link between an occurrence at work and subsequent disability, this issue must be carefully considered. Needless to say, familiarity with the requirements of the law in each clinician's jurisdiction, especially with regard to proving causation, should be assured prior to undertaking the evaluation.

b. Social Security disability insurance

Unlike workers' compensation evaluations, assessments of SSDI eligibility need not address causal factors (see Sec. II-C-4-b). Diagnosis is important, since SSA guidelines begin by inquiring into whether specified disorders are present. Reports should include sufficient detail concerning symptoms to allow corroboration of the diagnosis in the review process. Standard DSM criteria should be employed. A description of the history and current status of the mental disorder must be followed by consideration of the disorder's impact on the evaluee's ability to function at work. This should be structured to address the four areas specified by the regulations, as noted above (see Sec. II-C-4-b). Since the subject's residual functional capacity may become an issue in the review of her claim, data addressing the areas identified by SSA as relevant to this concept should also be included: understanding and memory, sustained concentration and persistence, social interaction, and adaptation. Documentation of the existence of disability over a 12-month period, or a prognostic statement concerning its likely duration for that period in the future should also be included. The American Psychiatric Association has developed useful guidelines for the presentation of SSDI evaluations (see Suggested Readings).

C. Technical considerations

1. INTRUSIONS ON THE PRIVACY OF THE FORENSIC EXAMINATION

Clinicians agree that the forensic examination is best done with patient and clinician alone together, absent concerns for the clinician's physical safety. However, occasionally requests are made to have other individuals (most commonly the patient's attorney, but sometimes another person) present or participating in the evaluation.

> ***Example 4:*** A female patient bringing suit for boundary violations and sexual misconduct by a previous therapist was being evaluated by the defense's male forensic expert. Not only was the session videotaped, but a request was made and granted that the patient's present female therapist be in the room during the evaluation to increase the patient's comfort. It was agreed, however, that the patient's therapist would sit back out of camera range and thus be unable to signal or otherwise communicate with the patient. The interview proceeded in a reasonable manner.

As many forensic practitioners can attest, however, there may be considerable problems with an attorney or other third party being present during a forensic examination. Interviewees may tend to "play to" the third party, "pitching" their material to advance their cause and "make their case." Alternatively, the third party, especially a lawyer, may interrupt the evaluation or attempt to influence the subject's responses. The interviewee's consequent manner of relating may lower the reliability of the interview.

This point seems so important as to require reiteration on each occasion that an attorney assumes that having an attorney present for the interview represents a "cost free" way of protecting due process rights. At least one court (*U.S. v. Byers*) has agreed.

The use of recording devices in the evaluation raises similar issues, but experienced forensic evaluators differ on the magnitude of their impact. Some clinicians routinely record all their evaluations, as a check on the reliability of their conclusions. Others believe that audiotaping or videotaping an assessment inevitably contaminates the evaluee's responses. Some empirical data have been generated on this question, but they are not conclusive. At this point, it is most reasonable to suggest that each evaluator follow the practices with which she is most comfortable, since that is likely to increase the skill with which she can perform the evaluation.

2. WRITING THE EVALUATION REPORT

In many jurisdictions specific questions or criteria are delineated for the forensic assessment at issue. In such cases the clinician's report should narrowly address those criteria with specific evidence from the evaluations. Some critical principles to keep in mind in reporting findings to the court are:

a. the importance of identifying the data bases and sources from which the information was derived and the evaluator's assessment of the reliability of those sources.

b. the need to qualify findings appropriately (e.g. difficulty of retrospective assessment; uncooperativeness of the defendant; conflicting statements of eyewitnesses; etc.).

c. the value of keeping a focus on the clinical findings, with the ultimate question of, say, criminal responsibility being left to the court. The sample reports in the Action Guide (See Sec. VI) provide models for the task.

3. REVIEW OF FINDINGS WITH THE EVALUEE

Although the evaluator is not the subject's agent, there are sound clinical reasons for going over the conclusions with her; some clinicians actually read the report to the subject; others discuss the findings more generally. This manner of including the subject in a process to which she is all too often a bewildered bystander demonstrates an ethical concern for the subject consistent with high standards of practice. The clinician should explain any areas that are unclear to the subject if asked to do so. The subject's agreement or disagreement should be listened to respectfully, but should not, of course, influence or alter the findings.

While a clinician may feel some trepidation concerning being the "bearer of bad tidings," this open approach is desirable because it includes the subject as a responsible participant in the process, regardless of agency. Additionally, such anticipatory discussion may protect the subject somewhat from traumatic effects of hearing the material in a public court room for the first time without preparation (see Suggested Readings—Strasburger).

D. Assessment of malingering

One of the most fundamental differences between clinical and forensic assessment is highlighted by the problem of malingering. The clinician treating a patient in therapy must always begin by attempting to see the world through the patient's eyes—non-critically, non-challengingly, non-judgmentally. A patient's description—of his insensitive boss, her sadistic parents, his unresponsive wife, her ungrateful children—should always be taken first at face value. The treating clinician must attempt empathically to adopt the patient's world view as her own.

In contrast, the forensic expert must always assume that an examinee may cherish covert goals, under the general rubric of "secondary gain," which inevitably attend most forensic evaluations. The defendant charged with a heinous crime may find it very much in his interests to be found incompetent to stand trial, thus postponing time in court until the memories of witnesses fade; or to be found criminally non-responsible, since prolonged hospitalization, though far from a picnic, may be more comfortable than prolonged incarceration in prison. The forensic expert appropriately questions every element of the data and remains attuned to the need for corroboration from external sources—the more unbiased and disinterested, the better. In sum, the treating clinician doing his job is credulous; the forensic expert doing her job is skeptical.

Malingering refers to the deliberate and conscious simulation of symptoms, disorders, or incapacities that are not authentic; this could be termed "clinical lying." The importance of this issue has generated a small literature (see Suggested Readings) whose rudiments should be familiar to forensic clinicians. While the subject cannot be treated exhaustively here, knowledge of some common characteristics of malingering may be helpful to the forensic evaluator.

1. CONTEMPORANEOUS DISCONFIRMATION OF CLAIMED SYMPTOMS OR BEHAVIOR

A defendant may claim to have been in a complete mental fog during the commission of a particular alleged crime. The testimony of contemporary witnesses, however, may portray this defendant as having evinced clarity and decisiveness, and as having made attempts to conceal evidence of the crime, as well as efforts to escape apprehension.

2. "THE WORDS BUT NOT THE MUSIC"

Students of malingering frequently look for evaluees' verbal subscription to symptoms without manifestations of the ordinarily attendant behavior. Thus, an evaluee claiming psychotic symptoms characteristic of schizophrenia may yet be perfectly cheerful, amicable and easy in relationships with evaluators and staff— a mode of relating usually inconsistent with that disorder.

3. SUBSCRIPTION TO ATYPICAL ENTITIES

Just as hysterical conversion symptoms often reflect a layperson's perception of neurology (and thus display glove or stocking anesthesia, findings inconsistent with actual denervation), so malingered psychotic symptoms may reflect laypersons' conceptions of psychopathology. Thus, individuals may endorse highly unusual or uncharacteristic symptomatology, as in a subject who responds affirmatively to the question, "Have you ever had the belief that automobiles are members of organized religion?"(example courtesy P. Resnick, M.D., and R. Rogers, Ph.D.).

4. INCONSISTENCY OF RESULTS

A subject may manifest, on mental status examination, a highly inconsistent picture, so that concentration, for example, appears high on one aspect of the mental status examination, yet low on another. Such inconsistency is especially meaningful where the disparity directly reflects the examinee's awareness of what is being tested for; thus, an examinee may be able to follow a reasonable conversation (showing concentration ability), but claim inability to perform even serial subtraction of 3's (a formal test of concentration).

While it is a truism that malingering should always be considered in every forensic examination, the diagnosis is, nevertheless, a stigmatizing one; hence, it should always be put forward with tact and respect for both the astonishing diversity of clinical conditions and the recognized limitations of available examination methods. Data emerging from the individual interview with the patient should always be augmented when possible with observations by other individuals (e.g., nursing staff for inpatient evaluations)—in particular, observations obtained when the individual is ostensibly unaware of being observed. Thus, the subject who appears catatonic and monosyllabic during an interview might be observed to be chatting amicably with an attractive patient of the opposite sex on the ward; such information should be correlated with the evaluator's opinion based on direct examination. Whenever possible, malingering should be an affirmative diagnosis, rather than merely a default position adopted when the evaluator is uncertain about the diagnosis or the assessment.

Structured instruments, including the MMPI, may be useful in detecting malingering in some cases (see Suggested Readings—Rogers).

IV. PITFALLS

A. Rescue

As in the second case example, for reasons deriving from the subject *or* clinician, the latter may misconceive her mandate as one that asks her to "rescue" the hapless subject from the grinding wheels of the uncaring judicial bureaucratic machine. While laudable in spirit, such an approach rarely does the subject an actual service and may interfere with the credibility and reliability of the forensic evaluation process, as well as with the smooth functioning of judicial due process for the subject's protection. The subject in such evaluations is best served by scrupulous care in the mandated determinations.

B. Reform

Inexperienced or overzealous clinicians, dismayed at the delay, duplicity, and entanglement of the criminal justice system, may misguidedly attempt to reform it through the medium of the court-ordered evaluation. One clinician-trainee, annoyed at "doing the court's dirty work" in evaluating defendants ostensibly referred for competence to stand trial evaluations, but really being sent for treatment and disposition, suggested finding *every* evaluee both competent and untreatable (regardless of their real condition) with the goal of flooding the courts with returned defendants without dispositions; such a move would allegedly force public attention to, and reform of, the failings of the judicial system.

Besides being naïve—judges are fully capable (and some are so disposed) of sending defendants en masse back to hospitals, ignoring all findings and recommendations—such an approach converts the evaluee into faceless cannon fodder hurled against nearly impregnable walls. The subject's individual situation must ever be the clinician's focus; on her own time, in political activism, or in the voting booth, the clinician should exert her efforts toward reform of the legal system by legislative remedies.

C. Requirement to make a finding

Clinicians asked to perform an assessment for criminal responsibility may be in danger of becoming preoccupied with the need to find relevant data to "make the case" for non-responsibility. It is essential to recall that the clinician is an objective observer who should hold himself apart from the defense attorney's unequivocal need to mount an insanity defense. The clinician should avoid feeling regret or even taking personal affront at the fact that the subject presents with some mild symptomatology of mental illness insufficient to meet local insanity criteria: this is not the clinician's problem. It is also fully defensible for the clinician to be unable to conclude unambiguously whether the subject does or does not meet criteria; subjects, after all, present with mixed clinical conditions—indeed, this is the rule in real life. Unambiguous cases either way, moreover, tend to be plea bargained out before clinicians ever become involved.

V. CASE EXAMPLE EPILOGUES

A. Case Example 1

The consultant pinpoints two areas of confusion that frequently arise with such referrals. First, the transfer from the criminal justice system to the psychiatric care system has been accomplished with minimal communication of relevant information. Second, both court and hospital appear to be confused about the purpose of the commitment. He urges the resident to contact the court directly, speaking first with the court clinic psychiatrist, then with the chief clerk, and if necessary with the judge to clarify the situation.

On calling the court clinic psychiatrist, the resident discovers that the case is quite complicated. The patient had indeed been arrested at the time of the crime more than a year previously. Because he was a first offender, however, his case was diverted before trial to an experimental program designed to rehabilitate rather than to punish those without previous criminal records. As part of his participation in this program, in exchange for which the charges against him were not prosecuted but were left pending, the patient was required to engage in outpatient psychiatric treatment in a community clinic and was required to take medication. He did this for a short period of time, but for the last two months he again had not taken his medication and had been missing his clinic appointments. His mother called the police when she felt that she could no longer take care of him and feared that, because of his wandering through the streets, he might be harmed.

The court, the psychiatrist confides, is not in the least interested in this patient's competence or criminal responsibility. Having diverted him from trial initially, they do not intend to prosecute him now. Rather, they have used the statute empowering them to order the pretrial hospitalization of defendants with pending charges as a means of getting the patient treated. If he has not recompensated by the end of the 20-day period, the court is willing to recommit him for an additional 20 days, as the statute empowers them to do, so that treatment can continue.

When this information is conveyed to the forensic consultant, he tells the resident that this is not an unusual state of affairs. Courts in this jurisdiction frequently use their powers to commit defendants who are genuinely in need of treatment under the only statute that they have available for the purpose, namely, the law covering competence and responsibility examinations. He advises her to perform the requisite forensic examinations to comply with the precise terms of the court order, but otherwise to approach this patient's care as she would any other patient's: seek to establish an alliance, begin treatment with medication if the patient consents, and try to develop an ongoing treatment plan to prevent rehospitalization. While the consultant said that he recognized that some psychiatrists are uncomfortable undertaking the treatment of patients committed under statutes ostensibly designed to provide only for evaluation, he himself felt that every patient committed to his care deserved the best treatment that he could provide, assuming that they consented to it, regardless of what other tasks he was additionally required to perform with them.

B. Case Example 2

The hospital legal consultant ushers in the resident and, seeing her evident distress, pulls up a chair and thrusts a cup of coffee into her hand.

After hearing the story, the consultant asks, "Who are you working for?"

The resident blinks in surprise. "The patient, of course."

The consultant holds up an admonitory forefinger. "There's the problem." He continues by explaining that the resident in this situation is an agent of the court, in its employ. While this arrangement does not entail ignoring the patient's needs, it does mean acknowledging the primacy of the mandate to assess the patient in this highly specific way.

The resident listens thoughtfully. "I guess I overidentified with him; I so much wanted to help."

"You can," the consultant observes. "From your story he seems like a guy who would lose his cool in court; let's tell that to his lawyer from the Legal Aid group so she won't put him on the stand. That will genuinely help his case. Now, let's go up and do a formal competency exam together; then we can write the court letter and discuss our findings."

C. Case Example 3

Deciding that his task as forensic evaluator is to give the most valid and honest assessment possible, no matter what the outcome, the psychiatrist puts great effort into writing an extremely detailed report. This report meticulously reviews the history of pre-existing difficulties, the subject's marginal functioning at the best of times, the dubious causal relationship between the robbery and subsequent claimed harms, the subject's insistence to many caretakers (as documented in the record) that the incident at age nine was the wellspring of all the difficulties, and the fact that the subject has a chronic disorder of presumptively genetic origin.

He concludes that the causal link between the robbery and subsequent injuries is a specious one unsupported by the weight of the data, thus he cannot take the position that the robbery was the cause of subsequent harms. With marked trepidation he mails the report to the attorney.

When no word follows, the psychiatrist calls the attorney in question, this time reaching the attorney directly instead of the paralegal. The psychiatrist is apologetic about how ineffective, perhaps even damaging, his report would be in mounting a case on the subject issue. To his surprise, the attorney is completely unruffled by the thrust of the report. Indeed, he confesses, it is quite clear the case was not meritorious in the slightest; however, for client good will, he needs a report from a psychiatrist to reinforce his position, since the client tends to throw enormous tantrums in the legal offices when confronted or thwarted in his often grandiose goals for litigation. The attorney thanks the bemused doctor for his time, promises prompt payment and hangs up.

VI. ACTION GUIDE

A. General Considerations in Court-Ordered Evaluations

1. *Establish* clearly the question of agency in court-ordered evaluation.
   a. *Define* employment (court, not patient).
   b. *State* limits of confidentiality at outset.
   c. *Repeat* definition of a and b, if patient appears to be moving into "therapeutic" mind-set or interview pattern.
2. *Identify* specific parameters of the evaluation at hand according to statute or policy.
3. *Obtain* objective data from court or elsewhere against which to evaluate patient's remarks.
4. *Offer* optimal treatment during course of evaluation as accorded to other non-court-referred patients.
5. *Resist* contamination of objectivity by economic pressures, previous knowledge of the patient, attempts to "second-guess" the court, slanting the evaluation, pressure from the attorney.
6. *Limit* scope of predictive aspects of evaluation report to those areas within predictive capacity; *employ* a "double negative" (e.g., "no contrain-dications") when feasible.
7. *Review* findings with patient.
8. *Beware* of potential difficulties interfering with the evaluation:
   a. Resentment of inability to influence patient admission,
   b. Rejection of patient as "different,"
   c. "Pre-conviction" of patient.
9. *Consider* malingering in all cases.
10. *Supervise* clinicians on misuses of court-ordered evaluation as:
    a. Rescue of the patient as victim,
    b. Attempts at reform of court system at expense of considering the individual patient,
    c. "Requirement" of positive finding.

B. Sample Report Outline for Competence to Stand Trial Evaluations

1. IDENTIFYING DATA

This should contain basic demographics in the standard clinical sequence: the subject's full name, as well as any aliases employed, age, sex, marital status, race, religion, employment status, date of birth, and social security number. In the case of an inpatient evaluation, this section should include the admission date, admission history (number of previous admissions), the name of the referring court or jurisdiction, a precise statement of the charges in statutory language, the date(s) of the alleged criminal act, and a brief statement summarizing the alleged criminal incident. For example, if the official charge is "Assault with a deadly weapon," the description might illuminate this by indicating that "it is alleged that, as a result of an argument Mr. Jones repeatedly struck his father with a tire iron on May 5, 1986."

2. RELEVANT STATUTORY CRITERIA

This again represents standard prose drawn from the actual statute or case used in the local jurisdiction.

3. ISSUES RELATING TO INFORMED CONSENT

This section should record precisely what the subject was told about the nature and purpose of the examination, the role and function of the examiner, the usual absence of confidentiality, and the subject's right to refuse to participate or to answer questions. The subject's apparent understanding or lack of same should be noted here, along with his consent to participate, if given.

4. DATABASE

Here, one records any additional sources of information that may have been utilized in the assessment (such as psychological testing), as well as the number of interviews or total time spent with the subject during the process.

5. CLINICAL HISTORY

While one could argue that the "snapshot" of the subject needed for the competence evaluation renders this kind of material irrelevant, certain determinations—for example, the patient's need for a secure setting or for treatment during the evaluation—may well be helped by these data. In addition, the clinical history can help to support the evaluator's conclusions about the presence or absence of psychopathology. Some jurisdictions may require that such material be contained only in the criminal responsibility assessment. Two important elements to include here, if not elsewhere, are the subject's suicide risk (relevant to questions of incarceration) and the subject's previous experiences with the legal system, the latter directly relevant to the subject's competence to participate in the process.

6. HOSPITAL COURSE

For inpatient hospitalization, a summary of the subject's hospital treatment history and response, relevant clinical observations substantiating diagnosis, and similar material would be included in this section. A summary of the subject's current mental status should be explicitly identified here in detailed descriptive terms, since such material will be directly relevant to the ultimate opinion flowing from this assessment.

7. DATA RELEVANT TO COMPETENCE TO STAND TRIAL

This section is, of course, the heart of the report and should address the data relevant to the forensic question being asked, those functions that contribute to the defendant's understanding of the nature and object of courtroom proceedings and of the charges and his capacity to participate in his own defense by cooperating with the attorney. Attention should be paid to the subject's capacity to endure the stress of the trial as well as any contingencies that bear on this capacity, for example: "Patient requires continuing medication at present doses in order to be able to tolerate the stress of trial in a non-psychotic manner."

Remember that ignorance is never identical to incompetence. Since the issues relevant to this determination represent a capacity to deal with a process, the finding of incompetence should occur only when the subject has demonstrated repeated inability to be instructed about the relevant matters.

8. CONCLUSIONS

a. The patient's clinical state

This section describes the patient's illness, functioning, and treatment issues. Some jurisdictions require a formal DSM-III-R diagnosis; others may require merely a statement about the presence or absence of a mental illness or disorder.

b. Competence to stand trial

Here, attention to the question of whether to address the ultimate issue becomes paramount. Some clinicians merely describe the patient as meeting the required criteria (example: "The patient appears to have the ability to cooperate with the attorney in her defense") and avoid an actual statement about competence. Others, after describing the specific statutory capacities, indicate that the patient possesses abilities "consistent with competence to stand trial." Judges (who do answer the ultimate question) vary in the degree to which they wish to have the conclusion made explicit by the clinician. Some feel that without an actual statement about the patient's competence the report is meaningless; others feel pre-empted when the clinician goes beyond the factual components.

c. Sample Report Outline for Criminal Responsibility Evaluations

1. Identifying data:

Same as above for competence.

2. Statutory criteria for criminal responsibility in this jurisdiction:

Comparable to above.

3. Issues relevant to informed consent:

Comparable to above.

4. Database:

Comparable to above.

5. Clinical history:

In circumstances where the competence and criminal responsibility reports are filed simultaneously it is permissible to refer to the competence report to avoid needless repetition.

6. Subject's version of alleged criminal act(s):

Here, the subject's account, as nearly verbatim as possible, should be recorded regarding the relevant actions. This should include not only physical actions and behavior, but also the subject's own statement of the varying states of mind, thoughts, fantasies, perceptions and the like that exist contemporaneous with the actions. For completeness, the subject's hindsight view of the experiences in question should also be recorded, although, of course, this has no direct bearing on the state of mind at the time of the event.

7. Official version(s) of alleged criminal act(s):

In this section should be included police and other investigative agency reports; reports of witnesses, bystanders, victims, family members, significant others; and all other relevant and contemporaneous assessments of the subject that may exist, including clinical material if the subject was in some clinical setting at the time.

8. Hospital course:

Same as above, including detailed present mental status.

9. Criminal responsibility:

Here the forensic evaluator should attempt a retrospective reconstruction of the subject's mental state at the time of the criminal behavior in longitudinal context. If the subject was experiencing a short-term alteration of mental functioning, that should be described; if the subject's behavior occurred in the context of a long history of significant mental illness, that longitudinal history should be placed in perspective, as it may have led up to and affected the present alleged offense.

The clinician should remember at all times that her task is not to prove a point nor to portray the examinee as responsible or not responsible. This implies that the clinician's narrative will include material factually and completely, no matter which side of the "case" such material may support. Thus, the subject's delusional expressions (appearing to support insanity) as well as the subject's attempts at concealment of the crime (seeming to support sanity) are all relevant to the report. The task in essence is not to "sell" the subject's insanity or lack of same, but to present a comprehensive (but not necessarily consistent) picture focused on the relevant determinations so that the ultimate fact finder can make an informed decision.

Remember to include the subject's level of cooperation and participation in the examination, the presence or absence of external corroboration, both the subject's behavior and internal mental state, any difficulties you encounter in constructing a retrospective case, and even the subject's persistent denial of his participation in the crime at all.

10. Conclusions:

Here again, review the subject's clinical condition and address the opinion evidence in an austere and restrained manner. Avoid both wild speculation and overly confident statements such as "the defendant is clearly insane" or "the subject should be found criminally responsible (or not responsible)." Instead, provide a distillation of the material in such language as: "incapacity to understand the nature and quality of his actions," "consistent with statutory criteria" or "appear to be able to appreciate the wrongfulness of the conduct."

d. Sample Report Outline for Determination of Emotional Harms

1. Identifying data

Comparable to above demographic information

2. Statement of the claim

Here, instead of statutory criteria, one provides the forensic question being addressed in the evaluation, using the language of the formal claim. Example: "Emotional harms, damages, humiliation, public embarrassment, conscious distress and suffering resulting from being inappropriately and negligently searched for falsely alleged shoplifting while leaving department store."

3. Issues relating to informed consent

As above. It is particularly important to inform examinees if one is working for the "other side" of the case (i.e., the defense) since many examinees will receive multiple evaluations and may not be sensitized to potential adversarial issues. If the examiner is also the treating clinician, care should be taken to explain the shift in agency.

4. Database

Comparable to above. Typical ancillary sources used here include neurological, psychological, and neuropsychological testing; previous medical and psychiatric or other clinical records (essential to determine pre-existing conditions and worsening); and reports, interview data, and deposition material from relevant parties. Note also the amount of time spent with examinee. If one is the treating clinician, supply data about the treatment. Example, "Mr. Jones was seen in weekly psychotherapy beginning June 17, 1987 for complaints of anxiety and sleeplessness and was formally evaluated in addition for six interviews related to his claim."

5. Clinical history

Again, a longitudinal picture up through the present is required to place the alleged harm-causing incident into perspective as exacerbating or having no particular effect on any pre-existing or underlying processes; clinically significant negatives should be articulated when relevant. Examples:

—"Prior to the alleged incident, Mr. Smith had nightmares extremely rarely, ca. once or twice a year";

—"Ms. Green's social isolation and withdrawal, consistent with her underlying chronic undifferentiated schizophrenia, are described in a comparable manner in her hospital records";

—"Ms. Wilson's chronic timidity was markedly increased to a full-fledged phobia by the accident";

—"Mr. Johnson's previous combat experiences were revived in a retraumatizing way by the alleged incident."

6. **Previous treatment and/or hospitalizations (if any)**

Note responses to treatment, successful or unsuccessful, and any possible exacerbating effects of treatment attempts.

7. **Conclusions**

The summary of your opinions given here should follow from the above material in a coherent and comprehensible way. Since it is a basic maxim of tort law that "the defendant takes the plaintiff as he finds him," the presence or absence of emotional harms should be described in relation to any pre-existing conditions or vulnerabilities—or, for that matter, strengths and personal resources—of the examinee. Some estimate of relative severity should also be attempted.

Remember to distinguish among harms, trauma, damages, and disorders. The examiner should be open to the fact that not all traumas produce full-fledged post traumatic stress disorder; some produce other conditions (anxiety disorders, depressions, other reactions) that represent no less valid harms, and some traumas have few lasting effects. Recall also that not all alleged harmful incidents are true; be sure to assess and comment on possibilities of malingering or delusional material presented as real. Examples:

—"Mr. White's previous childhood experiences of public humiliation by his father rendered him particularly vulnerable to the humiliating effect of the public 'stop and frisk' at the shopping center";

—"Ms. Brown's twenty-year history of chronic schizophrenia makes it nearly impossible to define an increase in social withdrawal and isolation as a result of the incident";

—"In the absence of outside observers' reports I am simply unable to determine if Mr. Black's account of the alleged incident is delusional or not, particularly since vaguely similar experiences are noted as delusions in the records of his 1980 hospitalization";

—"Ms. Carpenter's inadvertent admission of being coached to simulate the 'startle response' raises a clear question of malingering of the alleged post-traumatic stress disorder";

—"Although having the plane in which he was flying break apart on landing would seem fairly traumatic to anyone, Mr. Olsen's rather stolid and unimaginative character appears on examination to have insulated him from most of the expected symptomatic effects."

8. **Treatment recommendations**

If indicated, suggest useful treatment modalities. Since the costs of remedial treatment are a significant factor in litigating emotional harms, supply an estimate (backed up, if possible, by empirical data in the literature) of the length, intensity (frequency), duration, and likely cost of such treatment.

VII. SUGGESTED READINGS

A. COMPETENCE TO STAND TRIAL

1. Grisso, T.: *Competency to Stand Trial Evaluations: A Manual for Practice.* Sarasota, FL, Professional Resource Exchange, 1988.

2. McGarry, A. L., Curran, W. J. Lipsitt, P. L., et al.: *Competency to Stand Trial and Mental Illness.* Rockville, MD, National Institute of Mental Health, 1973.

3. Golding, S. L., Roesch, R. & Schreiber, J.: Assessment and conceptualization of competency to stand trial: preliminary data on the Interdisciplinary Fitness Interview. *Law and Human Behavior* 9:321–334, 1984.

4. Roesch, R. & Golding, S. L.: *Competency to Stand Trial.* Urbana, IL, University of Illinois Press, 1980.

5. Steadman, H. J. & Hartstone, E.: Defendants incompetent to stand trial, in Monahan, J. & Steadman, H. J. (eds.), *Mentally Disordered Offenders: Perspectives From Law and Social Science.* New York, Plenum Press, 1983.

6. Steadman, H. J.: *Beating a Rap? Defendants Found Incompetent to Stand Trial.* Chicago, University of Chicago Press, 1979.

7. Geller, J. L. & Lister, E. D.: The process of criminal commitment for pretrial psychiatric examination: an evaluation. *Am. J. Psychiatry* 135:53–63, 1978.

8. Lamb, H. R.: Incompetency to stand trial: appropriateness and outcome. *Arch. Gen. Psychiatry* 44:754–758, 1987.

9. Melton, G., Weithorn, L. & Slobogin, C.: *Community Mental Health Centers and the Courts: An Evaluation of Community-Based Forensic Services.* Lincoln, NE, University of Nebraska Press, 1986.

10. Davis, D. L.: Treatment planning for the patient who is incompetent to stand trial. *Hosp. Community Psychiatry* 36:268–271, 1985.

11. Pendleton, L.: Treatment of persons found incompetent to stand trial. *Am. J. Psychiatry* 137:1098–1100, 1980.

12. Geller, J. & Appelbaum, P. S.: Competency to stand trial: neuroleptic medication and demeanor in court. *Hosp. Community Psychiatry* 36:6–7, 1985.

13. Gutheil, T. G. & Appelbaum, P. S.: "Mind control," "synthetic sanity," "artificial competence," and genuine confusion: legally relevant effects of antipsychotic medication. *Hofstra Law Review* 12:77–120, 1983.

14. Winick, B. J.: Restructuring competency to stand trial. *UCLA Law Review* 32:921–985, 1985.

B. CRIMINAL RESPONSIBILITY

1. Simon, R. J. & Aaronson, D. E.: *The Insanity Defense: A Critical Assessment of Law and Policy in the Post-Hinckley Era.* New York, Praeger, 1988.

2. Goldstein, A. S.: *The Insanity Defense.* New Haven, CT, Yale University Press, 1967.

3. Morris, N.: *Madness and the Criminal Law.* Chicago, University of Chicago Press, 1982.

4. Fingarette, H. & Hasse, A. F.: *Mental Disabilities and Criminal Responsibility.* Berkeley, University of California Press, 1979.

5. Bonnie, R. J.: The moral basis of the insanity defense. *American Bar Association Journal* 69:194–197, 1983.

6. Insanity Defense Work Group: American Psychiatric Association statement on the insanity defense. *Am. J. Psychiatry* 140:681–688, 1983.

7. Morris, N. & Bonnie, R.: Debate: Should the insanity defense be abolished? *Journal of Law and Health* 1:113–140, 1986-87.

8. Slovenko, R.: The meaning of mental illness in criminal responsibility. *J. Leg. Med.* 5:1–61, 1984.

9. Steadman, H. J.: Empirical research on the insanity defense. *Ann. Am. Acad. Pol. and Soc. Sci.* 477:58–71, 1985.

10. Rogers, J. L., Bloom, J. D. & Manson, S. M.: Insanity defenses: contested or conceded? *Am. J. Psychiatry* 141:885–888, 1984.

11. Callahan, L., Mayer, C. & Steadman, H. J.: Insanity defense reforms in the United States—Post-Hinckley. *Mental and Physical Disability Law Reporter* 11:54–59, 1987.

12. McGraw, B. D., Capowich, D. F. & Keilitz, I.: The "guilty but mentally ill" plea and verdict: current state of the knowledge. *Villanova Law Review* 30:117–191, 1985.

13. Morse, S. J.: Undiminished confusion in diminished capacity. *J. Crim. Law Criminol.* 75:1–55, 1984.

14. Rogers, R.: *Conducting Insanity Evaluations.* New York, Van Nostrand Reinhold, 1986.

15. Homant, R. J. & Kennedy, D. B.: Subjective factors in the judgment of insanity. *Crim. Just. Behav.* 14:38–61, 1987.

16. Dietz, P. E.: Why the experts disagree: variations in the psychiatric evaluation of criminal insanity. *Ann. Am. Acad. Pol. Soc. Sci.* 477:84–95, 1985.

C. CIVIL COMPETENCE EVALUATIONS

1. McGarry, A. L.: Psycholegal examinations and reports, in Curran, W. J., McGarry, A. L. & Petty, C. S. (eds.): *Model Legal Medicine, Psychiatry, and Forensic Science.* Philadelphia, F. A. Davis Co., 1980.

2. Green, M. D.: The operative effect of mental incompetency on agreements and wills. *Texas Law Review* 21:554–589, 1943.

3. Green, M. D.: Proof of mental incompetency and the unexpressed major premise. *Yale Law.* 53:271–311, 1944.

4. Alexander, G. & Szasz, T.: From contract to status via psychiatry. *Santa Clara Lawyer* 13:537–559, 1973.

5. Spalding, W. J.: Testamentary competency: reconciling doctrine with the role of the expert witness. *Law and Human Behavior* 9:113–139, 1985.

D. EMOTIONAL DISTRESS AND MENTAL DISABILITY EVALUATIONS

1. Spalding, W.: Compensation for mental disability, in Michels, R., et al. (eds.), *Psychiatry.* Philadelphia, J.B. Lippincott Co., 1988.

2. American Psychiatric Association: Guidelines for psychiatric evaluation of Social Security Disability claimants. *Hosp. Community Psychiatry* 34:1004–1051, 1983.

3. Meyerson, A. T. & Fine, T. (eds.): *Psychiatric Disability: Clinical, Legal, and Administrative Dimensions.* Washington, DC, American Psychiatric Press, 1987.

4. Okpaku, S.: A profile of clients referred for psychiatric evaluation for Social Security Disability Income and Supplemental Security Income: implications for psychiatry. *Am. J. Psychiatry* 142:1037–1043, 1985.

5. Lamb, H. R. & Rogawski, A. S.: Supplemental Security Income and the sick role. *Am. J. Psychiatry* 135:1221–1224, 1978.

6. Perl, J. L. & Kahn, M. W.: The effects of compensation on psychiatric disability. *Soc. Sci. Med.* 17:439–443, 1983.

7. Goldman, H. H. & Gattozzi, A. A.: Murder in the cathedral revisited: President Reagan and the mentally disabled. *Hosp. Community Psychiatry* 39:505–509, 1988.

8. Platt, J. J. & Husband, S. D.: Post-traumatic stress disorder in forensic practice. *Am. J. Forensic Psychol.* 4:29–56, 1986.

E. TECHNICAL ASPECTS OF A FORENSIC EVALUATION

1. Goldstein, R. L.: Consequences of surveillance of the forensic psychiatric examination: An overview. *Am. J. Psychiatry* 145:1234–1237, 1988.

2. Goldstein, R. L.: Spying on psychiatrists: surreptitious surveillance of the forensic psychiatric examination by the patient himself. *Bull. Am. Acad. Psychiatry Law* 17:367–372, 1989.

3. Rachlin, S. & Schwartz, H. I.: The presence of counsel at forensic psychiatric examination. *Am. J. Forensic Sci.* 33:1008–1014, 1988.

4. Meister, N.: *Miranda* on the couch: an approach to problems of self-incrimination,

right to council and *Miranda* warnings in pre-trial psychiatric examinations of criminal defendants. *Columbia J. Law Social Problems* 11:403–30, 1975.

5. Strasburger, L.: "Crudely, without any finesse": The defendant hears his psychiatric evaluation. *Bull. Am. Acad. Psychiatry Law* 15:229–235, 1987.

F. MALINGERING

1. Rogers, R.: *Clinical Assessment of Malingering and Deception.* New York, Guilford, 1988.

2. Rogers, R. (ed): Malingering and deception: an update. *Behav. Sci. Law,* 8(1):1–104, 1990.

G. CHILD FORENSIC EVALUATION

1. Schetky, D. H. & Benedek, E. P.: *Child Psychiatry and the Law.* New York, Brunner/Mazel, 1980.

2. Schetky, D. H. & Benedek, E. P.: *Emerging Issues in Child Psychiatry and the Law.* New York, Brunner/Mazel, 1985.

3. Schetky, D. H. & Benedek, E. P.: *Clinical Handbook of Child Psychiatry and the Law.* Baltimore, Williams & Wilkins (in press).

7

Clinicians and Lawyers

I. CASE EXAMPLES

A. Case Example 1

Arriving one evening on an inpatient ward of a community mental health center, after transfer from the emergency room of a nearby general hospital, this 25-year-old nurse heads immediately for the public telephone on the ward. She is overheard saying, "This place is like a jail, I want to get out." After her phone call, she retreats angrily to her room, refusing to talk with staff members.

A few hours later, a young man describing himself as the patient's lawyer appears on the ward and, though visiting hours are over, demands to see her. When the staff initially refuses, he threatens to sue them all. Made nervous by his aggressive manner and persistent threats, they ultimately relent. After a brief conversation with the patient, the lawyer approaches the nursing station, insisting to the nurse in charge that the patient be released immediately into his custody. The nurse informs him that she has no power to release the patient but suggests that he call the psychiatrist in charge of the ward.

Speaking with the psychiatrist, the lawyer again demands that the patient be released, saying that he spoke with her, is satisfied that she is not mentally ill, and that therefore her involuntary admission violates her constitutional rights. The psychiatrist, having ascertained from the ward staff that the lawyer does in fact represent the patient, asks if he is aware of the circumstances surrounding her admission. Replying that he is, the lawyer says that the whole situation has been blown out of proportion. All that happened, he relates, is that the patient, a personal friend of his, accidentally took too many sleeping pills; she then had the good sense to call him, and he arranged for her to be taken to the emergency room. The psychiatrist responds that the emergency room psychiatrist felt that a far more serious and genuine suicide attempt had occurred and recommended emergency commitment. He suggests further that the patient remain on the ward overnight and that in the morning everyone involved gather to discuss the case. The lawyer reluctantly agrees.

B. Case Example 2

Ambling resignedly to the admissions office, a first-year resident goes to meet her newly admitted patient. Her lethargy vanishes abruptly when the admissions clerk, drawing her aside, hisses into her ear that her new patient is a lawyer, picked up by police for behaving erratically in the middle of an expressway, shouting at passing cars and attempting to direct traffic.

Clearing a suddenly dry throat, the resident introduces herself as the doctor to the patient, who is a pale but vigilant-eyed man in a dirty, torn, navy blue three-piece suit of expensive cut, mismatched with a Day-Glow orange tie. On hearing her name, the patient whips from an inside pocket a grimy notepad, the pages covered with scribblings and worn to translucency by much handling, and records the doctor's name; he then demands and records the name of the admissions clerk and of the two arresting officers who are standing uncomfortably in the doorway. Thrusting pad into pocket with an air of triumph, the patient fixes the resident with a baleful glare and snarls, "When I get you into court for this, you'll be lucky to have your gold fillings left."

Three days later, the patient, who has been roaming the ward haranguing all who will listen, has still not had admission blood work done, the morale of nursing staff lies in shambles, and the resident has twice checked with her insurer to be sure of continued coverage. Now, after a fellow patient has refused to lend him yet another cigarette, the lawyer-patient begins to assault the refuser. Staff are about to move in to restrain him, but the resident shouts, "Wait! He hasn't really hurt her yet, we can't stop him." The senior attendant, a seasoned veteran of many crises, grabs the lawyer-patient anyway and hustles him to seclusion. Returning, he shakes an admonitory forefinger at the resident and declaims, "You'd better check this case out with the attending, because this guy hasn't gotten one ounce of treatment since he arrived."

Angered by this unsought advice, but secretly agreeing with the attendant's assessment, the resident seeks out the staff psychiatrist who visits on the ward and presents the problem.

II. LEGAL ISSUES

A. Lawyers' perceptions of psychiatry

In contrast to the 1930s, forties, and fifties, when we witnessed a tremendous and sympathetic surge of interest in psychiatry on the part of the legal profession, more recent decades have seen many lawyers develop a decided antipathy to psychiatry. There are a number of factors that account for the development of this attitude, which ranges from wariness to hostility toward the methods and motives of the mental health professions.

1. DISAPPOINTED EXPECTATIONS

The expectations that psychiatrists aroused, and then disappointed, earlier in this century form part of the basis for lawyers' suspicions of psychiatry and the other mental health professions. In a variety of settings, psychiatrists seemed to promise to lend scientific certainty to many of the most difficult problems faced by the law. In the courts, following the turn of the century, psychiatrists and other mental health professionals began to participate in recommending alternatives to incarceration; in the prisons, they attempted to treat and rehabilitate criminals; in parole hearings, they offered opinions as to when prisoners should be released. All this activity was part of an attempt to deal with crime as a symptom of mental dysfunction, and, measured either by the development of internally consistent theories or the rates of recidivism of those treated, it failed.

Psychiatrists also became involved in the administration of the insanity defense, appearing to promise once and for all a definitive answer to the question of who should be deemed culpable for criminal acts. This attempt also failed, as equally renowned psychiatrists reached equally well-reasoned conclusions for opposite sides of the case (but see Chap. 8, Sec. II-C-2). In the civil courts, they tried to lend scientific certainty to child custody determinations, but again without success.

This overselling of psychiatry, and the consequent disappointments, left the legal profession with a lingering suspicion about the general validity of psychiatric theories and the utility of psychiatric practices. In lawyers' eyes, an unfortunate taint of charlatanism was seen to spread across the mental health professions.

2. EFFECTS OF LEGAL TRAINING

Certain elements of legal training also have contributed to lawyers' distrust of psychiatry.

a. The legal model

The law, above all, is a practical tool for maintaining order and resolving disputes in society. Rather than dealing with the infinite diversity and complexity of human beings (the aspects of human existence that most interest many clinicians), lawyers attempt to simplify the situation by postulating certain axioms and creating certain presumptions that redefine a more easily adminstered reality. The axioms include, "A man intends the natural consequences of his acts"; among the presumptions are that all individuals are competent to undertake their actions until proven otherwise. Psychiatric concepts complicate the work of the law by challenging these axioms and presumptions, while offering a competing system of explaining human behavior. The ideas of unconscious motivation and ambivalence, for example, cast doubt on exactly what any of us intend by our actions; the concept of regression suggests that in many situations, such as severe physical illness, human beings are *not* capable of acting as the competent, detached decision makers the law envisions them to be. To maintain intellectual consistency, most lawyers must ignore or disparage psychiatric formulations or else modify their legal conceptual framework. This latter, many lawyers are unwilling to do.

In addition, given the law's need to rely on observable verities, lawyers are trained to be suspicious of any attempts to take people's words and actions at other than face value. Most clinicians, on the other hand, are trained to understand behavior by assuming that people rarely say exactly what they mean. Any clinician who has ever tried to explain to a lawyer why her client's repeated entreaties to be released from the hospital actually represent a reaction formation against deep-seated and frightening desires to be cared for has probably experienced the profound disbelief engendered by such an attempt to counter one of the core assumptions of legal thought. (The effect on legal-psychiatric tension of legal devotion to an adversary model is discussed in Chap. 8, Sec. II-B.)

b. The "worst foot forward" effect

Unfortunately, the first professional contact most lawyers have with the medical and mental health professions comes in law school in their first-year class in torts, in which they are regaled with stories of medical and psychiatric negligence that have ended up in the courts. While this makes perfect sense from the point of view of legal pedagogy—one could hardly teach malpractice law by demonstrating the cases in which *no* grounds exist for suit—the cumulative effect is further destructive of trust between the legal and medical/mental health professions. Lawyers, unless their attitudes are leavened by personal experience, are led to expect malfeasance, often of a gross sort, as the norm of psychiatric behavior.

Courses on law and mental health in many law schools often compound this effect. Although many such courses are co-taught by law professors and experienced psychiatrists who can convey the complexity of clinical work and the need for a mutually sympathetic relationship between the psychiatric and legal systems, many are not. In either event, the casebooks used and the law review articles assigned again often focus on psychiatric incompetence or malevolence, and these frequently succeed in convincing idealistic students that only an aggressive attorney can truly assist the mental patient.

Even a teacher who can present the psychiatric perspective sympathetically is no guarantee against law students interpreting what they learn as evidence of the dangers represented by psychiatry. It has been pointed out that many of the most aggressive members of the mental health bar were trained by those few psychiatrists, usually analysts, who began teaching courses in law and psychiatry in some of the best law schools nearly three decades ago. The great wave of mental health litigation of the late 1960s and 1970s to some extent represented the coming of age of their students, whose eyes were first opened to the real and potential abuses of psychiatry in those pioneer courses.

c. Rights versus needs

The law's role as a system for settling disputes between parties requires it to be concerned with defining the legitimate rights that each party may express and with assigning priority when those rights come into conflict. So concerned is the law with adjudicating rights that it often neglects to consider the needs of the opposing parties (see Chap. 3, Sec. III-B-4). In most cases, this neglect is not fatal, because the rational exercise of rights is usually designed to satisfy needs. But the lack of attention to needs becomes crucial when one of the parties in question has lost the capacity to utilize his rights in that way, that is, when the expression of rights conflicts with the individual's basic needs.

A simple example of this situation arises when a psychotic individual is hospitalized, whether voluntarily or not, for treatment. His needs at that point are for the development of a trusting relationship with a capable professional who will administer efficacious treatment. To the extent that the individual's rights, whether the right to freedom, the right to due process, or the right to privacy, interfere with those needs, as by preventing hospitalization, creating an adversary posture with the therapist, or allowing medication to be refused, the conflict referred to arises.

The law, at least in the academic environment that many law students experience, tends to focus heavily on rights; the mental health professions tend to concern themselves almost exclusively with needs. Given the democratic nature of our system, in which the limitation of the individual's rights cannot be countenanced without convincing benefit, and even then never arbitrarily, it is clear that some accommodation must be reached between those who advocate unlimited rights and those who favor exclusive emphasis on meeting needs. But the tension between the two is productive of much friction across the law-psychiatry interface.

3. EFFECTS OF ANTIPSYCHIATRIC LITERATURE

The popular and academic literature of the last 30 years that has challenged most aspects of psychiatric practice also affects lawyers' attitudes. These works range from the classic descriptions of the effects of long-term hospitalization, to books that question whether mental illness actually exists, to works that challenge the basis for psychiatric diagnosis (maintaining that it is no more than a culturally determined label for deviance) and the need for psychiatric treatment (describing mental illness as a state of consciousness superior to mundane "normality"). (See Suggested Readings—Dietz.) Popular movies depicting gruesome scenes in psychiatric hospitals, such as the administration of ECT without anesthesia, or the effects of lobotomy, further heighten the sense that psychiatry is a brutal and sinister agent of the state that seeks to enforce conformity at the expense of the individual's freedom.

These works are less prominent now than they were two decades ago, when they were staples of college sociology and psychology courses. Many attorneys in practice today, however, still view psychiatry through lenses tinted by the accounts of Szasz, Laing, Goffman and the other "anti-psychiatrists." This is equally true of law professors, whose skepticism of the effects of the mental health system may be passed on to their students. Lawyers-to-be, of course, are particularly alert to evidence of such abuses as these works allege are commonplace in the practice of psychiatry, because their chosen profession has always seen itself as the means by which the oppressed can remedy their suffering. And, though some real abuses exist and were the basis for much of the antipsychiatric literature, the unfortunate conclusion drawn by many students who are exposed only to this side of the issue is that such abuses are universal. If one assumes that contact with psychiatry is inevitably harmful, it is only a short step to the further assumption that everything possible should be done to limit its scope and powers. Psychiatry's passivity

in countering such notions in the mass media has meant that many of the litiga-
tors of today have had little chance to temper their ideas about psychiatry with
any sense of the good done on behalf of the mentally ill by psychiatrists and other
mental health workers.

4. "SECOND GENERATION" LEGAL ADVOCACY

Notwithstanding the influences just mentioned, it seems clear that there has
been a shift more recently in the attitudes of many lawyers toward the mental
health professions, including some of the most radical and aggressive members
of the mental health bar. The reasons for this more positive approach to psychiatry are several, but the most important may be that the successes of the early
litigation designed to limit the scope and power of institutional psychiatry have
clearly not had the dramatic effects hoped for. Though it may be more difficult to
commit and treat mentally ill persons, only the most hard-hearted of advocates
would claim that the homeless mentally ill living on our streets have truly benefit-
ted from the change. It has become apparent to many mental health attorneys
that it is not enough to say as a matter of law what cannot be done to the mentally
ill; if their needs are to be met, one must also establish what must be done for
them.

Legal advocates who are part of this self-described "second generation"
thus pay increasing attention to finding ways to meet some of the needs of the
severely mentally ill. They battle for entitlements to disability payments, health
insurance, and community care. They oppose restrictive zoning provisions that
limit the development of community-based housing. They create innovative programs to find long-term housing options. This is advocacy on the importance of
which mental health professionals and the mental health bar can agree. If more
such areas of commonality can be found, it will bode well for the prospect of
harnessing mental health and legal energies in tandem on behalf of the mentally
ill.

B. The role of the lawyer in the mental health system

Despite the lack of trust that often pervades relationships between lawyers
and clinicians—and the effect of many clinicians' unfair stereotyping of all lawyers as intrusive, uncaring, money-hungry troublemakers should not be forgotten
as a contributing factor—it is clear that lawyers have an important role in the
functioning of the mental health system. Both patients and therapists will often
find themselves confronting situations in which legal assistance is indispensable.

1. WHEN THE PATIENT NEEDS A LAWYER

a. Situations related to psychiatric care

The day has passed when a patient could move from an emergency or
voluntary hospitalization to an indefinite involuntary commitment without both
a judicial hearing and legal representation at that hearing. Today, if the patient is
unable to afford an attorney's fees, all states will arrange for a public defender or
the equivalent to be available to the patient at no cost.

Beyond this minimal guarantee of representation at commitment hearings,
however, patients may face a variety of situations in which a lawyer's advice would

be helpful to them, but one is not automatically provided. Involuntary patients may wish to challenge the basis for their commitment by means of a writ of habeas corpus, either because they believe that their mental status has improved since the initial hearing, or on the grounds that their representation at that hearing was inadequate. (The latter, though infrequently a grounds for a second hearing, is all too common an occurrence in many publicly funded defender systems.) Patients may wish to object in court to involuntary and/or improper treatment, or to object to the conditions at the hospital in which they are held. If family members have filed a petition to have the patient declared incompetent, the patient may wish to oppose that motion.

b. Situations not directly related to psychiatric care

The status of a psychiatric patient confers no immunity from the varied exigencies of life that lead to legal entanglements. In fact, given the frequent instability of their lives, psychiatric patients may be more likely than most to require help with separation or divorce proceedings, child custody actions, eviction hearings, and civil damage suits. Pending criminal charges or the fear that such charges will be filed may also arise as a result of mental illness.

There are additional problems that often arise as a result of mental illness, but are not directly related to the treatment setting. These include establishing entitlement to welfare, Social Security (and its many permutations), Medicaid, Medicare, subsidized housing, vocational rehabilitation programs, and other social benefit programs designed to assist the disabled; arranging for the disposition of assets while hospitalized; opposing actions taken in the patient's absence by family, friends, or business associates that might be to the patient's financial detriment; and arranging for the temporary care of dependent children, while assuring that they will not be permanently removed from the patient's care. This list only covers the most common of the many situations, including many bizarre and unpredictable ones, that are related to patienthood.

c. Handling requests for legal assistance

Inpatient clinicians should consider it their obligation to help patients in obtaining legal assistance should the need arise; to fail to act is often to ensure that the patient's rights will not be advocated, since many inpatients will be unable to take any steps toward obtaining legal help beyond discussing the matter with the clinical staff. Even when the proposed legal action is not considered by the therapist to be in the patient's best interests, this situation is one in which clinical sensibilities should give way before basic rights. All citizens deserve legal representation, and to decline to aid an inpatient in obtaining it is effectively to deny her that right.

Of course, the situation is more intricate when the patient desires a lawyer's help to oppose hospitalization or treatment that the clinician believes is essential, or to sue either the therapist or the hospital. As difficult as it may be for the clinician, the obligation remains the same: the patient is entitled to representation and should be referred appropriately.

With outpatients, the situation may be even more complex. For a variety of therapeutic reasons, therapists might not want to become directly involved in assisting the patient to obtain a lawyer. But, at the very least, when it is clear that the patient is not able to obtain her own representation, the clinician should be sufficiently knowledgeable to be able to refer the patient appropriately.

d. Resources available

Private resources.   It is usually best for the patient to be represented by a private attorney if that is financially feasible. Attorneys working directly for their clients do not face the disincentives to devote sufficient time to the preparation of their cases that often stymie public defenders or legal aid attorneys. A check with the patient's friends or family may reveal that the patient has a private attorney who regularly handles his family's affairs. Failing that, a call to the local bar association should produce a list of lawyers with special knowledge in the particular area in question. Referring the patient to friends or acquaintances of the therapist is problematic; although it may be one way to ensure that he gets good representation, it may also raise the appearance of impropriety (i.e., that the clinician may be rewarded in some way for "steering" clients to the attorney) and may leave the patient uncertain about the crucial questions of confidentiality and conflict of interest. In general, it is probably better to avoid referrals to friends.

Protection and advocacy agencies.   The latest addition to the resources available to mentally ill people are the "protection and advocacy" (P&A) agencies established in all states with federal support. Based on a similar program for mentally retarded persons, the P&A's are charged with representing the interests of mentally ill persons who are receiving care in a broad array of institutional and community facilities. Representation may relate to the conditions of care or access to services, including welfare, disability, and other entitlement programs. The lawyers, para-legals and others who work for these programs can negotiate on behalf of patients, bring legal actions for them, or address broader issues through class action suits.

Although the potential utility of the P&A programs to patients is clear, it remains to be seen whether they will live up to their promise. Experience with earlier, similar models of legal services suggests they are most effective when negotiation, rather than litigation, is the main strategy employed. P&A's that rely on litigation to achieve their goals, or otherwise assume a hostile posture toward providers, only make things worse. Legal harassment is an added inducement to mental health professionals and administrators to abandon understaffed public facilities. To the extent that advocacy only results in shifting limited funds from one underserved group to another, its net effect is minimal; to the extent that a large number of persons are deprived to benefit a few, its net effect is detrimental. Efforts to assess the overall impact of P&A programs are clearly desirable.

Other nonprofit resources.   For patients without sufficient funds to hire a private attorney, another recourse is to the widespread network of privately or federally funded legal agencies. These go by various names in different cities, but are often called the Legal Aid Society or Neighborhood Legal Services. If a search of the telephone book proves unavailing, a call to the bar association should produce the appropriate number. Some of the agencies will not handle criminal cases, but should be able to make a referral to a public defender group to suggest a means of having a court appoint a lawyer.

Another set of resources that should not be overlooked is law school legal aid programs. Designed to provide hands-on experience for second and third year law students, these programs may handle all types of cases or may be restricted to a specialized area such as civil, criminal, prison, or mental health law. The students are supervised, though sometimes only loosely, by experienced attorneys, and often make up in enthusiasm what they lack in expertise. A caveat here: this is not the appropriate referral for complicated or potentially lengthy litigation.

The final option in areas in which none of the other resources are available is to fall back on the old system of lawyers volunteering their time to help indigents and to contact the local bar association for help.

2. WHEN THE CLINICIAN NEEDS A LAWYER

a. Malpractice

Although among the most feared of legal entanglements, the malpractice suit ordinarily raises few problems of representation for the therapist (see Chap. 4, Sec. III-B-2). Malpractice insurance companies automatically provide legal coverage for their clients, asking only that they be notified when even the threat of suit appears. Rarely, the clinician will require additional legal assistance. This is most likely to occur when the company is representing more than one defendant in a suit and the defense of one party depends on assigning blame to the other. The conflict of interest for the company is clearly unmanageable in such situations and the clinician who knows or suspects that such is the case should seek private consultation. The local medical or other professional society, or the local bar association, should be able to provide referral to experienced malpractice attorneys.

b. Consultation

The ever-expanding and ever-changing nature of legal regulation of clinical practice makes it almost a necessity for clinicians to have an attorney *knowledgeable in mental health law* available for consultation. When the subpoena arrives, when a patient demands to see her records, when a new state law outlining patients' rights is passed—in these and countless other situations, the clinician will want to know that there is an attorney who can provide assistance and advice. Often just being able to say to a court, to another attorney, or to a potential litigant, "I am doing this on the advice of my attorney," has a remarkable calming effect on all parties concerned.

Hospitals and large clinics have always had lawyers retained to represent them in negotiating contracts and handling financial matters or in litigation, but many are now adding to their legal staff an expert in mental health law to handle day-to-day problems. Medium or large-sized clinical practices might want to consider retaining the consultative services of a mental health attorney. Individual therapists may want to pool their resources with several colleagues to have such help available. Professional associations, including the American Psychiatric Association, now provide legal consultation services for a reasonable fee. At the very least, every practitioner should know where in her area she can turn for expert legal advice, even if this comes at a price. This means that in advance of trouble, the therapist should make contact with a capable attorney who will agree to respond quickly to the situations that are bound to develop. It should be noted that a good consulting attorney can often do more to protect patients' rights than the most aggressive of patient advocates, because in his position as an ally of the clinician his advice is more likely to be followed.

III. CLINICAL ISSUES

A. Dealing with patients' lawyers

Although accustomed by training and experience to dealing with the psychiatric patient, the clinician often finds himself *un*trained and *in*experienced in dealing constructively with the patient's lawyer. This condition can be highly demoralizing and may interfere with good patient care. Certain principles may help to smooth the potentially rocky road of clinician-lawyer interaction.

1. SEEKING THE ALLIANCE POSTURE

While they view the patient through different lenses and understand him by different models, clinician and lawyer share a common interest in the patient's welfare. Since the lawyer may be inclined to view the clinician as "the adversary" according to his legal model (see Sec. II), the clinician must often be the one to take the initiative in seeking an alliance based on this commonality of interests.

The clinician should not hesitate to be explicit about this shared interest in the patient's well-being, since some attorneys, especially less-experienced ones, have been so primed with antipsychiatric notions as to be astonished at the thought of collaboration.

2. EDUCATING THE LAWYER

Some suggestions about educating lawyers are detailed in Chapters 4 and 8. In general terms, the clinician must realize that the lawyer, although a professional in her own right, is usually a layperson in matters psychiatric. This point has several implications.

a. Permission

The clinician must remember that, from the patient's viewpoint, even the attorney is outside the bounds of clinician-patient confidentiality. Thus, the patient's permission (preferably written, but at least verbal) should be obtained before communicating with the lawyer; the usual emergency exceptions may apply, as described in Chapter 1.

Regrettably, the clinician may occasionally encounter some lawyers for whom confidentiality is a secondary consideration. The following example, although drawn from a fictional movie, captures the problem.

> *Example 1:* A law-firm partner asked a lawyer about an exciting and provocative case on which the lawyer was working. The lawyer protested that the information was privileged. The partner appealed, "Come on, you can tell me. *I'm* one of the privileged."

The clinician faced with an attorney of this persuasion may have to set limits with him, but should first seek the alliance position. The clinician might say: "Just as soon as we can obtain the patient's permission, I'll be happy to cooperate," rather than the misguidedly adversarial: "You're not getting a syllable out of me without a witnessed permission slip!"

b. Comprehension

Because of subtle (and less-than-subtle) "antipsychiatric" biases often found in the training of attorneys (see Sec. II-A), the clinician attempting to educate a lawyer must keep certain principles in mind to aid the informing process.

Disease versus myth. First, the clinician should clarify the "disease process" itself, recalling that the attorney may have been exposed to and accepted the philosophy that "mental illness is a myth." The signs and symptoms that constitute the syndrome in question and the typical course of the illness (both treated and untreated) should be outlined clearly. If any particular concerns are raised by the specific syndrome, they should be noted, as well. Examples are suicide in depressive states, homicide in paranoid states with violence, dissipation of property in mania, need for external controls in dyscontrol states, and need for isolation in states of vulnerability to overstimulation (see also Chap. 3, Sec. III-B-2 and Chap. 5, Sec. III-B). The clinician must clearly identify how apparently random combinations of symptoms or signs actually constitute clinical entities whose presence may have specific prognostic implications.

Mental illness and the need for care. That mental illness severe enough to result in hospitalization usually requires some form of care or treatment is generally so clear to the clinician as to verge on tautology, but it must be recalled that this association may be far from obvious to patients' lawyers. The clinician must, therefore, clarify how features of the illness may create specific needs for care and treatment: thought disorder, for example, may require treatment with phenothiazines; impaired capacity to adapt to the demands of everyday life may call for training in social skills. Even aspects of a patient's presentation that the attorney may interpret as variations of normality may actually represent manifestations of illness calling for treatment. For example, difficulty getting along with coworkers may be a manifestation of a "personality trait" or the result of a clinical entity—a paranoid disorder—that may respond to antipsychotic medication. Similarly, the pessimism that leads a patient to reject a chance at advancement may be not the result of a "bilious disposition," but the outcome of a predictable state of hopelessness in the treatable illness, depression.

In the case of the patient objecting to needed treatment, the clinician should attempt to explain to the patient's attorney exactly why he believes that the patient is not acting in her best interests. This is not an attempt to co-opt the lawyer, but rather an effort to convey the realities of the clinical situation to someone who may carry considerable influence with the patient. Although it is not rare for a lawyer who becomes convinced that the patient really requires further treatment to attempt to persuade the patient to go along with the treatment plan, even if that does not occur, the establishment of a good working relationship between clinician and lawyer conveys to the patient the idea that it is not a question of some people being "for" her and some "against" her; rather, at issue is a difference of opinions on how best to help the individual patient. This sense of everyone working on behalf of a common, ultimate goal, though often difficult to achieve, can be invaluable in ensuring proper follow-up care for the patient, regardless of the outcome of the case. It may also prove highly reassuring to the distressed patient.

Powers of prediction. Legal and psychiatric scholars are at present in accord on the general inability of psychiatry to make predictions as to patients' dangerousness (see Chap. 2, Sec. II-E-2). There are predictions, however, that psychiatrists are somewhat better at making. In the presence of a known clinical entity (e.g., bipolar disorder) in a patient who has had previous episodes of a similar sort, clinicians may be able to predict quite usefully the *consequences* of certain courses of action: treat or do not treat; petition to commit or release; begin immediate electroconvulsive therapy or wait for more delayed medication effect. Although absolute certainty is unattainable in medicine and in mental health care, the attorney should be made aware that a number of likely outcomes may ensue depending upon the course chosen.

Clinical conditions with legal implications.   The clinician should alert the attorney to those aspects of a patient's clinical picture that may have particular effects on legal matters. Many of these issues have been explored in Chapters 3 and 5; commonly encountered ones include: the effect of severe psychosis or depression on attitudes toward treatment, as well as on competence to consent to, or to refuse it; effects of fixed and/or progressive disorders like dementia on competence; and the highly varied and individualized relationship between illness, functioning, and committability, as reviewed in Chapter 2.

Particularly problematic are presentations of mental illness that exert a subtle but decisive effect on the patient's competence to make decisions in a particular area (see also Chapter Five and Suggested Readings for that chapter—Gutheil and Bursztajn). These subtle forms of incompetence are most often observed in: 1) paranoid states, which may significantly affect decision making but may leave cognitive ability—and therefore verbal fluency—intact; 2) mania or hypomania, where denial of serious deficit is a prominent finding; 3) depression, where the pessimism inherent in this disorder may cloud a patient's ability to perceive benefits of *any* kind in regard to a risk-benefit analysis for a treatment regimen; and 4) anorexia nervosa, where the patient may be significantly psychologically disturbed on the subject of food intake but quite rational in other areas.

The lawyer may also need education about the impact of the illness from which her client suffers on the lawyer-client interaction.

> **Example 2:** An agitated attorney sought out an inpatient's clinician and reported that her client, with whom she had had a long and positive relationship, had just insulted and verbally abused her, labeling her as an impostor, calling her by someone else's name, and accusing her of things she had not done. The clinician explained about paranoid states of misrecognition, much to the attorney's relief.

Finally, the clinician should adopt a tone in explaining matters to the attorney similar to that she would use for intelligent next-of-kin; this involves focusing on pragmatic rather than on theoretical aspects of the problem.

3. USE OF "HOUSE COUNSEL"

A growing number of institutions and other clinical settings have retained attorneys who specialize in consultation for mental health clinicians; in an institution, such an attorney colloquially may be called the "house counsel."

In addition to providing legal advice to the clinical staff, the house counsel may be supremely valuable in dealing with patients' lawyers, especially the overzealous and "thrusty" types. Indeed, when a psychiatrist and an attorney are arguing in the corridors of the hospital about, say, a patient's commitability, both are having "the wrong conversation" (see Suggested Readings—Gutheil and Magraw). This conversation properly should occur between the house counsel and the outside attorney. Moreover, attorneys on the strange turf of a mental hospital or clinic often feel more comfortable talking to another lawyer than to clinical personnel. Moreover, specious legal ploys and threats tend to be ineffective with the house counsel and thus are less likely to be employed.

Clinicians, therefore, should not hesitate to enlist the house counsel, when available, to assist in negotiations with the patient's lawyer. To make this collaboration succeed, clinical staff must be willing to spend enough time to inform the house counsel fully about the issues and the clinical data relating to the patient, and the counsel must be available on an impromptu basis.

4. SPECIAL REQUIREMENTS OF THE CRISIS SETTING

The demands of the patient's lawyer should not be allowed to take precedence over the emergent needs of the patient; for the patient's protection, responsible patient care must outweigh other considerations.

> ***Example 3:*** A lawyer called by the family barged onto the ward where an acutely psychotic patient was being evaluated and demanded his precipitous release. The patient, hearing this as a threat of being removed from a protected setting, panicked and began to assault nearby patients. When clinical staff moved in to restrain him, the lawyer screamed, "Stop! I forbid you to touch him." Staff hesitated, uncertain what to do, and the patient's dyscontrol escalated. A senior clinician on the scene ordered staff to intervene and the patient was safely secluded. The furious attorney was referred to the house counsel.

While one should attempt to avoid struggles and confrontations with patients' lawyers whenever possible, decisive action may be necessary when attorneys unaccustomed to psychiatric crises themselves "lose control," as in this example, and seriously impede patient care or endanger the patient's safety. Clinicians must "put the patient first," even in the face of threatened suit. Excessively intrusive lawyers, deaf to persuasion, may require hospital security or outside police to be summoned to remove them, although preferably as a last resort. Severe lapses of professional conduct should be documented, supported by written witness reports, and reported to the local bar association.

B. Dealing with lawyers for third parties

Problems in dealing with lawyers for third parties (e.g., families, employers, insurers, victims of the patient's actions) are often no different from problems that arise in dealing with anyone outside of the therapeutic relationship.

1. AGENCY

The clinician must recall that the patient, as her employer, commands her primary allegiance; the interests of other parties, except in emergencies, are secondary.

On rare occasions, attorneys may request clinicians to perform various tasks ostensibly in the patient's interest: writing letters to third parties, contacting various agencies, and the like. Clinicians can usually assume good faith on the part of attorneys but—whenever there is the slightest doubt—should check with their patients to be sure: 1) that the patient desires the clinician's assistance in the manner requested and 2) that the ends expected to be attained are part of the patient's plan. Such clarifying of consent can avoid significant conflicts that may arise by an attorney's misperception of what the patient "really wants."

2. PERMISSION FOR DISCLOSURE

The clinician must have the patient's permission for sharing any information relevant to the patient or his care, as described in Chapter 1.

3. OBTAINING LEGAL CONSULTATION

The clinician should seek legal advice from house counsel or her own attorney, when appropriate, to define her rights and responsibilities when these are in doubt or under attack.

C. Lawyers as patients

A lawyer-patient (especially an inpatient) presents challenges to effective clinical management similar to those of "VIP syndrome" (see Suggested Readings—Gabbard), in which the "specialness" of the patient operates to the detriment of good clinical care. (See the second case example for this chapter.) All the challenges cited below are dramatically intensified when the lawyer-patient presents with the borderline syndrome.

Before reviewing approaches to these challenges, we may outline them as follows:

1. PROBLEMS

a. Milieu anxiety

Free-floating fear of suit may raise collective anxiety among ward personnel, leading to a paralysis of action; familiar, time-tested treatment approaches may seem suddenly specious and indefensible in court, especially when applied to the lawyer-patient. Similarly, the clinician may feel severely inhibited in performing a variety of interventions, verbal and administrative (e.g., restricting the patient to the ward), even if these are necessary for the patient's care.

b. Avoidance of the patient

One maladaptive response to this anxiety is for staff and clinicians to avoid all but minimal contact with the patient—a classic phobic response. This does a severe disservice, of course, to the patient's clinical needs.

c. "A fool for a client"

The lawyer-patient, on the other hand, may attempt to deal with the stresses of illness and/or patienthood by wearing the professional mask and attempting to act as her own lawyer, even in relation to patently inappropriate matters. This inclination is as self-defeating as that of the physician-patient who attempts to self-prescribe medications during his own mental illness.

d. Legalism as defensive avoidance

Both lawyer-patient and clinical staff may take refuge from feared confrontation or from shared psychic pain by retreating into legalism, whereby conversations on legal quibbles replace serious grappling with treatment issues (see Suggested Readings—Gutheil). While legalistic acting out is not limited to lawyers (see Chap. 4, Sec. III-A-2-e), the defense assumes added force if a lawyer is initiating it.

2. APPROACHES

The approaches to the foregoing are those familiar to experienced clinicians from other problems of milieu countertransference; the basic principles to be followed in placing the patient's needs first are here reviewed.

a. Informed ward leadership

Strong, competent leadership for the clinical unit provides the necessary anchor against countertransference storms directed at the lawyer-patient; such leadership has a twofold function: to focus attention unfailingly on the clinical needs of the patient and to inform the clinical staff about the actual legal issues that arise, including their statutory or regulatory bases. By informing staff members about the realistic extent of their liability, energy used for unproductive and fearful speculation can be freed for patient care. In addition, senior staff must spearhead the corrective milieu process outlined below (Secs. b-d).

b. The toxicity of specialness

A patient may receive the label of "special" as a result of a number of factors; for a lawyer-patient these factors are commonly:

1. *Overidentification* with the lawyer (especially if comparable in age to treatment staff) as a "young professional, like me"—an attitude that may interfere with objectivity in assessment of the patient's needs and problems;
2. *Exaggerated perception* of the lawyer-patient as unduly litigious (regardless of whether this is accurate) and therefore threatening to the clinical staff;
3. *Reluctance* of front-line staff to use their own judgment in assessing the patient, coupled with an instinctive "upward transfer of authority" whereby front-line staff feel paralyzed to effect even needed interventions without sanctions from staff in ever more senior positions; thus the patient's care becomes "run from the top," a situation promoting schism, lowered morale, and resentment among the treatment team. The effective leader must often resist the complementary temptation to "jump in and take over" the care of the special patient—another move that worsens the situation. Instead, the leader should maintain normal delegation of authority, while staying fully informed about the case and remaining actively available for consultation. He may also have to "protect" the patient's treatment from well-meant but detrimental interferences from "above" (in the institution) or from extrainstitutional pressures, as occasionally occurs;
4. *Jettisoning* of usual procedures, assessments, interventions and their rationales because of some aspect of the "specialness."

Example 4: A lawyer-patient in a severe depression was fortuitously discovered in the ward seclusion room in the act of hanging himself with his belt; he was rescued at the last moment. In the post-incident review, staff discovered through discussion that several of them had independently subscribed to the same fantasy, namely, "This guy as a lawyer must be too smart to do a dumb thing like kill himself." The result of this shared, but tacit, belief was that they had not removed his belt, as time-honored procedure required, not wanting to "subject a professional to that indignity."

In sum, the above consequences of "specialness" in a patient may form a toxic synergy leading to avoidance and mismanagement of the patient's care. The remedy consists of active inservice education about the potential problems and about the importance of seeing the patient in need beyond the obscuring mist of "specialness."

c. The role of milieu group process

Much of the toxicity noted above can be mitigated by group discussion of the experience of working with the lawyer-patient and the difficulties and conflicts that may arise. Such opportunities, encouraged and catalyzed by the ward leadership, permit ventilation, consensual validation, and restoration of morale through sharing of experience—results that might have prevented the nearly tragic outcome of the case in Example #4, above.

d. Intervention against avoidance

Supervisory staff must remain alert to the factors noted above as they may affect the ability of staff to engage in a therapeutic relationship with the lawyer-patient; such defensive avoidances as described above (Secs. III-C-1-b, c) must be interpreted like other distancing maneuvers that prevent optimal involvement with the pressing life issues at hand. Front-line staff may need supervisory assistance in maintaining the proper clinical perspective in the face of pressures to engage in legalistic struggles.

In short, the attorney must be confronted as a patient instead of a lawyer, especially when legalizing the relationship is a ploy attempted as a resistance. A parallel might easily be drawn with the health professional who may attempt to take on a health professional role in her own care—a maneuver recognized as destructive by all clinicians.

IV. PITFALLS

A. Remaining the clinician

When legal and clinical issues are in tension (as described also in Chapters 3, 4, and 6), the clinician must let the patient's legitimate needs be the determinants of care. Even the patient who has a lawyer (or who *is* a lawyer) may need a clinician's help—help which is subverted if the clinician attempts to remove himself from his role and become lawyer-like.

B. Fear of suit

With reasonable preventive measures (see Chap. 4, Sec. III), the fear of lawsuit may become a peripheral concern; if this concern becomes central, it can obscure a clinical view of the patient, interfering with the quality of care. Fear of legal reprisals must then be worked out through supervision, administrative resolution, legal consultation, or a combination of these, lest therapeutic care be compromised.

C. Anger at lawyers

The clinician may develop anger at lawyers for a number of reasons, including their personal and professional styles (as depicted in the first case example for this chapter). Because this affect can also interfere with sound clinical functioning, the clinician must guard against its "side effects," e.g., getting angry at the patient in displacement because her lawyer is intrusive, hostile, obnoxious, obstreperous, provocative, or accusatory. Introspection, commiseration with colleagues, and other methods may maintain this affect within manageable bounds.

D. Overreaction

The impact of a lawyer in the picture may lead to overreaction in either direction on the part of the clinician: provocative, belligerent, grudging, or withholding behavior on the one hand; or, on the other, an overly submissive posture that leads to sacrifice of important clinical considerations merely for the sake of avoiding confrontation. Either extreme, of course, is potentially detrimental.

V. CASE EXAMPLE EPILOGUES

A. Case Example 1

Before meeting with the lawyer the following morning, both the resident to whom the case has been assigned and the psychiatrist in charge rapidly evaluate the patient. They agree that the patient, a bright, attractive woman, is a borderline personality, who, in the face of several interpersonal losses, had made a serious suicide attempt using sleeping pills. Only at the last minute did she change her mind, deciding to involve her friend, the lawyer, in rescuing her. She is not psychotic, nor does she appear suicidal at present, although given the lack of objects in her life, any subsequent reversal might predictably result in another suicide attempt. Nonetheless, she does not appear to meet strict commitment criteria at this moment. The psychiatrists believe that the preferred course of action would be to keep her in the hospital for up to two weeks to enable her to establish a treatment alliance with the resident, who will then follow her as an outpatient. They present this plan to the patient and to her lawyer.

Insisting that she is not suicidal and that the hospital is "worse than a zoo," the patient demands that she be released immediately. The lawyer supports this position, saying that to retain her any longer would violate her right to due process and that he will take responsibility for her safety if she is discharged into his care. If the hospital refuses to do so, he maintains that he will immediately go to court to seek a writ of habeas corpus.

Rather than risk turning the case into any more of an adversary issue than it has already become, thus losing whatever chance remains of gaining a working alliance with the patient, the psychiatrists agree to discharge her into the lawyer's care, on the condition that she return to see the resident on an outpatient basis. The patient concurs and discharge ensues.

For two weeks the patient comes to see the resident, continuing to insist that there is nothing wrong and that the resident cannot help her. When she misses the third appointment, the resident attempts, without success, to contact her. One week later, the lawyer calls the ward, in shock, to inform the staff that the patient's body was found in her apartment by a neighbor over the weekend. She had apparently taken a fatal overdose of the same sleeping pills.

B. Case Example 2

Hearing the description of the case, the staff psychiatrist observes that this patient, because of his profession, is receiving special treatment that is very much to his detriment, especially since the patient's manic picture demands firm and authoritative controls. The attending reminds the resident of the protections against suit afforded by careful documentation, frequent review with the chief resident and supervisors, and persistent seeking of an alliance posture even in the direct confrontations necessary to counter behavioral dyscontrol. In sum, the resident is enjoined to see the lawyer as a patient requiring treatment rather than as an attorney threatening suit.

The resident takes heart from this colloquy and proceeds; group discussions by ward staff also mobilize new resolve. Lab work, previously stymied by the patient's paranoid and grandiose refusals, is performed perforce and confirms the resident's suspicions that the patient is suffering a probable organic psychosis, mimicking mania, apparently produced by excessive corticosteroid intake, the result of a misread arthritis prescription. After the psychosis resolves, the patient describes the fearful feeling of being out of control and expresses gratitude at being restrained before he injured anyone.

VI. ACTION GUIDE

A. Checklist for Dealing with Patient's Lawyer

1. *Seek* alliance posture.
2. *Educate* lawyer on important clinical issues:
    a. *Remind* about permission for release of information even to attorney.
    b. *Inform* about clinical realities and conditions.
3. *Seek* assistance from house counsel and *refer* outside attorneys to house counsel as needed.
4. *Place* patient needs (especially in crisis setting) uppermost.
5. *Respond* to subpoena with presence, obtaining legal consultation.
6. *Attempt* to negotiate for patient's benefit instead of entering legalistic struggle.

B. Checklist for Dealing with Lawyer for Third Parties

1. *Recall* and *review* important factors:
    a. Clarity of agency,
    b. Permission for disclosures,
    c. Obtaining legal consultation.

C. Checklist for Dealing with Lawyer as Patient

1. *Recall* potential problem areas:
    a. Milieu anxiety and paralysis over "specialness" of patient,
    b. Phobic avoidance of patient,
    c. Lawyer's attempts to be own attorney,
    d. Legalistic avoidance as defense.
2. *Respond* to problems with:
    a. Ward leadership,
    b. Education of staff about "special patient" problems,
    c. Clarification of legal ambiguities,
    d. Encouragement of group discussion,
    e. Supervisory attention.
3. *Remain* alert to countertransference factors:
    a. "Remaining the clinician,"
    b. Excessive fear of suit,
    c. Anger at lawyers,
    d. Overreaction.

D. Utilizing Lawyers

1. *Obtaining a lawyer for the patient*
    a. *Obtain* attorney for inpatients (this is clinician's obligation); *use* discretion for outpatients.
    b. *Determine* if patient has private attorney; if so, *utilize* him preferentially;
    c. If not, *determine* if patient can afford private attorney.
    d. If patient can afford private attorney, *obtain* list of referrals through local bar association.
    e. *Do not refer* to personal acquaintances.
    f. If patient cannot afford private attorney, *refer* to:
        i. Legal Aid Society or Neighborhood Legal Services for most problems;
        ii. Law school legal aid programs, if available;
        iii. Nonprofit agencies specializing in mental health law, if appropriate to patient's problem;
        iv. If none of the above available, contact local bar association about availability of lawyers willing to volunteer time for indigents.
2. *Obtaining a lawyer for the clinician*
    a. In malpractice cases, insurance company will provide—*contact* them immediately.

    b. If conflict of interest appears possible (company insuring multiple defendants), *seek* private consultation—*obtain* referral from medical society, bar association.

    c. *Arrange* for availability of legal help for emergent problems in advance of their occurrence and for consultation—attorney must be knowledgeable in mental health law:

        i. Through hospital or clinic,

        ii. Through group practice,

        iii. By organizing several independent practitioners for the purpose,

        iv. By direct arrangement with a lawyer.

VII. SUGGESTED READINGS

A. LAWYERS' ROLES IN THE MENTAL HEALTH SYSTEM

1. Rubenstein, L. S.: Treatment of the mentally ill: legal advocacy enters the second generation. *Am. J. Psychiatry* 143:1264–1269, 1986.

2. Appelbaum, P. S.: The rising tide of patients' rights advocacy. *Hosp. Community Psychiatry* 37:9–10, 1986.

3. Lamb, H. R.: Securing patients' rights—responsibly. *Hosp. Community Psychiatry* 32:393–397, 1981.

4. Weicker, L.: Federal response to institutional abuse and neglect: The Protection and Advocacy for Mentally Ill Individuals Act. *Am. Psychol.* 42:1027–1028, 1987.

5. *Protection and Advocacy for Mentally Ill Individuals Act of 1986,* Public Law 99–319, 42 USC 10801.

6. Mowbray, C. T., Freddolino, P. P., Rhodes, G. L., et al.: Evaluation of a patient rights protection system: public policy implications. *Admin. Ment. Health* 12:264–283, 1985.

7. Brakel, S. J.: Legal aid in mental hospitals. *American Bar Foundation Research Journal* 1981:21–243.

8. Brakel, S. J.: Legal problems of people in mental and penal institutions: an exploratory study. *American Bar Foundation Research Journal* 1978:565–645.

9. Appelbaum, P. S.: Housing for the mentally ill—an unexpected outcome of a class-action suit against SSA. *Hosp. Community Psychiatry* 39:479–480, 1988.

B. CRITICAL PERSPECTIVES ON PSYCHIATRY

1. Dietz, P. E.: Social discrediting of psychiatry: the protasis of legal disfranchisement. *Am. J. Psychiatry* 134:1356–1360, 1977.

2. Scheff, T. J.: *Being Mentally Ill: A Sociological Theory.* Chicago, Aldine Publishing Co., 1966.

3. Szasz, T. S.: *The Myth of Mental Illness: Foundations of a Theory of Personal Conduct,* New York, Harper & Row, 1961.

4. Szasz, T. S.: *Law, Liberty, and Psychiatry: An Inquiry into the Social Uses of Mental Health Practices.* New York, Macmillan. 1963.

5. Laing, R. D.: *The Politics of Experience.* New York, Ballantine Books, 1967.

6. Klein, J. I.: Resistances to the care of the chronic patient: a lawyer's contribution. *New Directions for Mental Health Services.* No. 33, 87–93, 1987.

7. Kavaler, S. A.: Law versus clinical treatment: the case of L. C. *Am. J. Psychother.* 45:135–143, 1986.

C. CLINICAL ISSUES

1. Gutheil, T. G.: Legal defense as ego defense: a special form of resistance to the therapeutic process. *Psychiatr. Q.* 51:251–256, 1979.

2. Gutheil, T. G. & Magraw, R.: Ambivalence, alliance and advocacy: misunderstood dualities in psychiatry and the law. *Bull. Am. Acad. Psychiatry Law* 12:51–58, 1984.

3. Marzuk, P. M.: When the patient is a physician. *N. Engl. J. Med.* 317:1409–1411, 1987.

4. Colson, D. B., Allen, J. G., Coyne, L., et al: An anatomy of countertransference: staff reactions to difficult psychiatric hospital patients. *Hosp. Community Psychiatry* 37:923–928, 1986.

5. Gabbard, G. O.: The treatment of the "special" patient in a psychoanalytic hospital. *Int. Rev. Psycho-Anal.* 13:333–347, 1986.

8

The Clinician in Court

C. **Customs and demeanor in the "foreign land"**
 1. THE ROLE OF THE WITNESS: WHAT IT IS AND IS NOT
   a. Informing
   b. Arguing
   c. Preaching
   d. Advising
 2. TECHNICAL CONSIDERATIONS
   a. Clearing time
   b. Oral presentation of material
   c. Credentials
 3. SUBJECTIVE ASPECTS
   a. Impugned expertise as narcissistic assault
      i. *"Rules of the game"*
      ii. *Realistic limitations*
      iii. *Defense mechanisms*
 4. STRUCTURAL ASPECTS OF TRIAL PRESENTATION
   a. Direct examination
      i. *Laying a foundation*
      ii. *Hypothetical questions and follow-ups*
   b. Cross-examination
   c. Redirect and recross
D. **The "foreign language" of the courtroom**
 1. STRUCTURAL ASPECTS OF COURTROOM LANGUAGE
   a. The scope of the question
   b. "I don't know"
   c. Reasonable medical certainty
 2. SUBSTANTIVE ASPECTS OF COURTROOM LANGUAGE
   a. Describe versus interpret
   b. The qualities of an expert witness's answers
 3. TECHNICAL ASPECTS OF COURTROOM LANGUAGE
   a. Tips on responding to queries
      i. *The value of delay*
      ii. *Unanswerable questions*
      iii. *The context of the question*
      iv. *Qualifiers*
      v. *Metaphors and analogies*
   b. Consideration for the subject's presence
   c. Some common maneuvers by attorneys in court
      i. *Fee as focus for attack*
      ii. *"Never say never"*
      iii. *The lulling series*
      iv. *The use of literature as authority*
      v. *Inaccurate quotations*
      vi. *Simple harassment*
      vii. *Testifying about preparing to testify*
      viii. *Incomprehensible questions*
E. **Summary**

IV. **PITFALLS**
 A. **Remaining the clinician**
 B. **Maintaining humility**
 C. **Taking it personally**
V. **CASE EXAMPLE EPILOGUE**

I. CASE EXAMPLE

Without warning, a therapist receives a subpoena to testify in court the following week. At first, she is sure that a mistake has been made, because she has never been involved in the treatment of offenders or in performing evaluations for the courts. When, at the suggestion of a colleague, she calls the office of the attorney whose name appears at the bottom of the subpoena, she is told by a secretary that the case in question is an action for damages following an auto accident in which the condition of the plaintiff prior to the accident is a prime issue of contention. The secretary says that it is her impression that the therapist is being subpoenaed because she has been treating the plaintiff.

Looking more closely at the subpoena, the therapist recognizes the married name of a current psychotherapy patient who usually uses her maiden name. The patient had begun treatment only three months previously under the stress of impending marital separation. Although patient and therapist have touched on many issues together, their sessions have focused on the patient's relationship with her husband, an extramarital affair about which the husband does not know, and her feelings about her father, who had died when she was only six years old. The accident has not been mentioned.

After the passing of her initial shock at being subpoenaed, the therapist becomes concerned at the prospect of having to testify. She worries about the time it would take for her to appear in court. The amount of money that she stands to lose is substantial, but she is also concerned about the effect of such an abrupt cancellation of appointments on some very unstable patients. In addition, she fears that the testimony that she could be forced to give in court might damage her therapeutic relationship with her patient, leading the patient to withdraw from therapy at a time when she especially needs the support that the therapist could provide. Finally, it is unclear to the therapist just what role the court expects her to play. She does not feel that she knows enough about the legal issues involved or about how the accident affected the patient to contribute in any meaningful way to the court's decision. On the other hand, she is fearful that some of the information that she might reveal, particularly concerning the extramarital affair, might needlessly damage her patient's life.

Faced with this confusing array of issues, the therapist decides to call her patient to inform her that the subpoena has arrived. The patient is distraught at the news and says that she will contact her lawyer immediately. She confirms the therapist's impression that she does not want her to testify in any way concerning her mental state. Quite uncertain about how to protect the multitude of interests that she now sees endangered, the therapist approaches a colleague whose practice is largely devoted to forensic work to ask his advice.

II. LEGAL ISSUES

A. The role of the expert witness

Mental health professionals are finding themselves increasingly called upon to serve the legal process in the role of expert witnesses. Sometimes this role is voluntarily assumed, as in the case of those forensic clinicians whose practice is almost entirely devoted to evaluations and courtroom testimony; sometimes, however, clinicians find themselves unwillingly drawn into the adversary process. This may occur when a patient requires commitment; or when the contact that a clinician had with a patient and the opinions that he formed become relevant to nonmental health litigation, such as a child-custody case or a suit for psychic damages following a negligent act. Thus, all clinicians are susceptible to unexpected subpoenas and ought to be aware of the formal and informal rules governing their participation in courtroom proceedings.

1. DEFINITION OF AN EXPERT WITNESS

Wigmore's classic legal treatise on evidence defines an expert as someone who has the "skill to acquire accurate conceptions." That is to say, in those circumstances in which the bare facts of a situation are inadequate to lead the average person to an informed judgment, the expert has the capacity to draw meaningful conclusions from those facts. An expert need not be possessed of a formal degree; for example, a self-trained ornithologist, whose expertise has come to be widely recognized, might qualify as an expert in a case in which the identification of a particular species of bird were relevant. In cases of alleged mental illness, however, the courts—abandoning their historic position that even a layperson can tell if someone is crazy or not—have turned more and more to mental health professionals for help in interpreting individual behavior.

The status of expert can be granted in two ways. The legislature can determine that groups of professionals should be considered experts for a given purpose. Along these lines, in many states physicians and psychologists are allowed to provide expert testimony at commitment hearings, while other clinicians, even those who may be quite familiar with mental disorders, are excluded. In most cases, though, it is the court that is hearing a particular case that decides if an individual should be deemed an expert on the issue in question. For issues related to mental health, the tendency of late has been for courts to exclude nonpsychiatric physicians from expert witness status while being more liberal about allowing psychologists and occasionally social workers to testify as experts.

The use of mental health experts and the admissibility of their testimony appears to be increasing in both civil and criminal cases. On the civil side, for example, as the courts have become more receptive to claims of negligent infliction of emotional distress (see Chap. 6, Sec. II-C-3), mental health testimony has become more prevalent. In criminal cases, the U.S. Supreme Court has recognized that the assistance of a psychiatrist may be essential to the preparation and presentation of a defendant's case, even when she is not invoking the insanity defense. The Court's ruling in *Ake v. Oklahoma* established the constitutional necessity of making mental health experts available to indigent defendants at the state's expense.

2. THE SCOPE OF EXPERT TESTIMONY

The expert is allowed greater flexibility within the usually strict rules of evidence than the nonexpert witness.

a. The opinion rule

In general, witnesses are permitted to testify only to *facts* relevant to a given case; *opinions* are excluded. Thus, a witness may be allowed to state that the defendant drove his car through two red lights prior to the accident. Should the witness insert an implicit opinion about the defendant's driving, however, as by saying that the defendant "drove through those lights like he didn't give a damn," that would be stricken from the record as a violation of the opinion rule. The rule is based on the belief that it is the job of the jury, not of the witness, to evaluate the factual information presented; to the extent that the witness has no greater ability to do so than does the jury (or the judge), her opinions are irrelevant to the trial process.

On the other hand, the expert is allowed to state an opinion in situations in which the average person would be unable to form a meaningful opinion from the facts of the case. The information that an individual was talking rapidly, had not slept for three nights, and was fearful that his plan for bringing peace to the Middle East might be sabotaged by the CIA is, to most people, a confusing collection of interesting but bizarre facts. Only a clinician is capable of bringing order to those facts by offering an opinion that they may represent manifestations of a manic episode, for example, with attendant grandiosity and paranoia.

Expert testimony is permitted only when the judge determines, as a matter of law, that the facts in question cannot be properly analyzed by a layperson. In some cases, an expert might be allowed to offer an opinion on one aspect of an individual's behavior but not on another, because the judge feels that the latter (for example, a demented person's confusion) is susceptible to determination by the untrained mind.

b. The hearsay rule

Ordinarily, an individual's testimony is permitted to be based only on facts that she has directly perceived. Anything else is considered to be "hearsay." In practice this means that if a patient has threatened to harm someone to that person's face, the latter can testify to the reality of the threat. If the threatened person has told the patient's psychiatrist about the threat, however, the psychiatrist may not offer the threat as evidence, because that would be hearsay. The rationale for this is that it is improper to admit evidence that cannot be subjected to cross-examination.

As the example suggests, even experts usually are bound by the hearsay rule. There is one exception relevant here. While an expert cannot introduce hearsay evidence to establish a fact—for example, that the threat was made—she is permitted to offer hearsay testimony in support of her opinion. Thus, if the psychiatrist has concluded that the patient is dangerous and in need of involuntary commitment, she may introduce her second-hand knowledge of the threat as a basis for that opinion. Of course, the fact that the opinion is at least partially based on hearsay may serve to weaken it under cross-examination.

c. The hypothetical question

The expert witness has the right to answer a hypothetical question, a function that ordinary witnesses, whose testimony is limited to the recounting of observations, cannot fulfill. The hypothetical question is useful in obtaining the expert's opinion about a factual situation other than the one he presumes to have existed. Since the jury is under no obligation to accept the expert's version of the facts, a hypothetical allows both sides of a case to place the expert's opinion on record with regard to any one of a number of factual situations that the jury might determine to have been present.

Hypotheticals sometimes stretch the bounds of the expert's imagination, but they do allow the attorneys to probe more carefully the basis for the expert's opinion by altering one element of the history at a time to determine the crucial variable. The fallacy in many cases, and one that any alert expert should point out in responding, is that psychopathological signs and symptoms often appear in conjunction as syndromes, so that to alter one or another element of the presentation may present an artificial picture that has no correspondence to reality. Nonetheless, the expert may not refuse to answer hypotheticals, and the well-prepared expert will have anticipated them and thought through potential responses in advance.

d. The weight of expert testimony

Many clinicians may naively assume that, having been summoned into court to testify as an "expert" in a given case, their opinion will be the decisive element in its resolution. Although that may sometimes be true—empirical studies of commitment hearings, for example, have shown that unopposed psychiatric testimony is usually accepted without challenge and psychiatric recommendations are usually followed—in most instances, for a variety of reasons, the expert's testimony is not the decisive factor. First, in many important cases, both sides will have obtained their own experts who will often offer contradictory testimony. It will then be up to the judge or the jury to decide which expert or set of experts to believe.

But even when expert testimony is uncontradicted, the legal finders of fact are still free to disregard it. The expert is expected not only to offer an opinion, but also to state grounds on which that opinion has been formulated. To the extent that those grounds are unpersuasive the testimony will be ignored. While this may appear to the expert witness to be farcical, since the basis for her being called to testify in the first place was the assumption that the members of the jury were not able to draw their own conclusions about the evidence, this approach is supported in jurisprudential theory by differentiating between scientific and legal truths. Whereas scientific truth is concerned only with objective reality, legal truth reflects judgments of policy as seen by the judge or jury. Thus, despite expert agreement that a defendant was unlikely to have been criminally responsible at the time of a particularly heinous crime, a court might find him responsible and guilty because the values of the community are such that it will not let the perpetrator go unpunished. Though frustrating to the expert, such flexibility is said to allow the system to express the moral sentiments of society.

3. DISCREDITING EXPERT TESTIMONY

As with all evidence offered in court, the opinion of an expert may be subject to the most rigorous cross-examination. Some lines of attack are common to all challenges of expert witnesses. Opposing attorneys will often challenge the expert's credentials, either as an individual (e.g., his training was insufficient) or as a member of a group (e.g., no psychiatrist can expertly testify about future dangerousness). The expert's objectivity may be questioned by asking how much money he is receiving for his testimony, in a manner that implies that his opinion is for sale to the highest bidder. The adequacy of his examination, the validity of the conclusions, even the theoretical basis on which his opinion was drawn—all are open to attack.

Psychiatric witnesses, moreover, are particularly vulnerable in a number of these areas. Given the profusion of schools of thought in mental health, it is easy for an enterprising attorney to find professional literature that flatly contradicts almost any theoretical assumption on which an opinion may rest. Guides have been published to alert attorneys to these issues of controversy and to steer them to the relevant citations (see Suggested Readings—Ziskin and Faust). Particularly vulnerable are an expert's opinions about the nature of the defendant's diagnosis (given studies showing low reliability of diagnoses among raters), the presumed psychodynamic bases for the patient's behavior (given the panoply of anti-Freudian literature), and a prediction of dangerousness (given studies showing that psychiatrists are poor predictors). Challenges may also be launched against the relevancy of medical school training to assessing psychological problems, the reliability of information gathered in the clinical interview, the presumed effect of experience as contributing to the ability to make a more accurate diagnosis, and the propensity of psychiatrists to seek unnecessarily protective environments for their patients.

Any mental health professional who is going to testify regularly in court, or even in a single, particularly important case, should familiarize himself with a book such as Ziskin and Faust's, anticipate the arguments that are most likely to be offered, and gather references to refute them. Of special note is the fact that many of the studies that showed psychiatric diagnosis to be unreliable were performed several decades ago, and took into account neither the recent heightened awareness of psychiatrists to conditions such as manic-depressive illness, nor the effect on reliability of the specific criteria for diagnosis listed in *DSM-III* or *DSM III-R*.

There are two advantages, though they are small ones, that the expert possesses in this struggle. First, an expert cannot be made to answer a question with a simple "yes" or "no" when he feels that further qualification is needed. Second, no textbook or other published work can be used to challenge an expert's opinion unless the expert either explicitly has relied upon that work in formulating his opinion or acknowledges it as an authoritative work in the field.

4. THE VICISSITUDES OF EXPERTDOM

a. The unwilling expert

In those cases in which the expert has agreed to undertake an evaluation for forensic purposes, there is usually no question about the expert's willingness to present the data in court. Therapists who attain expert knowledge about patients in therapeutic situations, however, and are then asked to testify about that knowledge for trial purposes are usually less than eager witnesses. The reasons for their reluctance may range from an unwillingness to spend time away from their work to a fear of the impact of such testimony on their former or current patient, to a dislike of courtroom procedures and of aggressive attorneys.

Nonetheless, experts who have been properly subpoenaed, and whose patients have waived privilege or where privilege is inapplicable (see Chap. 1, Sec. II-C-5), cannot legitimately avoid testifying. Lawyers are often warned to shun the unwilling expert, for fear that the disgruntled witness will torpedo their case by placing even favorable information in an unfavorable light. Despite this, experts are frequently called against their will because their testimony is perceived as crucial to the outcome of the case. The only solace for the unwilling expert is that he can bill the side that subpoenaed him for a reasonable expert's fee, in addition to expenses.

b. The "nonexpert" expert

As was noted in Sec. 2-a above, the court is free to define the extent to which any individual may speak with expert status on the facts of a case. This means that a professional who is in reality an expert in mental health may be called to testify as an ordinary witness. This will obviously be true when the clinician has witnessed an event, a bank robbery, for example, unrelated to her field of expertise. But the professional can similarly be called to testify only to the facts of an occurrence on an inpatient ward, as when one patient assaults another, without being asked for an expert's opinion on the matter. Clinicians are frequently in this situation when called to the stand to introduce into evidence clinical records of a factual sort, like medication logs that they themselves have compiled.

While relieved of the evidentiary and ethical burdens of the expert witness, the "nonexpert" expert is at something of a disadvantage when it comes to reimbursement for her time. Ordinary witnesses are reimbursed at a standard rate for travel and lost time, usually amounting to several dollars a day. To the professional who loses hundreds of dollars as a result of abandoning clinical activities for the time involved it is often cold comfort that our system of justice relies on such sacrifices from all of us to perform its fact-finding function.

c. The expert "discovered"

An expert who agrees to testify in court can find herself answering questions in quite a different setting, as well. As part of the procedures for equalizing the contest between parties in a civil suit, the courts have developed a set of elaborate pretrial investigative routines that are encompassed by the term "discovery." The discovery process permits each side of a case to summon and interrogate the principals and witnesses for the opposing side before the case reaches the trial stage. Thus, an expert who conducts a psychiatric examination for the plaintiff in a psychic damages case may find herself subpoenaed to present the results of her examination to the lawyers for the defense.

Discovery can take several forms. The questions to which the opposing party wants answers can be transmitted in writing and responded to in kind ("a written interrogatory") or the witness can be summoned to an attorney's office to answer questions in person ("an oral deposition"). Additionally, documents such as hospital records or objects can be requested, or the opposing party may demand that her expert be permitted to perform a physical, psychiatric, or psychological examination of the plaintiff. While each side can always challenge the other's requests for information, courts are generally quite liberal about granting the desired access. One exception is material that may be privileged in court, such as the information conveyed in clinical sessions in some states (see Chap. 1, Sec. II-C-3), which is similarly privileged in discovery and should not be revealed without the patient's waiver or a judicial order abrogating the privilege.

Discovery has been subjected to some criticism of late because of its use in malpractice and other tort suits that have been filed without adequate reason to believe that negligence occurred; an aggressive use of discovery can then be employed in a legal "fishing expedition" designed to uncover enough adverse facts to justify going to trial.

For the expert witness, the most important point is that testimony obtained by means of pretrial discovery can be as potent and critical as anything said in court. Discovery, whether oral or written, takes place under oath, and—although it ordinarily cannot be introduced at trial in lieu of a witness's testimony—it can be used to challenge and discredit testimony that does not correspond to the account that the witness gave earlier during discovery. The rules that a careful witness should observe, therefore, are identical to those that should govern trial testimony (see Sec. III-C); the witness should, above all, present her responses in a thoughtful manner that reflects her final conclusions on the subject. A careless comment at the taking of a deposition can completely destroy a witness's effectiveness.

B. The adversary system

The culture shock that so frequently accompanies the entry of a mental health professional into the courtroom setting derives from some very profound differences in the orientations of the legal and mental health professions. Nothing so typifies this divergence in approaches as the assumptions that underlie the adversary system.

1. THE THEORY OF THE ADVERSARY SYSTEM

It has long been the presumption in Anglo-American jurisprudence that truth can only be ascertained by witnessing the combat of minds, each attempting to prove the falsehood of the other's position. So important is this belief that a large part of procedural law is devoted to enhancing the ability of the contesting parties to attack each other as vigorously as possible. Such rules in civil cases as pretrial discovery, and in criminal cases as the constitutional rights to notice of the charges, speedy and public trial, confrontation of witnesses, power of subpoena, and representation of counsel, were all devised to equalize and maximize the ability of each side to prove its point.

There are, of course, other approaches to truth. The collaborative model, in which all the involved parties pool their data and share their insights, is the more familiar schema in scientific and clinical work. But the law generally rejects such methods as insufficiently protective of individual rights. An exception to this general practice of eschewing nonadversary approaches occurred from the early years of this century until roughly the late 1960s in both juvenile and mental health proceedings. Reasoning that the wayward young and the mentally ill were not really criminals and could benefit more from the collaborative efforts of the courts, the professions, and the state, legislatures relaxed the ordinarily strict procedural guidelines in such cases. Hearings were held informally, hearsay was accepted as evidence, counsel were excluded, cross-examination was shunned, and the goal was generally framed not so much to assign blame as to settle upon the most desirable and therapeutic outcome.

The difficulty with this ostensibly humane approach to juveniles and the mentally ill was that what seemed desirable from the point of view of the court was not necessarily equally desirable for the individual. The *parens patriae* assumption that the state knows better than the individual what is in his best interest (see Chap. 2, Sec. II-D-2-b), while used to justify such procedures, was called into serious question when it was recognized that juveniles and mentally ill alike were being committed to facilities that were underfunded, understaffed, custodial at best, and brutalizing at worst. When the legal profession recognized that their abandonment of the adversary model was in part responsible for the commitment of so many to such institutions, the quick-step march began to reinstitute the safeguards. Juvenile law and mental health law both have been dominated in the last several decades by the reimposition of an adversary framework.

While the return of the adversary approach may be regretted, it can certainly be understood in this light. Although clinicians are uncomfortable with the adversary system, its replacement in the future (at least insofar as the mentally ill are concerned) will be dependent on not only the goodwill of those involved in the courts of law, but also on the willingness of society to validate the paternalistic approach by providing adequate resources to construct truly beneficent dispositions. At the present time, that seems unlikely.

2. THE ROLE OF THE LAWYER

The key to the effectiveness of any adversary approach to truth is the performance of the advocate—in this case, the attorney. If adversary theory is fully applied, the lawyer can have only one approach to his work: an unflagging and undeviating devotion to proving that his client's position is correct. In those cases in which the lawyer actually believes this to be the case, or in many civil suits where honest differences of opinion can arise about the issues at stake, this presents few problems for attorneys. The lawyer not only attempts to construct as solid a case as possible for his client, but also to contest at every point the assertions of the opposition. A number of ethical problems, however, arise in two instances: (1) in civil and criminal cases in which the attorney believes his client to be wrong; and (2) in cases for which the goal of the hearing is not to punish or reward, but to treat or protect.

a. Criminal cases

Lawyers' codes of ethics are complicated documents that struggle with these problems, but inevitably provide no entirely satisfactory solutions. The vigorous defense of those the lawyer believes to be guilty is justified both by establishing certain procedural safeguards (lawyers are not allowed to present, or to let their clients present, deliberate falsehoods, for example), and by arguing that insofar as the system requires an adversary confrontation to establish the truth, it would be impossible (and unconstitutional, as well) to deny the assistance of counsel to some defendants who are believed in advance of trial to be guilty without making a mockery of the entire adversary system. Yet the fact that lawyers must exert their full efforts to defend the guilty is still a troubling matter for many of them. One suspects that the reluctance of so many of the graduates of the finest law schools to enter criminal law is, in part, related to this issue.

b. *Parens patriae* proceedings

A different set of ethical issues is raised by legal proceedings ostensibly designed to benefit their subjects. Many juvenile court hearings and most mental health proceedings (except for commitments initiated under a pure "dangerous-ness to others" rationale) fall into this category. To the extent that the subjects of these hearings are less capable than the state to decide wherein lie their best interests (the basis for any *parens patriae* action), it appears at first glance some-thing of an anomaly to encourage lawyers to defend their client's wishes as forcefully as possible. If the best interests of a psychotic individual obviously require hospitalization, the lawyer who successfully persuades a judge to release his client to the fortunes of the street may well wonder what good his pleadings have accomplished. In fact, it was just this line of logic that led to periods of relaxation of adversary procedures in the early part of this century and again in the 1950s.

What has induced the current reversion to stricter adversary proceedings has been the previously noted perception that, theory aside, the actual disposi-tions of the mentally ill—in most cases in state hospitals—were not clearly in their best interests. Of course, many would argue that commitment to even the less-well-run state hospitals was preferable to allowing psychotic people to roam the streets, but the impact of the social theorists of institutional life, the labeling theorists, and the diverse arms of the antipsychiatry movement has been to convince many members of the legal system otherwise. Few ethical problems bother attorneys who doubt if mental illnesses exist or who consider psychiatrists to be mere agents of social control. They might be expected to approach every hearing with the aim of preventing their client from being hospitalized.

Other attorneys, often those with more experience in practical mental health law or those who have had a chance to observe the natural course of mental illness, recognize a tension between their charge from the system to "defend" their clients maximally and their desire to see their clients get the help they need. This tension is frequently resolved by their subverting the adversary component of their work, acting instead in what they perceive to be their clients' best interests. Involved here may be such steps as perfunctory challenges to psychiatric credentials and testimony, waivers of certain procedural niceties, and even the utilization of questions designed to display their client's level of psycho-pathology. Almost every study of commitment proceedings has uncovered such behavior, but it is usually chalked up to incompetence on the part of the attorney or insufficient time or remuneration to prepare a case. Both of the latter factors are undoubtedly often important, but even efforts to train attorneys to perform more aggressively in circumstances in which these factors are minimized have failed. As long as the adversary nature of the system appears to work against the needs of the mentally ill for assistance, many attorneys will take what seems to them to be the common-sense approach to dealing with the problem.

3. THE ADVERSARY SYSTEM AND THE EXPERT WITNESS

Foremost among the complaints of most novice expert witnesses is that they were subject to a cross-examination that seemed to resemble the name-calling games of their childhood more than a dispassionate search for truth. The likely content of this attack was outlined above (see Sec. II-A-3), but the emotional impact must be taken into account, as well. A respected professional whose expertise, competence, and integrity are questioned, and sometimes shaken, before an audience of nonprofessionals may feel as violated as the victim of a mugging on the streets. Some leading forensic experts claim to relish the combat of minds involved in a cutting cross-examination, but for most professionals, it is often the low point of their careers.

4. DISCOVERING THE TRUTH IN COURT

Platitudes from civics class aside, one of the most startling revelations for novice witnesses is that the judicial system's dedication to the pursuit of truth is not always its preeminent value. Some examples of this slighting of truth in favor of other values have already been alluded to. The rules governing hearsay evidence, for example, are enforced even in cases in which the evidence can be shown to be quite reliable, because the value of preserving the adversary system itself takes precedence over the discovery of truth in any given case. A clinician who is barred from testifying about threats reported by a patient's family because he himself did not hear them, with the result that a patient who he feels is dangerous is released, may be bewildered at this apparent failure of the legal system. Clinicians, of course, tend to be pragmatists, willing to adopt any stratagem or to abandon any theory if the patient at hand will be helped thereby. But the legal system often sees things differently and needs to be accepted on its own terms if mutual bitterness is not to be the inevitable result of interaction between psychiatry and law.

These sorts of compromises with the unfettered pursuit of truth may seem more reasonable if viewed in a slightly broader perspective. Breaching the confidentiality of the psychiatrist-patient relationship may aid the search for truth in many instances, but because society values the benefits that derive from such relationships, it is forbidden in many states (see Chap. 1, Sec. II-B-3). Similarly, forcing a defendant to testify about his own activities, even to the point of torture, may produce the most reliable evidence of what actually occurred, but forced self-incrimination is precluded by our Constitution. In these and comparable instances, it is not an exaggeration to say that when truth and justice compete with each other for preeminence in court, the avowed goal of the system is to assure that justice prevails.

C. Ethical issues for expert witnesses

1. THE "HIRED GUN" PROBLEM

Most expert witnesses are hired not by the court, but by one side or the other in a given case. This frequently leads to confusion in the expert's mind as to the extent of her obligation to those who are paying her fee. Should the expert try to support the point of view her employer is espousing when the evidence for it is weak to nonexistent? How much "prepping" before trial with the attorney for the side that hired her is legitimate? When confronted in court with evidence that seems to negate the basis for her opinion, how obstinately should the expert stick to her original conclusion? In short, is the expert a "hired gun" who is being paid to express only the opinion that would favor her employer's case, or does she owe allegiance to some loftier principle?

a. Skills for sale

These issues can begin to be resolved by focusing on exactly what the expert is selling in the bargain struck with an attorney. The honest expert is offering a set of skills, a way of analyzing the problem at hand, and the means of presenting that analysis in court. He should most emphatically not be mongering an opinion, for sale to the highest bidder and amenable to influence by the power of pecuniary suggestion. The court expects the expert to reach an opinion by an impartial exercise of the relevant skills and to present the opinion with as diligent a regard as possible for the uncertainties inherent in the evaluation process. It is, strictly speaking, for the time that it takes to reach a conclusion and to appear in court for which the expert is being paid, not for the vector of the conclusion.

b. The evaluation process

As a consequence of this approach, an expert witness who agrees to conduct an evaluation should do so with the explicit understanding that the conclusion may not conform to the outcome desired by the attorney. A corollary is that the expert should always arrange to be paid the same amount for the evaluation (usually depending on the time involved) whether or not the attorney decides ultimately to use it in court. Many experienced expert witnesses feel that payment of a retainer in advance lessens the psychological pressure on them to reach the "right" conclusion, although the poor track record of many attorneys in paying their experts is probably a more persuasive reason to arrange for such a retainer.

With that understanding, the potential expert witness should approach the evaluation as he would any other clinical task, attempting to reach the most accurate assessment possible. Because of the subtle influences on clinicians in these situations to resolve doubts in favor of the side on whose behalf they have been asked to testify, the expert should search assiduously for contradictory evidence and consider it as seriously as possible before reaching a conclusion. This will often mean going beyond the direct assessment of the individual whose status is in question, seeking evidence from family members, friends, and others who have come into contact with him. Where such corroborative evidence is necessary but unavailable, or the attorney refuses to allow the expert to interview other informants, the expert may want to consider withdrawing from the case on the grounds that a truly "expert" opinion is unattainable.

c. Pretrial preparation

Having performed the evaluation as described, the expert is obligated to convey her findings as precisely as possible to the attorney. This includes noting the basis for the opinion, its strengths and weaknesses, the reasonable opinions that other consultants might reach and their strengths and weaknesses, and the confidence with which the expert will be able to uphold the opinion in court. If the opinion is not useful to the side for which she was asked to do the examination, her participation may end here. Assuming the attorney agrees that the expert's unvarnished opinion will be of use to his case, however, it is legitimate for the expert and the attorney to rehearse its presentation in detail and for the expert to reveal ways of buttressing her testimony in court. Involved here is a switch from the role of impartial assessor to a position as a pretrial consultant, in preparation for the situation in court in which once again the expert will assume the neutral role.

d. Testifying

On arriving in the witness stand, the expert is again expected to testify to the truth as he perceives it regardless of which side called him into court. Of course, the very fact that the witness has arrived at this point implies that his opinion fits the expectations of those who are paying his fee. Nonetheless, he should not overstate the certainty of the conclusions he has reached, understate the likelihood that alternative interpretations are correct, or—in the face of new evidence that was previously unavailable to him—resist changing his opinion if that seems called for. Hypotheticals should be answered honestly, even if doing so would seem to weaken the case he is supporting. The wise attorney will recognize the advantages of this neutral approach to expert testimony: the more independent-minded, reasonable, and open to input the expert appears to be, the more likely it is that his testimony will be respected by a jury.

This composite system of performing the role of the expert, though difficult to fulfill in that it requires several complicated psychological shifts in perceived allegiance, can serve to obviate many of the ethical issues in expert testimony. A residuum of difficulty will always remain, of course, because of the natural desire to please those with whom one is working; but, unless expert testimony is to be discarded altogether on these grounds, this desire to please must be overcome insofar as possible by constant attention to the possibility of bias that it creates.

2. THE BATTLE OF THE EXPERTS

Among those mental health professionals who advocate complete abstention from courtroom proceedings, the most common rationale is that the diversity of expert views that can be observed in many cases does nothing but degrade the professions in the eyes of the public. This phenomenon of the "battle of the experts" creates the impression, they continue, that expert clinicians are for sale to the highest bidder and that there is no common store of knowledge on which any of their opinions rest.

Unfortunately, it is sometimes the case that opinions can be bought, whether the sale takes place consciously or unconsciously in the mind of the expert. More often, expert witnesses develop ideological biases that shape their testimony in individual cases, this resulting in the phenomenon of the psychiatrist who always testifies for the defense in criminal responsibility cases or one who always testifies that the mental patient needs to be committed. Interpersonal factors are also of importance. Even without realizing the effect of a developing relationship with the attorney who employs her, the expert may find herself drawn toward the attorney's position out of reluctance to disappoint a "friend." Many attorneys recognize this tendency and cultivate personal relationships with their expert witnesses.

The most common reason for a difference of expert opinion, however, is simply that those cases that reach the trial stage are frequently so laden with complicated factual elements that it is not difficult to find professionals who honestly can express differences of opinion about their interpretation. Naturally, the considerable uncertainties and gaps in psychiatric knowledge contribute to this process. But seen in this light, the much-deplored battle of the experts differs little from the vigorous disputes that take place at many grand rounds presentations, or—for that matter—disputes that might well arise between experts in engineering, architecture, or geology concerning complex issues that might have forensic impact in those fields. Unless one sees a value in hiding from the world at large the fact that psychiatry is not an exact science, a revelation that is unlikely to surprise most educated laypeople, there seems little reason to shun courtroom confrontations of opposing experts.

3. NONADVERSARY APPROACHES

Given all the previously cited reasons for professionals' reluctance to get involved with the adversary system, it is not surprising that the suggestion is frequently made to abandon it in favor of nonadversary approaches. The most common scenario that is offered is as follows: the court appoints *one* expert to examine the individual or group of individuals (in child custody cases, for example) whose condition is in dispute; all sides cooperate in making evidence available to the expert consultant, whose opinion serves as the sole basis for the argumentation of both sides in the case. While this proposal does not remove the need for vigorous cross-examination, it does remove the pressures toward partisanship that many experts feel and the trauma of opposing a fellow professional in court.

As appealing as the nonadversary approach may be (and as much as it was utilized, in practice if not in theory, in the juvenile and mental health systems for many years), there are sound reasons for both lawyers and clinicians to reject it. Foremost among these reasons is the spurious sense of certainty that a single opinion may tend to convey in a field that is still in its scientific infancy and is therefore riddled with uncertainties. Much of the venom that lawyers and judges direct at psychiatry today is a result of the unwarranted self-assurance with which it welcomed the task of participation in decisions about sentencing, rehabilitation, and prediction of recidivism in the earlier part of this century. A return to the pretense that there is only one psychiatric approximation of truth will do neither the legal system nor psychiatry much good.

In addition, to disallow the side that is disenchanted with the neutral expert's findings the right to enlist experts of its own to challenge the assumptions and procedures employed and the conclusions reached is not only quite likely unconstitutional, but on a pragmatic level will serve to encourage sloppy assessments and to attract the least competent practitioners into the field. Although it is the constitutional due process issues that probably ensure that such nonadversary procedures will not become the norm, it is doubtful that, even from the clinician's point of view, they would, in the end, be desirable.

4. THE PROBLEM OF CAUSING HARM

One of the trickier ethical issues for mental health professionals relates to the consequences of their participation in court proceedings. Ordinarily, clinicians comfort themselves with the thought that they are devoted entirely to the welfare of their patients and to the principles of beneficence (doing good) and non-maleficence (not doing harm). The courtroom setting, however, clearly calls these presumptions into question.

When testifying in court, mental health professionals may contribute directly to harming the people whom they have evaluated. Testimony, for example, about a defendant's mental state at the time of the crime may lead to his being convicted, rather than being found not guilty by reason of insanity. Evidence of a low likelihood of responding to treatment may lead to the imposition of a harsher sentence. Even in civil proceedings, testimony that benefits one side will harm the other, often including the person who has been the subject of the clinician's evaluation.

Is this acceptable? Can clinicians (especially psychiatrists, whose ethics derive from a long tradition of medical adherence to the principle of *primum non nocere*—first do no harm) legitimately testify in ways that may cause harm to the people they have assessed? Some clinicians answer this question in the negative and shun all forensic work as a result. But this seems too extreme a conclusion. In their clinical roles, clinicians in fact must seek the best interests of the people they evaluate and treat. Their functioning in the forensic setting, however, is guided by a different set of principles, emphasizing the pursuit of truth, within the limits of fairness. This is not problematic, as long as the forensic evaluator makes clear the distinctions between his clinical and forensic roles. In this non-clinical task, it may still be obligatory to avoid needless harm to subjects, but harm resulting from the disclosure of information in proper legal settings is not ethically problematic.

III. CLINICAL ISSUES

A. The courtroom as a foreign country

The clinician called into court for the first time to testify on his own or another's behalf commonly regards his entry into this novel arena, so different from his own "turf," as something akin to parachuting unarmed into enemy territory; this view, however romantic, is usually a derivative of the clinician's ignorance of the language and customs of the courtroom, and thus confounds the unfamiliar with the threatening. Such an approach, although understandable, lends neither comfort nor assistance to the beleaguered therapist.

A more useful approach may be to view the courtroom as a friendly, potentially interesting foreign country that one has occasion to visit. Although the language, garb, and customs of the inhabitants may appear startling to the first-time tourist, potential rough spots of such a visit can be smoothed by: (1) careful attention to preparation; (2) learning a bit of the language in advance; and (3) acquiring some familiarity with the customs one is likely to face, especially those governing sensitive areas of behavior and demeanor. Different kinds of courts may use different rules, but the following review of information for the clinician in court is organized on the fundamentals suggested above to help the relatively inexperienced traveler.

B. Preparation for appearance in court

This topic has two facets: preparation for appearance in court as the defendant in a malpractice suit and preparation for participation as an expert witness. The former, described in Chap. 4, Sec. III-B, will be largely guided by one's attorney; the latter will be discussed below.

1. USE OF CHARTS AND RECORDS

The data base for the expert witness in forensic psychiatry consists of several categories of information. The most familiar source of data is a hospital's, clinic's, or individual practitioner's records relating to a particular case. These are examined not only as to significant form and content as reviewed in Chapters 1 and 4, but as to omissions, ellipses, and ambiguities in relation to the question at hand (negligence, child custody, assessment of disability or damages). Further information may be sought from other appropriate sources or obtained from direct examination of the subject (see below) or others.

It is often wise for the expert witness to make, then familiarize herself with, her own notes and summaries on the material she reviews, with the intent of taking these to the witness stand in place of the original materials; not only are these notes easier to manage and retrieve information from than are the voluminous documents that are part of most cases, but they offer no invitation to the cross-examining attorney to seize gratuitously upon words or phrases read out of context from the record.

Particular attention should be paid (for records of inpatients) to nurses' notes, medication records, and similar parts of the chart often overlooked in casual review. These can be critical in discovering from eyewitnesses what occurred. Consistency or inconsistency should be determined; for example, does the nurse's note on the 11-to-7 shift report the incident in the same way as the doctor's progress note written the same *calendar* day but actually the next morning, when new data and the benefit of hindsight provide additional perspective?

Lab slips and test results of all types should also be scrutinized with care, since the results may not necessarily be recorded within the body of the chart's progress notes; important bases for a decision made by the treaters may not otherwise be explicit or even comprehensible.

It is entirely appropriate, though not always possible, for the expert witness to interview caretakers or relevant parties directly, first obtaining their permission and explaining clearly both her task and the "side of the case" that she represents. (If the expert is employed by neither side, this, too, should be made explicit.)

In malpractice cases, the data gathered from these multiple sources should be organized in terms of a "decision tree"; that is, since clinical treatment consists of innumerable decisions where one path is chosen over another, the expert should arrange the information in such a way as to reflect the data available to the treating clinicians at the time the decision was made. The expert must be alert to the alternatives: what would have been the outcome of "the road not taken"?

Was the chosen path consistent with good clinical practice? These and related queries must be thrown against the backdrop of the unique aspects of the case and the consensus of the profession on guidelines for sound treatment.

> **Example 1:** An expert witness, testifying in a suit for wrongful death following the suicide of an inpatient, noted from the record that the depressed patient had been attempting in a relentless manner to strangle herself with her own clothing. A course of antidepressants had been initiated. Given the patient's documented suicidal press, the expert realized that the pivotal questions were: why was electroconvulsive therapy (ECT) *not* used? What conditions might have militated against its use? Was the failure to use it a mark of negligence, or were other factors significant in this decision? Was ECT considered, and did the chart evince a careful weighing of the pros and cons?

2. DIRECT EXAMINATION OF THE SUBJECT

As outlined in Chapter 6, subjects being examined for court-related matters deserve clear and candid explanations, before examination, about the clinician's agency (i.e., for whom the clinician is working) and about the purpose to which the information may or will be put. The subject should be informed that he need not answer any question if he does not wish to do so: if he is uncertain about the ground rules governing his participation, he should be encouraged to contact his attorney. The expert witness should also explain that his task is to deliver an opinion, no more or less, and that, while other opinions may or may not be vouchsafed, the judge and/or jury will be making the actual decision. This last is an important point to make explicit since a number of naive subjects view the interview with the expert witness as resulting in the decision itself.

Embarking on the interview, the expert must bear in mind both the unique professional skills of inquiry and investigation that he brings to the task *and* the limitations of any examiner of whatever skill in determining some of the information that judges and juries wish to obtain. The "one, true, correct" treatment decision, a person's fitness to be a parent, the actual past dangerousness of a person examined long after the danger has passed—all these issues tax, if not exceed, the capabilities of even experienced interviewers, by virtue of their complexity, their variability from person to person, and the inevitably retrospective viewpoint of the examiner.

For example, can one truly assess fitness as a parent without seeing the relationship with the child over time, and would not even that assessment be powerfully influenced (if not distorted) by the very presence of the observer?

The existence of these difficulties should not preclude the examination nor should it necessarily invalidate the results; rather, such problems demand from the witness a keen awareness of the necessity for being explicit about the data from which his conclusions are drawn and the limits of such data. Few types of testimony are more damaging to the case, to the witness, or to the credibility of the profession than sweeping, final, and confident conclusions, drawn from unsupported "intuition" and "experience."

The actual interview should conform to the information-gathering, rather than the treatment, model; however, the importance of rapport with the subject, patience, tact, and respect remain unchanged from the clinical setting. In addition to exploring the key area in question, the clinician should elicit background material as to functioning in other related areas, general psychological strengths and weaknesses, and the subject's manner of relating in the interview. With proper introduction, a full mental status examination should be performed; time and again this exam reveals unexpected psychosis, cognitive disturbance, memory defects, and the like. As many interviews as needed should take place.

A detailed record of the interview should be made as soon thereafter as possible. Repeated interviews may be necessary and should be anticipated, since a subject's mental state may fluctuate, or a subject may communicate more freely with someone seen more than once; additional questions or uncertainties, moreover, frequently arise at the point when the clinician writes or reviews the notes from his first interview.

The report, if written, should be organized along the general lines of a case presentation: general background including the questions to be addressed and the circumstances of the examination; present and past historical data obtained from interview and other sources; family and social history, where appropriate; mental status examination report, including verbatim queries and responses when indicated, especially in critical areas where the demonstration of a patient's understanding or capacities is significant; notation of areas where data could not be obtained and/or conclusions would not be supportable; and finally, a summary of impressions and conclusions, together with the summarized data on which they are based. (See sample reports in Chap. 6, Sec. VI.) Other ways of organizing reports for the court have been suggested; the expert should settle on a format that she finds comfortable and will use consistently. Experienced witnesses often include some comment about their own assessment of the validity or reliability of the examination and conclusions; for example, "The absence of psychotic symptomatology at this point, five months after the alleged onset of the psychosis, would not imply that use of medication at *that* time was inappropriate."

3. Literature review

Because attorneys engaged in mental health litigation routinely attempt to gather information from mental health literature to develop their cases, the expert witness should certainly review current professional work on any subject not within the purview of her area of major activity, interest, or research. The purpose of such a review is largely to diminish the disconcerting impact of surprise questions; in practice, no clinician can be expected to keep absolutely *au courant* with all developments, even within a specialized area of her field. Clinicians should also review their own writings on the subject in question, paying particular attention to conclusions that might seem to contradict their current testimony.

4. Preparation of "your" attorney

The traveler abroad develops a two-way communication with her guide, on one hand learning from him the significance of the terrain, signposts, and landmarks, the expectations of proper behavior and customs, on the other hand imparting a sense of her interests, her capacities and strengths, and such information as she may already have assimilated. Similarly, an essential part of preparation for appearance in court is establishment of just such a two-way communication with the attorney representing one's side of the case.

a. The role of education

Educating one's lawyer about various aspects of the psychiatric profession, including diagnosis, treatment practices and the like, represents one of the most vital functions of the expert witness, especially in the early preparation of the case; the amount, level of complexity, detail, and extent of this education, of course, are directly related to the attorney's experience and familiarity with the subject.

> *Example 2:* A deposition that had been confusing to the attorney was submitted to an expert witness; the case involved a patient with schizophrenia who had at one point been depressed. The expert witness realized (and explained) that the word "depression" was being used in three ways, all carrying different connotations in psychiatric parlance. The defendant physician meant the transient mood disturbance; the opposing attorney meant the full-fledged syndrome; and the *Physicians' Desk Reference* (from which the attorney was quoting) meant the decrease in central nervous system electrical activity (as in "CNS depressant").

The educative process, of course, is a two-way street. The capable attorney reciprocally prepares the witness as to what to expect in court, probable lines of direct and cross-examination, strengths and weaknesses of the case, and the pivotal legal issues.

b. Handling unrealistic expectations

Less experienced attorneys do not differ from laypersons in general in sharing unrealistic expectations and misconceptions of the abilities, capacities, and predictive or retrospective powers of mental health as a field and of psychiatrists in particular; as might be expected, many expectations are wishful, deriving from attorneys' desires for certainty in areas of inherent and inescapable ambiguity.

A typical unrealistic expectation portrays the clinician as a human lie detector, able to detect insincerity, fabrication, or malingering on the basis of an examination. While inconsistencies may, indeed, emerge over the course of one or several interviews, the clear and convincing determination of lying lies beyond the clinical sphere.

Another expectation limns the clinician as an evoker of speech. Clients who refuse to speak or answer questions when their own attorney asks them will not necessarily become garrulous when confronted by a mental health professional.

A third view depicts the evaluator as possessed of a time viewer or "retrospectoscope"—a mythical instrument capable of detecting by examination, a year after the fact, a patient's mental state during the commission of an alleged crime.

A fourth expectation is based on the failure to appreciate such human factors as ambivalence, the role of the unconscious, and the operation of defenses in mental life. Thus, a parent may overtly press for custody of his child as though of one mind about it, but, harboring profound ambivalence about the outcome, may unconsciously sabotage his own case; a psychiatrist, asked by an angry, frustrated, or bewildered attorney to determine the genuineness of the parent's desire for custody, would not be able to give a yes-or-no answer.

A fifth legal expectation skirts the fringes of unethical behavior. Attorneys may exert pressure on the clinician to suppress or ignore certain events that have actually taken place. For example, an attorney, having sent a particular letter to the clinician, may ask her to pretend she never received it, or the attorney may try to dissuade the clinician from retaining his private notes of an interview. Clearly clinicians should resist any attempts that would have, as an ultimate consequence, lying under oath. The clinician must acknowledge receipt of all documents and all records and leave it up to the attorneys to fight over whether some material is inadmissible or privileged as a work product. When attorneys attempt to solicit unethical behavior from clinicians, clinicians should withdraw from the case.

> **Example 3:** A psychiatrist indicated to an attorney that he had retained certain written notes of an interview whose content might prove somewhat problematic for the case the attorney was attempting to advance. The attorney nudged the psychiatrist conspiratorially with his elbow and muttered, "Psychiatrists don't always keep those notes, you know."

Certainly there is no inherent ethical problem in discussing or negotiating with attorneys over the particular phrasing of certain points in ways that do not compromise the basic opinion; but attorneys who attempt to enter into an argument over the clinician's objective views should be gently but firmly resisted.

> **Example 4:** A forensic psychiatrist examining a patient for dangerousness in consideration of his release from a hospital obtained a fairly benign picture from the patient himself, but found, on reviewing the old charts, a terrifying record of dangerous child molestation (which the patient had denied). The psychiatrist explained to the attorney that this history precluded present release. The attorney began to complain about the problem with psychiatrists' always getting into history, and asked why they can't take a patient as he stands. The psychiatrist gently but firmly held his ground on the point.

Another common expectation arising out of a wish for certainty is the demand for an absolute diagnosis—the production of which is a problem for the profession itself, needless to say, a fact often very hard to grasp for the novice counselor. The fact that a patient with highs and lows (mood swings) may have not only manic-depressive illness but schizophrenia, organic brain disease, an intercurrent drug habit, a personality disorder, or a variation of normalcy often bewilders attorneys unfamiliar with the diagnostician's dilemma in the field.

While this list cannot be exhaustive, it may convey a sense of the problem; the expert witness's job includes clarifying for his attorney the manner in which some expectations cannot be realized. Of course, a similar task of "reality testing" may have to be performed on the witness stand.

Most attorneys experienced in this area are cognizant of these difficulties and appreciate the lack of certainty that characterizes much of clinical evaluation and treatment; for the attorney who is unaware of these elements, the expert witness should clarify the matter during pretrial collaboration.

5. CONCLUSIONS IN PSYCHIATRIC EVALUATION

The section just above on uncertainty in the field should be kept in mind by the expert witness in presenting the conclusions of the evaluation (either pretrial or in court). The truism that there is more than one way to skin a cat is eminently applicable to the clinical sphere: there is more than one way to diagnose or treat a patient, interpret a finding, or view an outcome of a case. This realization should evoke humility in offering an opinion, recognizing the presence of human fallibility and bias, rather than presenting it as an omniscient, unitary, and absolute finding.

C. Customs and demeanor in the "foreign land"

While courtroom etiquette has been touched on in Sec. II of this chapter, it will be discussed from a different perspective here. The psychiatrist traveling to court must first dismiss her visions of courtroom drama drawn from the Perry Mason television show and similar fictional scenarios. These dramas often include a scene in which the cross-examining attorney, breathing fire into the face of the crumbling witness, snarls or bellows question after question, reducing the witness to rubble before the opposing counsel can even shout "Objection!"

In reality, counsel may not physically approach the witness and would be severely enjoined from any such histrionics. But the fact remains that the witness's knowledge of certain guidelines that do apply to demeanor in court can considerably aid her effectiveness on the stand.

1. THE ROLE OF THE WITNESS: WHAT IT IS AND IS NOT

If the clinician-witness, unfamiliar with the courtroom role he will play, seeks to draw on some familiar model to guide his participation, the best such model might well be his teaching experience. In that arena, the goals are to inform the audience; to impart information in the most readily assimilable way; to maintain the audience's interest and attention; and to field difficult, challenging, or provocative questions on what is being taught.

These precepts closely parallel the guidelines for the witness. The best teachers know the secret that among the most powerful forces in fine pedagogy is the audience's perception of the teacher's *wish* to convey the material, and the eagerness and effort expended on this goal; this is also true of reaching a judge and jury.

These goals may be readily distinguished from other infelicitous intentions, inconsistent with optimal presence on the stand—intentions also to be eschewed by the traveler in a foreign land. The undesirable aims include the wish to be admired and to impress others by showing off one's vast knowledge and erudition; the wish to win the case through intimidation of one's audience by one's arrogant, authoritarian demeanor; the wish to fawn upon, flatter, or seduce the jury; or the wish to patronize, or condescend to one's audience from a position of superiority. All these approaches are alienating, self-defeating, and ineffective. The seasoned expert witness is aware, moreover, that judges and juries may *feel* that these attitudes are present even when they are not, just as the foreigner's motives may be misunderstood by the natives; therefore, he avoids even the semblance of such inappropriate aims.

a. Informing

The tasks of the witness, beyond delivering an opinion based on the data gathered as described above (Sec. III-B), is to inform judge and jury about the area of psychiatric knowledge under question; this would be the case regardless of whether there is one expert only or one on each side of a case. The informing function must be distinguished from arguing.

b. Arguing

The witness who provokes or is drawn into argument with counsel or judge betrays her function and undermines her position on the case. The view has been frequently expressed that juries decide more on the basis of dictates from the viscera than from the cerebral cortex, and the argumentative witness is viscerally less convincing.

c. Preaching

The role of the witness is not to advance the cause of psychiatry, deplore legal blindness and ignorance, propose statutory reform or—in sum—to confuse the witness stand with a soapbox. Again, the blurring of the role also may alienate the jury.

d. Advising

The witness must recall that to judge and/or jury belongs the task of deciding and concluding on the basis of the information provided. The witness who preempts this task may face stern reprimands since—while judges vary in their tolerance for flexibility in courtroom conduct—they rarely relish having their decisions "made" for them in public.

> **Example 5:** An overenthusiastic witness was testifying at a hearing on the committability of a suicidal patient for whom a writ of habeas corpus had been filed. He stated, at the end of his response to a question, "This patient should clearly be committed since the law states that patients dangerous to self through mental illness should be committed." The judge stared in disbelief, then announced through clenched teeth that that decision was the substantive issue before the court and was therefore something that he alone would decide. The crestfallen witness was dismissed.

2. TECHNICAL CONSIDERATIONS

a. Clearing time

Legal personnel are mindful of physicians' and other clinicians' schedules and usually cooperate with choosing a date and time for the witness to appear in such a way as to maximize convenience. However, many courtroom events are of unpredictable duration. The experienced witness therefore clears a generous amount of time and brings work or recreational reading along. The witness who is preoccupied with a patient yet to be seen that day as the trial drags on and the clock ticks inexorably away has made her situation more difficult and her preoccupied, hurried, or distracted court appearance far less effective, as well as having earned the displeasure of the patient(s) kept waiting.

b. Oral presentation of material

In the entire history of jurisprudence, no expert witness ever spoke too clearly, audibly, or comprehensibly; this axiom should be borne in mind. Teaching or lecturing experience is invaluable here; absent this background, some "dry runs" or rehearsals with an objective audience would be excellent preparation, since the witness who mutters, mumbles, or speaks too softly markedly reduces his credibility, no matter how impressive his credentials.

c. Credentials

The "battle of experts" is sometimes influenced, if not decided, by the respective credentials of the two parties; in some jurisdictions, specific case law permits judge or jury to weight testimony differentially, based on differing levels of expertise, however determined (e.g., by extent of direct clinical experience with the type of problem at hand).

When one side's expert has more powerful or impressive credentials, certain tactical approaches by counsel commonly come into play. The opposing side attempts immediately to concede the witness's expert status, thus preventing the judge and/or jury from hearing the witness intone the lengthy catalog of her stellar achievements. Counsel on the expert's side attempts (with equal celerity) to insist that the minute details of the expert's curriculum vitae be read into the record precisely for their impressive effect. The outcome of this struggle is usually settled by the judge.

3. SUBJECTIVE ASPECTS

a. Impugned expertise as narcissistic assault

More than any aspect of the foreign country of the courtroom, it is the cross-examination of the expert witness by the opposing side that causes clinicians to turn pale and shudder when they hear the phrase "appearing in court."

This reaction stems in part from the fact that in clinical settings experts frequently and freely disagree, but usually (though not always) with preservation of mutual respect, maintenance of a diplomatic mode of conveying disagreement, and awareness that the complexity of the field allows for differing views. In stark contrast, the cross-examination in court may hew single-mindedly to a given viewpoint, in most *un*diplomatic terms, with apparent gross disrespect of the witness.

This last point is essential in understanding the experience of personal narcissistic assault so commonly described by clinicians who have served as experts in court. While the process of cross-examination is, more often than not, carried out with reasonable respectfulness in calm tones of voice, on occasion the opposing attorney opts to direct his attack, as a legitimate courtroom tactic, against the expertise, competence, character, motivation, or corruptibility of the witness, rather than against his conclusions per se. In clinical settings, social surroundings, and formal debating procedures, it would be unfair, inappropriate, self-defeating, and proof of dubious conviction of righteousness to resort to an *ad hominem* attack (that is, an attack on the person rather than on the substance of the issues); in court, however, such impugning of the witness's personal features is simply part of the repertoire of techniques used by counsel to discredit the witness (see Sec. II-A-3 above).

The mistake commonly made by the novice witness under such a barrage is to assume that this personal attack is personally intended. In his native land of clinical practice, the clinician would readily grasp that personal abuse may represent the adolescent's need to test, the paranoid's need to project, or the borderline patient's need to torture the object; such an understanding permits him to maintain perspective in the service of the clinical work. The disconcerting effect of such assault in court stems from the fact that its perpetrator is a nonpsychotic adult lawyer whose undisguised (and *apparently* unmotivated) hostility, hatred, and contempt utterly bewilder the clinician. The assault is all the more demoralizing for the expert because it is (1) public, (2) unanswerable in the courtroom conditions of question and answer, and (3) so markedly in contrast with the awestruck veneration accorded by his *own* attorney to his pronouncements just moments ago.

The primary succor to the beleaguered expert in such a situation derives from these sources:

"Rules of the game." The expert must understand that even so personal an attack is merely a tactic, representing one approach by an attorney to doing her job: attempting to put her own side of the case in a favorable light by derogating the opposing testimony. In a well-functioning adversary system, the lawyer should be viewed as playing the role prescribed for her, one that she considers essential to the attainment of justice.

Realistic limitations. An attorney may attack a witness for the uncertainty of his conclusions or may impugn the data base ("Doctor, do you mean you base your opinion on a mere four hours of examining the patient?"). The nonexistence of certitude should be accepted in clinical matters and should not distress the witness; if the time spent was adequate for the determination, this should be stated (the expert having, it is hoped, determined the adequacy of this amount of interviewing time before trial).

Defense mechanisms. One means of surviving the assault is to call into play the high-level defense mechanisms of humor, rationalization, and intellectualization. Just as a therapist deals with the pointed thrusts of an angry borderline patient by attempting to understand the dynamic issues that lie beneath the angry exterior, so the clinician in court can analyze the nature of the legal attack on her previous testimony. While this is not to claim that utter humiliation can be an enjoyable experience, lesser degrees of insult can be made more tolerable if the witness can psychologically step back from the proceedings to recognize the nature of the process. At times this perspective is materially aided by such common courtroom scenes as the attorney who, after trial, sincerely compliments the same witness against whom (during the process) she was directing disparagement, scorn, and scathing contempt.

4. STRUCTURAL ASPECTS OF TRIAL PRESENTATION

The expert witness will go through at least two and perhaps four stages of the trial process in presenting her testimony.

a. Direct examination

In this phase, the attorney for "her side" of the case will ask specific questions, usually designed to be answered "yes" or "no," or to require a brief narrative response, with the goal of presenting to judge or jury the expert's contribution in a manner both systematic and persuasive.

Laying a foundation.   In developing the material for presentation, the attorney must create a hierarchy of statements that justify or substantiate the conclusions to be drawn before the latter are addressed. For example, in a negligence suit about bad effects from medication, an expert witness may be examined as to the appropriateness of that medication for the illness in question. The questioning does *not* begin in this manner:

Example 6

ATTORNEY: Doctor, should this medication have been used for this patient?
DOCTOR WITNESS: In my opinion, based on review of the case plus my own extensive experience, I would say, yes.

Instead, each of the several components that make up the witness's answer—an outline of her experience and her expertise, a summary of the issues, and the opinion itself—must be buttressed by previously established facts or affirmations (i.e., the foundation), some or all of which may be challenged by opposing counsel. In a condensed form, the direct examination may evolve in this manner:

Example 7

ATTORNEY: Doctor, please state your name and address.
DOCTOR-WITNESS: (Does so.)
ATTORNEY: Describe your training, please.
DOCTOR-WITNESS: (Describes in moderate detail.)
ATTORNEY: Doctor, do you have an area of particular expertise?
DOCTOR-WITNESS: (Witness, who has several, understands that the attorney is referring to the subject in question and lists publications, awards, and association memberships in psychopharmacology, after which counsel asks for her acceptance as an expert, which is unchallenged.)
ATTORNEY: Doctor, in the course of your practice, do you have occasion to treat patients directly?
DOCTOR-WITNESS: Yes, I do.
ATTORNEY: Do some of these patients suffer from schizophrenia?
DOCTOR-WITNESS: Yes.
ATTORNEY: About how many?
DOCTOR-WITNESS: About one-third.
(Opposing attorney objects, noting that this gives no idea of the actual numbers; objection is sustained.)

ATTORNEY: How many of such patients is that, Doctor?

DOCTOR-WITNESS: About 50 a year for the last 10 years.

ATTORNEY: And do you ever have occasion to prescribe medication for some of these patients? (This rather redundant question, again, serves only to lay a foundation for the key question that will cap the sequence of queries.)

DOCTOR-WITNESS: Yes, I do.

(Further questions establish the frequency of drug treatment decisions made by the expert, her familiarity with the medication's effects and side effects, her wide consultative experience, and the like.)

ATTORNEY: Doctor, have you had occasion to review the case of Mr. _____?

DOCTOR-WITNESS: Yes.

ATTORNEY: And have you formed an opinion, based on your experience and said review, as to the appropriateness of the medication for this patient?

DOCTOR-WITNESS: Yes, I have.

ATTORNEY: And what is that opinion?

DOCTOR-WITNESS: That it was appropriate.

The denouement of this prolonged series of questions is identical to that in Example 6, though a hundredfold longer and more painstakingly detailed; yet this meticulousness allows the final opinion to carry the greater force. Rather than appearing as a self-styled expert "off the street," the witness has been characterized carefully for judge and jury as having *specific* experience, training, and expertise that should lead to her opinions being considered with care.

Hypothetical questions and follow-ups.   Hypothetical questions and follow-ups, the rationale for which is outlined in Sec. II-A-2-c, often pose a problem for the novice witness. Strictly speaking, hypothetical questions should be based only on material previously introduced into evidence; the witness should be alert to any changes from her view of the facts of the case that might affect her answer. Follow-up queries, either in the direct examination, or more commonly in the cross-examination, are designed to consider alternative possibilities, and to determine which elements are decisive to a particular outcome. Since their function is often speculative, hypotheticals may delineate a fantasy world that bears no relation to the case at hand. Failure to grasp this point can lead to embarrassment:

Example 8

ATTORNEY: Doctor, is it possible that this patient's psychosis resulted from taking angel dust or PCP?

NOVICE WITNESS: (Heatedly) But he *didn't* take it!

Here, the witness has failed to go along with the "what if" intention of the query, and has forgotten that the judge and/or jury have the final decision as to which of the alternate universes of hypotheses will be considered to apply to the case. Although the attorney may have asked the question merely as a tactic to implant doubt about the diagnosis in the jurors' minds (even though previous testimony may have excluded any possibility of PCP being involved), the fact is that even a psychosis with classically functional symptoms may be caused by a host of factors. A response that said just that would be the appropriate one.

b. Cross-examination

After one attorney has developed the expert's opinion by direct examination, the opposing counsel takes over the questioning for cross-examination, the heart of the adversary process (see Sec. II-A-3 above); the function of this stage is to put to the proof the assertions of the witness and the supporting data. Some specific pointers on this phase of testimony will appear in Sec. III-D, below. The critical consideration for the expert is the realization that, although until now one attorney has been attempting to showcase her expertise and competence in a very supportive (and, it is hoped, persuasive) manner, the opposing attorney has an equally legitimate goal. He must attempt to invalidate, derogate, discredit, or even ridicule her testimony—in order to induce disbelief in the minds of the jurors—by leading her to display doubt, self-contradiction, or confusion.

This intention of the cross-examining counsel should alert the witness to the need for caution in replying, care in weighing the question and its impact, and thoughtful anticipation of the direction in which the line of inquiry may go. The cross-examiner may also lay a foundation and employ hypothetical questions to establish the position he wishes the jury to perceive.

c. Redirect and recross

As the names suggest, these stages permit the expert's attorney and the opposing counsel respectively to have their final opportunity to elaborate or challenge any points that may have emerged during the first two stages of the testimony. On occasion, these last two stages are waived. After that point, the witness is usually dismissed, although on occasion (especially if new developments supervene) the expert may be recalled.

D. The "foreign language" of the courtroom

In the clinician's native land, two kinds of language prevail: narrative, the language of the case presentation, lecture, textbook, article, or clinical report; and dialogue, the language of the interview, case discussion, team treatment planning session, or consultation.

In the courtroom, narrative is brief, if present at all, and the dialogue evinces certain peculiarities and unique locutions that make it seem a foreign language to the clinician's ear; these peculiarities may be divided into structural aspects, substantive aspects, and technical aspects. The clinician bound for court, like the experienced traveler, does well to familiarize himself with the language of the land.

1. STRUCTURAL ASPECTS OF COURTROOM LANGUAGE

a. The scope of the question

In many clinical settings, questions addressed to the consultant (expert) are open-ended; a question like "Do you think that this patient's diagnosis was correct?" might, with full appropriateness, call forth a 15-minute response covering diagnosis, precipitants of the clinical reaction, and dynamic formulation of the case, each with corroborative material, anecdotes, personal associations, and examples from the consultant's practice. In contrast, the examining attorney's question is usually "closed-ended," directed to a brief response or even to a "yes" or "no" answer. The expert witness is strongly advised always to stay within the question addressed to her.

This constraint poses several difficulties. First, many clinical questions (perhaps most) cannot be answered in this manner but require qualifications. The expert may then state that the question requires a qualified yes (or no), on which occasion the attorney (or the opposing counsel) may ask about the qualification; some questions are so phrased as to evoke "It depends" as the only possible answer.

While being asked questions, the expert may wonder if the answer is germane to the case or even admissible as evidence. This matter should be left to the attorney; the witness should concern herself only with the question before her. This restraint should entail avoiding volunteering information; unlike the situation in clinical settings, the usual courtroom question is not an invitation to discourse. The exception, of course, is the question specifically aimed at a discursive answer, such as, "Tell us the purposes of the mental status examination."

In answering, the witness must recall the structure imposed by the need to lay a foundation as outlined above. Thus, when the attorney asks, for example, "What—if any—treatment did you administer?" the "if any" is not a snotty disparagement of the witness's wish to treat the ill; rather, it is a locution designed to avoid appearing to assume that treatment *was* administered before this had been established.

b. "I don't know"

A major pitfall for the novice witness is equating "expert" with "omniscient." The witness should candidly acknowledge ignorance when she does not know the answer to a particular question or when the phrasing of the question —because of vagueness, infelicitous choice of words, or irrelevance—makes it impossible to answer knowingly.

> *Example 9:* A cross-examining attorney was attempting to shake the expert witness's testimony as to the value of the use of seclusion for a patient in a particular case; the witness had been established as an expert on seclusion. The attorney asked, "What would be the effect of seclusion on a normal person?" The witness realized that the problem with this disarmingly simple question lay in the fact that normal people are never secluded in psychiatric inpatient settings; hence, there are no theoretical or clinical data on this situation. Overcoming her anxiety at admitting ignorance to so deceptively simple a query, the witness replied, "I don't know." The attorney feigned astonishment and asked further questions, to which the witness gave the explanation alluded to above.

Clinicians should also remember that some information is simply not knowable by any clinician, no matter how gifted. For example, a member of a racial minority with schizophrenia commits an apparently racially motivated crime while drunk, in a setting in which there were no reliable witnesses, contemporaneous police reports, or other objective observers. He later disavows any recollection of the event. A clinician evaluating that person for criminal responsibility could not be expected to give an assessment of his mental state at the time of the offense, nor of the respective roles quantitatively played in the crime by the defendant's schizophrenia, intoxication, or response to racial slurs. A clinician asked such questions may wish to consider pointing out (although perhaps not in the actual courtroom itself—better in depositions or in conferences with the attorney) that some material is simply not clinically knowable.

c. Reasonable medical certainty

In most civil litigation, experts will be expected to testify that their opinions are accurate to a "reasonable medical certainty" (or sometimes "reasonable medical probability"). (Psychologists will be held to a "reasonable psychological probability.") If they fail to express this minimum degree of confidence in their judgments, their testimony may be excluded from consideration by the finder of fact (i.e., judge or jury). Thus, in a malpractice case, after a foundation has been laid, an expert may be asked, "Doctor, do you have an opinion *to a reasonable degree of medical certainty* as to whether Dr. Jones conducted his practice with that degree of care and skill required of a reasonable psychiatrist at that time and in those circumstances?" (See Suggested Readings, Sec. VII-B—Rappeport.)

There has been some considerable degree of confusion, however, over just what constitutes a reasonable medical certainty. Some jurisdictions have case law that clarifies this issue, but many do not. Reasonable medical certainty may mean a 51% likelihood or "more probable than not." Alternatively, it can be conceptualized as that degree of confidence in her opinion that a physician would need before undertaking treatment of a patient. Prior to testifying, an expert who is uncertain of the meaning of the standard in her jurisdiction should clarify this with her attorney. If no clear standard exists, there is some value in the expert herself specifying the meaning that she gives to it. For example, she might begin her response to the question above by saying, "If by reasonable medical certainty, you mean more likely than not, then I do hold my opinion to that degree of certainty."

Novice experts are occasionally disconcerted when a question is put to them in the form of "possibility" rather than reasonable medical certainty. Asking a question in terms of possibility (since this is not the requisite standard of proof) is, in most cases, an attorney's ploy to place some image before a jury that will compete in the jury's minds with the image proposed to a "reasonable medical certainty." Thus an attorney, working for the plaintiff in a suicide case where it is doubtful that negligence actually occurred, might well ask the question: "Doctor, is it possible that a psychiatrist might miss the suicidal thinking in a patient?" This question, of course, is irrelevant since 1) *anything* is "possible"; 2) the issue is not possibility but reasonable medical certainty; and 3) the question should focus on *this* case rather than some hypothetical case. Regardless, the attorney may be attempting to plant a picture in the jury's mind of the doctor missing something.

Experienced witnesses simply take questions about possibility at face value. Since anything is possible, the answer to a possibility question is generally "yes." The opposing attorney may, of course, object to the effect that possibility is irrelevant to the matter under consideration. Clinicians should not get into a struggle about this and should simply answer questions about possibility in the affirmative, leaving it to the pertinent attorney to straighten out the questions of standard of proof.

2. SUBSTANTIVE ASPECTS OF COURTROOM LANGUAGE

a. Describe versus interpret

The witness in court should remember the first lesson of microscopic pathology: *first* describe, *then* interpret. This brings the audience (judge and/or jury) into the sequence of data gathering leading to certain conclusions and demonstrates the substantiation process. Direct observations, examinations, and measurements should be identified as such and distinguished from inferences, intuitions, impressions, and hypotheses drawn from clinical experience or "hunches."

b. The qualities of an expert witness's answers

The point has been made by Halleck that after the swearing-in process, the psychiatric witness should abandon his role as advocate for one side of the case and become, in effect, an advocate for clinically founded truth. This fundamental principle contains certain implications for the content of the witness's answers:

- The answers should be true to the best knowledge of the witness.
- They should be germane to the issue at hand.
- The answers should embody objectivity in examination and evaluation, and austerity in expression. Prolix or opinionated responses should be avoided.
- The responses should be clear, as simply expressed as possible, with attention paid to making the answers comprehensible to a lay audience.
- In this vein, the answers should be expressed in a manner designed to avoid provoking or alienating the audience. Often this principle is best served by total avoidance of jargon. It is a fact of courtroom life that everyday lay language, spoken in a noncondescending manner, is more convincing by far than a profusion of polysyllabic terminology aimed at conveying vast erudition.

3. TECHNICAL ASPECTS OF COURTROOM LANGUAGE

The substance of this section might be described as "tips and traps," a phrase referring to the fact that certain hints can make testifying easier and more effective, while awareness of certain well-known snares set by attorneys may prevent the informed witness from being caught therein.

a. Tips on responding to queries

The value of delay.   The habit of pausing a moment before answering can be of significant value to the witness, because it allows time to check on whether one understands the question, to replay the question in one's head, and to weigh and choose one's answer. In addition, it allows the nonquestioning attorney to object if desired, thus perhaps preventing compromising or inappropriate answers from being expressed. If the witness realizes that the query will require considerable reflection, he should ask for a moment to think over the question—a move that tends to reduce the audience's impatience at the delay.

Unanswerable questions.   Certain questions that are phrased in perfectly good English are yet unanswerable on clinical grounds, for example, "Would a patient with schizophrenia be likely to assault his mother?" The response "I don't know" is not nearly so apposite as "I can't answer that question"; the inability to answer a question phrased confusingly or without qualifications (schizophrenia per se being irrelevant to the patient's likelihood of assaulting his mother) should be freely and frankly admitted. Ideally, the judge will direct rephrasing the question, or the attorney will spontaneously do so.

The experienced witness can convey certain hints to his attorney that aid in the elucidation of the testimony.

> ***Example 10:*** In a case involving a violent patient, commitment had been sought based on violent behavior that had occurred just *prior* to hospitalization. The attorney asked the expert witness (who had supervised the case only in the hospital) a question including the phrase "violent while under your care." The witness replied, "I can't answer in that time frame." The alert attorney realized the problem and broke down the query into subsidiary questions that clarified the timing of the violent behavior in relation to the petition for commitment.

In a similar manner, such responses as "I can't answer that phrasing" or "I can't answer without qualifiers" may aid the attorney in developing the point at issue.

The context of the question.   While second-guessing the attorney can lead to serious difficulty for the witness, the astute expert will attempt to tune in to where the question is coming from, on what assumptions it is based, and in which direction the question is headed. This approach permits forethought and diminishes surprise.

The expert witness should remain alert to the possibility that the questioning attorney may reveal by the phrasing or content of a query that she is confounding distinct entities; for example, the attorney may treat insanity as inherently equivalent to incompetence, irresponsibility, or committability, or psychosis as identical to a schizophrenia. If such a confusion appears to exist, the witness should protest an inability to answer the question and hope that the opportunity will be provided to clarify the matter.

Qualifiers.   Especially when being cross-examined, the witness is well advised to be alert to qualifying phrases in his response. The reason for this is that the attorney may "stop the question" when the answer he desires has been given.

> ***Example 11:*** In reply to a question as to whether a certain situation could occur, the witness wanted to respond, "Yes, but that situation is very rare and unlikely, in fact, to occur." However, as soon as he had uttered the "Yes," the attorney said briskly, "Thank you, doctor; no further questions," and the judge intoned, "Witness may step down." The expert was, in essence, turned off with little recourse short of causing a disturbance in court.

In anticipation of this difficulty, the witness should develop the habit of leading with qualifying phrases; opposing counsel will be motivated to permit completion of the response since the desired portion will not have been stated until the end.

Example 12: In the same situation as Example 9, the witness might respond, "While that situation is rare and quite unlikely, it is theoretically possible."

Metaphors and analogies.   Although these rhetorical devices may be immeasurably useful in clarifying a point for the jury, due care must be exercised in judicious use thereof, and the limitations of even the aptest analogy must be delineated.

Example 13: Attempting to distinguish data based on his single evaluation of a patient from data that could be obtained over a period of time, a witness characterized the former as being like a snapshot. Opposing counsel proceeded to begin each subsequent query with, "Now, regarding this—this *snapshot* you took, Doctor . . ." With each repetition of the metaphor the expert's examination was more embarrassingly trivialized, so that by the end of cross-examination the expert felt (and appeared) like an incompetent dilettante in photography rather than like a competent psychiatrist!

b. Consideration for the subject's presence

In most if not all cases, the subject of the examination is present during the proceedings. With this in mind, the witness should remain the clinician by exercising tact and consideration in choosing diplomatic (yet accurate) ways of expressing her opinions or findings. It is preferable to state, for example, "The defendant revealed a history of antisocial acts over 10 years," rather than, "The defendant is your typical common thug of the 'born-loser' type."

Indeed, the psychiatric literature (see, for example, Suggested Readings—Strasburger) suggests that intense negative reactions can occur when the subject feels that his innermost thoughts are being revealed.

Example 14: In the case described in the above article, the subject stated ". . . I had the feeling [upon hearing your testimony in the courtroom] I was on an operating table and you had a dissecting knife and you just opened me up wide for everyone to see . . . [it was] frightening, positively frightening . . . [I] just wanted to be dead, I didn't want to be in that room."

This subject further described struggling with severe, acute suicidal feelings after the testimony.

On an ethical basis it might be argued that clinicians have a duty to explain to attorneys the potential negative impacts of such disclosures in their client's presence.

c. Some common maneuvers by attorneys in court

Attorneys vary, of course, in their approaches to a witness from respectful to abusive and over all points in between. Certain familiar traps should be watched for because of their ubiquity.

Fee as focus for attack.   As suggested in Sec. II-A-3 above, attorneys attempting to impugn the integrity of the witness may fix on the fee as a vehicle for doing so. The most common provocative question is, "How much are you being paid for your testimony, Doctor?," a remark that implies that the witness is corruptly vending his *testimony* instead of his time. The witness should come to terms with a reasonable fee earned for time spent (as well as time lost from usual professional activity) and should state the fee if asked about his *time.*

The following example from an actual deposition captures how this might occur in real life.

Example 15

QUESTION [Examining attorney]: What year was this that you gave your testimony (in a particular case)?

ANSWER [Expert witness]: Three years ago, maybe, roughly.

Q: Were you paid for your testimony in that case?

A: No.

Q: You did that for free?

A: No.

Q: Then how do you explain that inconsistency?

A: I was paid for my time. My testimony cannot be bought.

Q: Are you being paid for your time in this case?

A: I certainly hope so.

Some experienced witnesses, asked about their charges, respond disarmingly, "It depends how long y'all keep me here." Others, asked if they are being paid for their services, assume a worried expression and say, as above, "Gosh, I certainly hope so!" Such ingenuous remarks usually defeat the attorney's attempt to taint the witness with the suspicion of venality. Interestingly, these ploys are usually reserved for juries; attorneys arguing before a judge alone (as sometimes occurs) rarely resort to such gimmicks, since judges are rarely impressed with them.

"Never say never."   Attorneys may attempt to build queries around "always" and "never"—two referents that rarely fit any real clinical situation. The expert should not worry about seeming indecisive or unsure but should stick to the realities of experience, uncertain though they may be.

The lulling series.   An opposing attorney may ask a series of questions, all calling for a "yes" answer, for example, after which a question requiring "no" is unobtrusively inserted, in the hope that the witness is so lulled into the rhythm of assenting that momentum alone, as it were, will generate an inadvertent "yes" to the last query. The obvious remedy is alertness and use of the time lag alluded to earlier in responding to allow individualized attention to each question.

The use of literature as authority.   The expert's view in court may be challenged by references to the psychiatric literature. Though this may be an intimidating encounter, the novice expert should be aware that the citation (book, article, or monograph) must first be recognized as an authority *by* the expert before it can be used to challenge her testimony (see Sec. II-A-3). While this principle may lead to disclaimers redolent of *hubris* ("Freud had *his* theories, I have mine"), the expert is best advised to be reluctant to award authority to any work except possibly her own published material; even in the last case, the expert still may determine whether the cited point applies to the present case. Commonly employed authorities are the *Physicians' Desk Reference*, the *Comprehensive Textbook of Psychiatry*, and, at present, *DSM-III-R*.

DSM-III-R carries a disclaimer noting that the diagnostic criteria it contains are not necessarily synonymous with legal definitions of mental disorder. In particular, since *DSM-III-R* is designed to maximize interexaminer reliability of diagnosis, cases that are in some way atypical are often left without a category into which they can fit. This limitation on the use of the manual in legal contexts, however, is frequently neglected, as attorneys attempt to equate a plaintiff's or defendant's failure to meet all the criteria required for a particular diagnosis with the absence of legally relevant mental disorder.

Given this situation, experts legitimately can make diagnoses other than those contained in *DSM-III-R* (e.g., simple schizophrenia), or can assign diagnoses covered by the manual even when patients do not meet all the *DSM-III-R* criteria, as long as they acknowledge that they are departing from the standard nomenclature and are prepared to justify and explain the bases for their conclusions. Within the diagnostic system itself, the category of disorders denominated "atypical" or "not otherwise specified" provides considerable flexibility for cases that depart from typical presentations.

Inaccurate quotations.   The expert should be wary of questions that begin "Doctor, you testified earlier, did you not, that . . ." It is a common attorney's dodge to alter the previous testimony slightly in quoting it, so that the misquoted remark may be used to throw the witness's testimony into contradiction. The expert should always critique such queries in her mind to see if they are accurate. In the last analysis, the stenographic record may be consulted if there is doubt and if the point is critical.

Simple harassment.   Attorneys on occasion resort to certain locutions designed to needle and thus rattle the witness. Examples are: "Now, Doctor—it *is* 'Doctor,' isn't it?"; referring to the witness as "Mister" rather than "Doctor"; referring to a psychiatrist as a psychologist and vice versa; or employing heavy sarcasm and disparagement concomitant with the examination.

The best counter to those ploys is a deadpan, strictly factual response to the substance of the question. The attorney who harps on "Mister" more than a few times soon begins to sound petty and foolish and will normally cease before alienating the jury. The witness who becomes irritated, contentious, or sarcastic in turn, of course, is in danger of vitiating the force and credibility of his testimony.

Testifying about preparing to testify.   Another point of attack for the attorney trying to discredit the witness is the pretrial preparation, alluded to in Sec. II-C-1-c. While review of anticipated testimony and some "rehearsal" of possible cross-examination is customary practice, this rehearsal may be painted by opposing counsel as "coaching," implying that the witness is simply mouthing preformed testimony supplied by counsel for her side.

On the stand, the witness should acknowledge that time was spent reviewing the case and her testimony. Some experienced witnesses disarm the imputational tack by saying, for example, "Counsel recommended that I tell you the truth," or "The attorney told me to answer your questions as honestly as possible."

As usual, the ethical balance here pivots on the autonomous functioning of the witness who offers independent conclusions based on unbiased evaluation. The clinician who permits counsel to dictate her testimony has, in fact, sold out to the law.

Incomprehensible questions.   Some questions are put to the witness in a form so grammatically complex or maladroitly worded that even a correct answer, somehow arrived at, would only heighten the preexisting confusion. A rewording may be respectfully requested; alternatively the witness may simply want to state that she doesn't understand the question or the wording. Consider this real-life example:

> *Example 16*
> QUESTION [Examining attorney]: Would it be speculative on your part to give an opinion as to whether or not therapy and treatment wouldn't have been effective even if she had not attempted this suicide?
> ANSWER [Expert witness]: I'm sorry. I got lost in the double negatives.
> OTHER ATTORNEY PRESENT: Me, too.

Another form of incomprehensible question is one in which the attorney attempts to ask several questions at once, as it were, in an effort to either confuse the witness or render the witness apparently befuddled.

> *Example 17:* A malpractice case where a patient had killed his girl-friend turned upon the question of whether the patient should have been committed. The patient, however, was with his family, and with-out any professional observers present at the critical moment. The following dialogue occurred in the courtroom.
> QUESTION (Examining attorney): At the time the patient was with his parents, was this patient committable?
> The expert paused a moment to think about this question since the patient's committability would have been difficult, if not impossible, to assess in the absence of professional observers accustomed to think-ing in terms of the statutory standards. As he paused a moment, the examining attorney declaimed, dramatically:
> QUESTION: Do you mean you even have to *think* about it? That's a yes or no question.

Predictably the other side's attorney objected to this question. The single question really has three components: first, the question of the patient's commit-tability in the absence of observers trained to make that legalistic assessment; second, the question of whether a witness under oath should, indeed, have to or be allowed to think about answers given in that context; and third, the question (disguised as a statement) as to whether in fact so complex an issue is answerable with a simple yes or no.

In the real-life example, following the objection the questions were broken down and answered separately. However, the expert might have had several op-tions, assuming the opposing attorney had not objected, which are presented below.

Option 1: ANSWER: That's three questions, counselor. If you'll just choose the one you'd like me to answer first, I'll be glad to take a crack at it. [This response is useful for whenever multiple questions are asked at once].

Option 2: ANSWER: Of course, I have to think about it, I take being under oath very seriously and I think about every answer I give you, just as I think about every question you ask me. Why is that so surprising to you?

Option 3: ANSWER (expert turns to judge): Your honor, I would need your guidance on what to do. It seems I've been asked three questions at once; what's the appropriate procedure for a witness under these circumstances?

All these responses permit a rapid reaction to the attorney's question by the expert, but allow the full duplicity of the examining attorney's multiple queries to stand out (while conceivably gaining some sympathy and support from the judge in the last example).

E. Summary

The citizen in his native land may be able to muster sufficient glibness to talk a traffic policeman out of a ticket, where both share the language and culture; in a foreign country, this becomes a task far less likely of success.

Similarly, in the foreign land of the courtroom, the setting is different, as are the assumptions and the culture. The witness, then, should attempt to familiarize herself with these cultural determinants as thoroughly as possible in advance to permit making a useful contribution not only to the case at hand but to the role of the psychiatric profession in due process.

IV. PITFALLS

A. Remaining the clinician

As in the cases reviewed in Chapter 6, the clinician may be tempted to "turn lawyer" for the duration of the courtroom experience. This temptation should, of course, be resisted because no other person is in a position to consider and attend to the clinical issues.

B. Maintaining humility

A number of factors conspire to encourage an attitude of humility in the clinician bound for court: the imprecise nature of the clinical field; the "foreign land" of court; the need for the expert's testimony to inform the court; and the importance of avoiding alienating the jury by the use of jargon, pomposity, or self-righteousness.

C. Taking it personally

As earlier noted, the best witness is the calm, dispassionate witness off whose back rolls the most barbed, scathing, and defamatory harangue.

V. CASE EXAMPLE EPILOGUE

The colleague she consults confirms in part the bad news. She will have to honor the subpoena, he says, even if that involves cancelling a number of appointments. On the other hand, since she is being called to testify as an expert witness on her patient's mental state, the therapist is entitled to reimbursement of a reasonable expert's fee.

With regard to her fear of damaging her patient, either by provoking a termination of the relationship or by revealing sensitive information, the forensic psychiatrist she consults has equally gloomy news. He explains that, unless state law stipulates otherwise, all citizens are required to testify about any information that might be relevant to a given case. While this state has a statute that provides for limited psychotherapist-patient privilege in civil cases, it does not apply to cases in which the plaintiff specifically raises the issue of psychic damages. Therefore, if it were specifically requested, the therapist might have to provide detailed information about her patient's life. The consultant reviews with her the legal issues involved in tort suits, especially the points that the lawyers questioning her would be seeking to prove.

From the tone of her friend's questions, however, the consultant senses that she is asking for something beyond just information. Since in her training she had never been prepared for courtroom testimony, and after entering practice she has assiduously avoided cases in which she might be called to testify, he assumes that she is quite anxious about the unfamiliar courtroom setting. He offers to tell her something about what to expect in court, how court procedures work, and some of the simple things that she could do, such as carefully preparing her testimony in advance, that might make the experience easier for her. He directs her to readings that outline techniques of coping with cross-examination and point to likely lines of attack. In addition, he suggests that, once she knows what she intends to say, they sit down together and role-play, he playing judge and lawyer, and she rehearsing her testimony.

At the role-playing session, the consultant surprises his colleague with the vigor of his attack on her credentials and background, but she stands her ground and answers to the point. The consultant explains that this may occur in the courtroom setting, where the opposing side may attempt to discredit the testimony by discrediting the witness.

In court the therapist is, indeed, forced to discuss her patient's life and background in detail and to give an opinion on whether, in a hypothetical case, the personality of a woman with a background similar to the patient's could have changed markedly following the accident. Since she honestly feels that this outcome is unlikely in this case, and so states, her own patient's attorney is the one who attempts to tear down her credentials and to suggest that her theoretical claim is unsupported by empirical data. Although shaken by this attack from an unexpected quarter, the therapist is able to answer most of the questions confidently, since she has reviewed the literature relevant to her presentation before coming to court. The issue of her patient's extramarital affair is never raised.

The therapist cannot say afterwards that she enjoyed the experience, but she does feel that, because she presented the information in a reasonable and knowledgeable way, she is satisfied with her performance.

VI. ACTION GUIDE

A. Checklist for Preparing to Testify in Court:

1. *Review* relevant data, charts, and records in detail.
2. *Interview* directly the patient, witnesses, caretakers.
   a. *Alert* patient and others to agency and purpose of interview.
   b. *Explain* that judge and/or jury make actual decision.
   c. *Include* formal mental status exam.
3. *Record* results of above determinations for court, then *condense* into easily carried notes.
4. *Review* pertinent current literature on contested subject, especially papers you have written.
5. *Prepare* "your" attorney.
   a. *Educate* attorney about clinical elements of case.
   b. *Correct* unrealistic expectations:
      i. Lie detection by clinician,
      ii. Evocation of speech from mute patient,
      iii. Retrospective assessment of state of mind long before evaluation,
      iv. Attempts to subvert opinion,
      v. "Absolute" diagnosis.
6. *Avoid* absolute and invariant conclusions in report.

B. Checklist for Testifying in Court:

1. *Recall* role of witness: to inform the court.
2. *Clear* sufficient time in schedule to permit unhurried participation in proceedings; bring work or reading.
3. *Present* testimony clearly, audibly, and comprehensibly; *avoid* jargon.
4. *Attempt* to have impressive credentials spelled out and entered into the record.
5. *Avoid* responding to discrediting cross-examination as personal attack.
6. *Recall* the stages of presentation: direct examination, cross-examination, redirect, recross.
   a. *Anticipate* attorney's laying a foundation.
   b. *Move* readily with questions into the new "what if" situation.
7. *Attend* to specific question and *remain* within its scope in answering.
8. *Accept* that "I don't know" is perfectly appropriate answer when called for.
9. *Remember* concept of "reasonable medical certainty."
10. *Describe* data first, *interpret* meaning or conclusions later.
11. *Tell* truth as best known, regardless of "side" of case.
12. *Delay* a moment before answering to permit reflection, weighing of answer, and objection by counsel.
13. *State* when question cannot be answered.
14. *Remain* alert to context, direction, and implications of question.
15. *Beware* of qualifying phrases, metaphors, and analogies.

16. *Exercise* consideration for patient's presence by judicious choice of language. *Educate* attorney about impact of testimony on subject.
17. *Remain* alert to attorney's maneuvers:
    a. Focusing attack on fee.
    b. Use of "always" and "never."
    c. Series of lulling questions with a sudden reversal.
    d. Use of literature as authority.
    e. Inaccurate quotations.
    f. Simple harassment.
    g. Implication of "coaching."
    h. Incomprehensible questions.
18. Above all, *remain* cool under fire.

VII. SELECTED READINGS

A. THE CLINICIAN IN COURT: THEORY AND ETHICS

1. Special Issue on the Ethics of Forensic Psychiatry. *Bull. Am. Acad. Psychiatry Law* 12(3), 1984.
2. Rappeport, J. R.: Differences between forensic and general psychiatry. *Am. J. Psychiatry* 139:331–334, 1982.
3. Bonnie, R. J. & Slobogin, C.: The role of mental health professionals in the criminal process: the case for informed speculation. *Virginia Law Review* 66:427–522, 1980.
4. Morse, S. J.: Failed explanations and criminal responsibility: experts and the unconscious. *Virginia Law Review* 68:971–1084, 1982.
5. Brent, R. L.: The irresponsible expert witness: a failure of biomedical graduate education and professional accountability. *Pediatrics* 70:754–762, 1982.
6. Appelbaum, P. S.: In the wake of *Ake*: the ethics of expert testimony in an advocate's world. *Bull. Am. Acad. Psychiatry Law* 15:15–26, 1987.
7. Slovenko, R.: The lawyer and the forensic expert: boundaries of ethical practice. *Behav. Sci. Law* 5:119–147, 1987.
8. Fitch, W. L., Petrella, R. C. & Wallace, J.: Legal ethics and the use of mental health experts in criminal cases. *Behav. Sci. Law* 5:105–117, 1987.
9. Shuman, D. W.: Testimonial compulsion: the involuntary medical expert witness. *J. Leg. Med.* 4:419–446, 1983.
10. Zusman, J. & Simon, J.: Differences in repeated psychiatric examinations of litigants to a lawsuit. *Am. J. Psychiatry* 140:1300–1304, 1983.
11. Kennedy, D. B., Kelley, T. M. & Homant, R. J.: A test of the "hired gun" hypothesis in psychiatric testimony. *Psychol. Rep.* 57:117–118, 1985.
12. Kaplan, L. V. & Miller, R. D.: Courtroom psychiatrists: expertise at the cost of wisdom? *Int. J. Law Psychiatry* 9:451–468, 1986.
13. Weinstock, R.: Controversial ethical issues in forensic psychiatry: a survey. *J. Forensic Sci.* 33:176–186, 1988.
14. Appelbaum, P. S.: The parable of the forensic psychiatrist: ethics and the problem of doing harm. *Int. J. Law Psychiatry* (in press).

B. PRACTICAL ASPECTS OF TESTIMONY

1. Resnick, P. J.: The psychiatrist in court, in Michels, R., et al. (eds.), *Psychiatry.* Philadelphia, J. B. Lippincott, 1986.
2. Ziskin, J. & Faust, D.: *Coping with Psychiatric and Psychological Testimony,* 3rd ed. Venice, CA, Law and Psychology Press, 1988.

3. Faust, D. & Ziskin, J.: The expert witness in psychology and psychiatry. *Science* 241:31–35, 1988.

4. Goldstein, R. L.: Psychiatrists in the hot seat: discrediting doctors by impeachment of their credibility. *Bull. Am. Acad. Psychiatry Law* 16:225–234, 1988.

5. Rappeport, J. R.: Reasonable medical certainty. *Bull. Am. Acad. Psychiatry Law* 13:5–16, 1985.

6. Strasburger, L. H.: "Crudely, without any finesse": the defendant hears his psychiatric evaluation. *Bull. Am. Acad. Psychiatry Law* 15:229–233, 1987.

7. Tanay, E.: The expert witness as a teacher. *Bull. Am. Acad. Psychiatry Law* 8:401–411, 1980.

8. Halpern, A. L., Ciccone, J. R. & Stone, A. A. DSM-III in court: ask the experts. *Newsletter of the American Academy of Psychiatry and the Law,* 11:6–8, 1986.

Index